Rules and Guidance for Pharmaceutical Distributors 2022

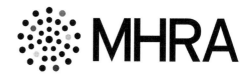

Rules and Guidance for Pharmaceutical Distributors 2022

Compiled by the MHRA

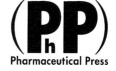

Pharmaceutical Press

Published by Pharmaceutical Press

66–68 East Smithfield, London E1W 1AW, UK

© Crown Copyright 2022

 Medicines & Healthcare products Regulatory Agency

Medicines and Healthcare products Regulatory Agency,
10 South Colonnade,
Canary Wharf,
London E14 4PU UK.
Stay connected: mhra.gov.uk/stayconnected
Information on re-use of crown copyright information can be found on MHRA website: www.mhra.gov.uk

Designed and published by Pharmaceutical Press 2022

(**P.P**) is a trade mark of Pharmaceutical Press

Pharmaceutical Press is the publishing division of the Royal Pharmaceutical Society

First edition published in 2007, second edition 2014, third edition 2015, fourth edition 2017, fifth edition in 2022, reprinted in 2023

Index by Lyn Nesbitt-Smith of LNSIndexing, Brighton, UK

Typeset by Newgen Knowledge Works, Chennai, India

Printed in Great Britain by TJ Books Limited, Padstow, Cornwall

ISBN 978 0 85711 441 9 (print)

Contents

Brokering of Medicines   219

Manufacture, Importation and Distribution of Active Substances 239

Future UK rules and guidance

The UK left the EU on the 31 January 2020. EU legislation was carried forward during the transition period to provide stability to industry as well as time to implement necessary mitigations. After the transition period expired on 31 December 2020, Northern Ireland (NI) continues to comply with EU law as per the Northern Ireland Protocol (NIP) whilst GB (England, Scotland and Wales) does not.

The EU published (in December 2021) a package of measures designed to remove barriers to NI supply of medicines. The package includes an extension to the existing grace period to provide time to put in place long term legislative solutions and new legislative proposals which seek to resolve NI issues permanently to come into effect in 2022.

The extension to the grace period means that existing flexibilities for medicines supplied to NI will remain in place until the permanent solutions can be legislated for.

The MHRA has published guidance online which is regularly updated and can be accessed here: https://www.gov.uk/government/collections/new-guidance-and-information-for-industry-from-the-mhra#importing-and-exporting.

Preface to the 2022 edition

This is the 2022 edition of Rules and Guidance for Pharmaceutical Distributors (the "Green Guide"). This is the fifth edition of the guide and the first after the UK left the EU. Despite leaving, UK wholesalers, brokers of medicines and distributors of active substances are still required to comply with EU guidance on Good Distribution Practice and Good Distribution Practice of Active Substances. In this revised edition EU legislation has been removed but the good practice guidance has been retained.

This edition has revised sections on:

- MHRA (Overview of MHRA, MHRA Innovation Office, Compliance Teams, Applications and Registrations, Defective Medicines Report Centre, Importing unlicensed medicines – import notifications, Criminal Enforcement Unit, and Compliance Management and Inspection Action Group)
- amended extracts from the Human Medicines Regulations 2012 relating to:
  - wholesale dealing
  - brokering medicine and
  - importing and distributing active substances
- UK guidance on complying with the guidelines on Good Distribution Practice for wholesale distributors and brokers of medicines and importers and distributors of active substances
- UK guidance on
  - risk-based inspections
  - conditions of holding a wholesale dealer's licence, a broker registration and an active substance registration
  - a Responsible Person for import
  - controls on certain medicinal products.

There is new guidance on pharmacovigilance for wholesalers, the naming of sites on a licence, self-inspection and the Responsible Person for import.

This revised edition brings together in one chapter Good Distribution Practice guidance and the MHRA's expectations for compliance. There is also a new flowchart for the registration of handling active substances.

The 2022 version is available online, as part of "Medicines Complete" – a subscription-based database of leading medicines and healthcare references and in e-reader formats.

The *Green Guide* 2022

I am pleased to introduce the fifth edition of the Rules and Guidance for Pharmaceutical Distributors, also known as the Green Guide, issued by MHRA. This is the first edition since 2017 and includes significant updates on UK guidance on complying with the guidelines on GDP for distributors and brokers of medicine and importers and distributors of an active substance, and the conditions of holding a wholesale dealer's licence, a broker registration and an active substance registration. There are also new sections on pharmacovigilance for wholesalers, the naming of sites on a licence, self-inspection and the Responsible Person for import. There is also an extended flowchart for active substance registration.

I am pleased that the Green Guide continues to satisfy a demand for information in one authoritative and convenient place. I hope that this edition in its revised layout will continue to be useful, but the publication team very much welcome feedback so we can continue to improve this, and our other publications. See section on Feedback for details.

Dr Laura Squire OBE Chief Healthcare Quality and Access Officer
January 2022

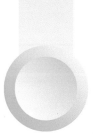

Acknowledgements

To the European Commission for permission to reproduce the 1995–2017 text of the Directives (only European Union legislation printed in the paper edition of the Official Journal of the European Union is deemed authentic), Regulations, Guidelines and associated documents.

To the Heads of Medicines Agencies for permission to reproduce the names and addresses of other human and veterinary medicines authorities in Europe.

To Cogent for permission to reproduce the new Gold Standard role profile for the Responsible Person.

To HMSO and the Queen's Printer for Scotland for permission to reproduce extracts from the Human Medicines Regulations 2012 [SI 2012/1916] as amended. Contains public sector information licensed under the Open Government Licence v3.0.

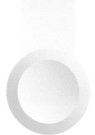

Feedback

Comments on the content or presentation of the Green Guide are encouraged and will be used to develop further editions. Your views are valued and both the MHRA and Pharmaceutical Press would appreciate you taking the time to contact us. Please visit the feedback page at http://www.pharmpress.com/orangeguide-feedback or send your feedback to the address below:

"The Rules and Guidance for Pharmaceutical Distributors 2022"
Customer Services
MHRA
10 South Colonnade
Canary Wharf
London E14 4PU
United Kingdom
Tel.: +44 (0)20 3080 6000
Fax: +44 (0)20 3118 9803

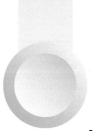

Introduction

The distribution network for medicinal products has become increasingly complex and now involves many different players.

The obligation on the UK government to ensure that pharmaceutical wholesale distributors are authorised is stated in the Human Medicines Regulations 2012 [SI 2012/1916] which requires all authorised wholesale distributors to have available a Responsible Person (RP) and Responsible Person (import) (RPi) where required and to comply with the Commission guidelines on Good Distribution Practice (GDP). These Regulations also set out requirements for registration and obligations of brokers of medicines and importers and distributors of an active substance.

This publication brings together the Commission guidelines on GDP, UK guidance on wholesale distribution practice and UK legislation on wholesale distribution, which wholesale distributors are expected to follow when distributing medicinal products for human use. It is of particular relevance to authorised wholesale distributors and to the RP and RPi, who have a responsibility for ensuring compliance with many of these regulatory requirements. Wholesale distributors are required to appoint an RP and/or RPi who has the knowledge and responsibility to ensure that correct procedures are followed during distribution. Updated notes on the qualifications and duties of the RP and RPi are included in this publication to assist this.

This publication is also of particular relevance to all brokers of medicines because it brings together UK guidance on brokering medicines and UK legislation on brokering, which brokers are expected to follow when brokering medicinal products for human use.

It is also of relevance to importers and distributors of active substances. The manufacture of active substances for use in a licensed medicinal product must be in compliance with the relevant Good Manufacturing Practice (GMP). Active substances imported from outside the EEA must have been manufactured in accordance with standards of GMP at least equivalent to those in the EU.

There are principles and guidelines for GMP for active substances, GDP guidelines for active substances and guidelines for the formal risk assessment process for excipients.

This guide brings together guidance and legislation on the importation and distribution of active substances, which importers and distributors of active substances are expected to follow when supplying active substances for use in licensed medicinal products for human use. For completeness, this guide also includes matters on what manufacturers of active substances have to comply with in order to provide further background information for importers and distributors of active substances.

The aim of GMP and GDP is to assure the quality of the medicinal product for the safety, well-being and protection of the patient. In achieving this aim it is impossible to over-emphasise the importance of individuals, at all levels, in the assurance of the quality of medicinal products. The great majority of reported defective medicinal products has resulted from human error or carelessness, not from failures in technology. All individuals involved with the distribution of medicinal products should bear this constantly in mind when performing their duties.

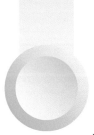

Glossary of UK Legislation

UK Legislation

The Human Medicines Regulations 2012 [SI 2012/1916]

The Regulations set out a comprehensive regime for the authorisation of medicinal products for human use, for the manufacture, import, distribution, sale and supply of those products, for their labelling and advertising, and for pharmacovigilance.

For the most part the Regulations implement Directive 2001/83/EC of the European Parliament and of the Council of 6 November 2001 on the community code relating to medicinal products for human use (as amended). They also provide for the enforcement in the United Kingdom of Regulation (EC) No 726/2004 laying down Community procedures for the authorisation and supervision of medicinal products for human and veterinary use and establishing a European Medicines Agency.

The Medicines (Products for Human Use) (Fees) Regulations 2016 [SI 2016/190]

These Regulations make provision for the fees payable under the Medicines Act 1971 and other fees payable in respect of EU obligations including those relating to authorisations, licences, certificates and registrations in respect of medicinal products for human use.

The Unlicensed Medicinal Products for Human Use (Transmissible Spongiform Encephalopathies) (Safety) Regulations 2003 [SI 2003/1680]

Regulates the importation and marketing of unlicensed medicinal products for human use in order to minimise the risk of the transmission of transmissible spongiform encephalopathies via those products.

Medicines and Healthcare products Regulatory Agency

1

Medicines and Healthcare products Regulatory Agency

Contents

Medicines and Healthcare products Regulatory Agency

The Medicines and Healthcare products Regulatory Agency regulates medicines, medical devices and blood components for transfusion in the UK.

About the Medicines and Healthcare products Regulatory Agency

Our purpose is clear: to protect and improve patient health by enabling the earliest access to, and high-quality supply of, safe, effective and innovative medical products through proportionate, data-driven assessment of risks and benefits.

We aspire to be a leading global example of delivering excellence in public health and patient safety, enabled through regulation and at the forefront of innovation. Delivering our vision relies on our ability to act as one agency and to relentlessly pursue the delivery of meaningful outcomes for the patients we serve.

This means drawing together our scientific rigour and regulatory expertise to address the challenges faced by the life sciences sector and health service; how best to develop new regulatory frameworks and quickly realise the benefits that new therapies, artificial intelligence and innovative healthcare products can bring to patients, while still ensuring the right levels of safety, quality and efficacy. It also means more systematic engagement with patients and putting patient outcomes at the heart of what we do.

How we operate

We are a government body that regulates medicines, medical devices and blood products for transfusion in the UK, underpinned by science and research.

We do this by making sure that the products we regulate — from painkillers to pacemakers — work properly and are acceptably safe; and by responding quickly and effectively when new concerns come to light.

No product is completely free of risk, but by using an array of evidence, we provide a critical appraisal of whether a healthcare product's benefits outweigh its risks and is suitable for use in the UK. Where some lower-risk medical devices are regulated by third party organisations, we set the regulatory requirements that define when those products can be approved for use in the UK.

To help the life sciences industry to develop effective and innovative healthcare products, we also engage proactively in the early stages of development.

We advise on the designs of clinical trials to ensure patient involvement and patient safety, and we advise on the evidence of safety and impact that developers will need to demonstrate for each product, to help products reach patients as quickly as possible while maintaining high levels of safety and quality.

Following our appraisal decision, we work with manufacturers to help them to comply with expectations of quality for their product to ensure they are safe to use.

We also monitor trends in data from a wide range of different sources, which enables us to quickly identify safety concerns.

Where these arise, we investigate and take a decision, using independent expertise, on the best course of action which could lead to products being removed from the UK market.

Our responsibilities

The Medicines and Healthcare products Regulatory Agency is responsible for:

- ensuring that medicines, medical devices and blood components for transfusion meet applicable standards of safety, quality and efficacy;
- ensuring that the supply chain for medicines, medical devices and blood components is safe and secure;
- promoting international standardisation and harmonisation to assure the effectiveness and safety of biological medicines;
- helping to educate the public and healthcare professionals about the risks and benefits of medicines, medical devices and blood components, leading to safer and more effective use;
- supporting innovation and research and development that's beneficial to public health; and
- influencing UK, EU and international regulatory frameworks so that they are risk proportionate and effective at protecting public health.

All licensed human medicines available in the UK are subject to rigorous scrutiny by the MHRA before they can be used by patients. This ensures that human medicines meet acceptable standards on safety, quality and efficacy. It is the responsibility of the MHRA and the expert advisory bodies set up by the Human Medicines Regulations 2012 [SI 2012/1916] to ensure that the sometimes difficult balance between safety and effectiveness is achieved. MHRA experts assess all applications for new human medicines to ensure that they meet the required standards. This is followed up by a system of inspection and testing that continues throughout the lifetime of the medicine.

As the UK government's public health body that brings together the regulation of human medicines and medical devices, science and research, the roles of the MHRA are to:

- license medicines, manufacturers and distributors;
- register brokers of finished medicines and manufacturers, importers and distributors of active substances;
- register websites that offer medicines for sale or supply to the public;
- regulate medical devices;
- approve UK clinical trials;
- monitor medicines and medical devices after licensing;

MHRA: LICENSING, INSPECTION AND ENFORCEMENT

- ensure the safety and quality of blood;
- tackle illegal activity involving medicines, medical devices and blood;
- promote an understanding of the benefits and risks;
- facilitate the development of new medicines;
- support innovation in medicines and medical devices;
- be a leading provider of data and data services for healthcare research;
- work with international partners on issues; and
- provide a national voice for the benefits and risks of medicines, medical devices and medical technologies.

Our priorities are outlined in our Delivery Plan Delivery Plan 2021-2023: Putting patients first: a new era for our agency. The plan ensures we keep a constant focus on delivering meaningful outcomes for patients, protecting public health through excellence in regulation and science and becoming a truly world-leading, enabling regulator. The plan sets out 14 objectives grouped into 6 central themes:

- Scientific innovation
- Healthcare access
- Patient safety
- Dynamic organisation
- Collaborative partnerships
- Financial sustainability

You can find the Delivery Plan 2021-2023 on our website: www.gov.uk/mhra

Compliance

The MHRA is responsible for ensuring compliance with the standards that apply to the manufacture and supply of medicines on the UK market. This is achieved by licensing, inspection and enforcement across the full lifecycle of medicines, including manufacturers, wholesale dealers and importers of medicines, and by inspecting clinical trials, toxicology laboratories and pharmacovigilance systems.

Compliance Teams and Applications and Registrations

Compliance Teams

Compliance comprises of dedicated teams of Inspectors for Good Manufacturing Practice (GMP), Good Distribution Practice (GDP), Good Laboratory Practice (GLP), Good Clinical Practice (GCP) and Good Pharmacovigilance Practice (GPvP).

Good Manufacturing Practice (GMP)

GMP Inspectors conduct inspections of pharmaceutical manufacturers and other organisations to assess compliance with EU guidance on Good Manufacturing Practice (GMP) and the relevant details contained in marketing authorisations and Clinical Trials Authorisations. They ensure that medicines supplied to the UK and its mutual recognition partners meet consistent high standards of quality, safety and efficacy. Overseas manufacturing sites to be named on UK marketing authorisations are also required to pass an inspection prior to approval of the marketing authorisation application. Following approval, a risk-based inspection programme maintains on-going surveillance of UK and overseas manufacturing site compliance with EU GMP.

GMP Inspectors are responsible for inspecting and authorising a range of manufacturers of sterile and non-sterile dosage forms, biological products, investigational medicinal products, herbal products and active pharmaceutical ingredients, in addition to certain analytical laboratories. The manufacture of unlicensed medicines by holders of Manufacturer "Specials" Licences in the UK NHS and commercial sector is also inspected on a routine basis to assess compliance with relevant legislation and GMP.

The safety and quality of human blood for transfusion, or for further manufacture into blood-derived medicines, is ensured through inspections of relevant collection, processing, testing and storage activities at Blood Establishments and UK Hospital Blood Banks. These inspections assess compliance with specific UK regulatory requirements, which take into account the detailed principles of GMP.

GMP Inspectors serve on a number of UK and international technical and standards committees, and provide help and advice to senior managers, Ministers and colleagues across the Agency, as necessary. Support and expertise is also provided to the inspection programmes of the European Medicines Agency (EMA), European Directorate for Quality of Medicines (EDQM) and the World Health Organization (WHO).

Good Manufacturing Practice: gmpinspectorate@mhra.gov.uk

Good Distribution Practice (GDP)

GDP Inspectors conduct inspections of sites of wholesale dealers to assess compliance with EU guidelines on Good Distribution Practice (GDP) and the conditions of a wholesale dealer's licence set out in the Human Medicines Regulations 2012 [SI 2012/1916].

Inspectors will ensure that medicinal products are handled, stored and transported under conditions as prescribed by the marketing authorisation or product specification.

Inspections are undertaken of new applicants and then subsequently on a routine schedule based on a risk assessment of the site.

Good Distribution Practice: GDP.inspectorate@mhra.gov.uk

Good Laboratory Practice (GLP)

GLP Inspectors conduct inspections of UK facilities that carry out non-clinical studies for submission to domestic and international regulatory authorities to assess the safety of new chemicals to humans, animals and the environment. These inspections are designed to assure that studies are performed in accordance with relevant regulation and the Organisation for Economic Co-operation and Development (OECD) principles as required by OECD Council acts relating to the Mutual Acceptance of Data. The range of test facilities to be monitored include those involved in the testing of human and veterinary pharmaceuticals, agrochemicals, food and feed additives, industrial chemicals and cosmetics.

Good Laboratory Practice: gxplabs@mhra.gov.uk

Good Clinical Practice (GCP)

The GCP Inspectorate is responsible for inspecting clinical trials for compliance with Good Clinical Practice (GCP). Compliance with this good practice provides assurance that the rights, safety and well-being of trial participants are protected, and that the results of the clinical trials are reliable.

The function of the GCP Inspectorate is to assess the compliance of organisations with UK legislation relating to the conduct of clinical trials in investigational medicinal products. This is achieved through carrying out inspections of sponsor organisations that hold Clinical Trial Authorisations (CTAs), organisations that provide services to clinical trial sponsors or investigator sites.

Clinical Practice: ctdhelpline@mhra.gov.uk

Good Pharmacovigilance Practice (GPvP)

Good Pharmacovigilance Practice (GPvP) is the minimum standard for monitoring the safety of medicines on sale to the public in the UK. The MHRA's Pharmacovigilance Inspectorate conducts inspections of marketing authorisation holders (MAH) to determine whether they comply with pharmacovigilance obligations established within the UK. GPvP inspections are scheduled as part of the MHRA's national inspection programme according to a risk-based approach, largely founded on the risk factors listed in EU statutory guidance (Good Vigilance Practice [GVP] Module III), as modified

by the Exceptions and modifications to EU guidance on good pharmacovigilance practices that apply to UK MAHs and the licensing authority.
Good Pharmacovigilance Practice: gpvpinspectors@mhra.gov.uk

Applications and Registrations

Manufacturers' and wholesale dealers' licence/authorisations

Manufacture of and wholesale dealing in medicinal products are licensable activities in the UK. These licences are referred to as process licences and include a wide range of licences covering diverse activities listed below:

- licences for the manufacture/importation of licensed medicinal products for human use, commonly abbreviated to MIA;
- "Specials" licences for the manufacture/importation of unlicensed medicinal products for human use, commonly abbreviated to MS;
- authorisations for the manufacture/importation of Investigational Medicinal Products for human use, commonly abbreviated to MIA(IMP);
- authorisations for the manufacture/importation of licensed medicinal products for veterinary use, commonly abbreviated to ManA;
- "Specials" licences for the manufacture of unlicensed medicinal products for veterinary use, commonly abbreviated to ManSA;
- authorisation for the manufacture of Exempt Advanced Therapy Medicinal Products, commonly abbreviated to MeAT;
- licences for the wholesale dealing of medicinal products for human use, commonly abbreviated to WDA(H);
- licences for the wholesale dealing/importation of medicinal products for veterinary use, commonly abbreviated to WDA(V);
- Blood Establishment Authorisations, commonly abbreviated to BEA.

The MHRA makes use of computer technology to process all applications for new licences, variations to existing licences, changes of ownership, terminations and cancellations, as well as suspensions and revocations on the instructions of the Inspection Action Group (IAG). It is also responsible for issuing Certificates of Good Manufacturing Practice (GMP) and Good Distribution Practice (GDP) on behalf of the GMP and GDP Compliance Teams.

Registrations

The Human Medicines Regulations 2012 set out requirements that certain activities require registration and that a minimum of information be published on publically accessible registers. These activities include:

- Brokering of finished human medicines;
- Manufacture, importation and distribution of active substances.
- Internet sales of medicine in Northern Ireland to the public

The MHRA process all applications for registration, variations to existing registrations and annual compliance reports, terminations, cancellations, suspensions and revocations, making extensive use of computer technology to do so.

Export Certificates

The MHRA is also responsible for issuing certificates in support of the World Health Organization (WHO) scheme on the quality of pharmaceutical products moving in international commerce (often referred to as export certificates):

- Certificate of a pharmaceutical product (CPP). The certificate shows details including:
  - the marketing authorisation holder;
  - the active ingredients and excipients;
  - the manufacturing, packaging and batch release sites;
  - whether or not the product is on the market in the UK.
- Certificate of licensing status (CLS). The certificate of licensing status is for importing agents who must screen bids made by an international tender for licensed or unlicensed products (excluding specials). The certificate has a limit of 10 products and one country for each certificate. The product name, dosage form, active ingredients and amounts should be the same as the medicine's product licence (if it is licensed).
- Certificate of a pharmaceutical product (unlicensed). The drug must have been manufactured in the UK and you must have a manufacturer licence for the drug.
- Certificate of manufacturing status (CMS). The certificate confirms the named sites on a specified manufacturer licence meet Good Manufacturing Practice requirements. All or any of the sites named on the manufacture licence can be listed on the certificate. The certificate will not show any product-specific information.
- Certificate for the importation of a pharmaceutical constituent (CPC). The specific active ingredient or excipient must be in either a:
  - current licensed human medicine;
  - national or international pharmacopoeia (official standards for pharmaceutical substances and medicines).

The manufacturing site must hold a valid certificate of inspection from the Medicines and Healthcare products Regulatory Agency (MHRA). The certificate is country and ingredient specific. A certificate can only be for one site function, e.g. manufacture, packaging or batch release. You can apply for a certificate for each function.

Defective Medicines Report Centre (DMRC)

The role of the Defective Medicines Report Centre (DMRC) is to minimise the hazard to patients arising from the distribution of defective medicines by providing an emergency assessment and communication system between manufacturers, distributors, regulatory authorities and users.

It achieves this aim by:

- receiving and assessing reports of suspected defective medicinal products for human use;
- advising and monitoring necessary actions by the responsible Licence Holder;
- communicating the details of this action to relevant parties as necessary.

The DMRC is staffed by suitably trained and experienced personnel with backgrounds in pharmaceutical quality assurance and Good Manufacturing Practice in hospital pharmacy and/or the pharmaceutical industry.

The pharmaceutical assessors are supported by administrative staff. Experts in specialist areas can be consulted when needed, e.g. experts in biological products, medical risk assessments or specific manufacturing techniques such as freeze-drying.

The DMRC operates a telephone line (020 3080 6574) from 08:45 to 16:45, Monday to Friday, except for public holidays, and can also be contacted directly via email at DMRC@mhra.gov.uk. Outside normal working hours, in an emergency, a MHRA Duty Officer (DO) can be contacted (07795 641 532). If needed, the DO will contact the relevant professional (pharmaceutical or medical) for further advice.

Where a medicinal product recall is required, the decision is taken in consultation with the relevant Licence Holder. It is the Licence Holder's responsibility to ensure that a recall is carried out effectively throughout the distribution chain to the appropriate level. If necessary, the DMRC will issue a Recall Notification to support action taken by the Licence Holder.

Medicines Recall Notifications are issued by the DMRC to a number of contacts for onward cascade to healthcare professionals in the public and private sectors.

Medicines Recall Notifications are also copied to various professional and trade organisations and journals. Medicines Recall Notifications are published on the MHRA website usually within 1 working day of issue. A cumulative list of Licence Holder-led recalls of UK licensed products and Medicines Recall Notifications is maintained on the MHRA website.

All existing centrally authorised product marketing authorisations (MAs) have been automatically converted into UK MAs, effective in the UK (only) and issued with a UK MA number on 1 January 2021. These UK MAs are referred to as "converted EU MAs". As a result of the implementation of the Northern Ireland Protocol, existing centrally authorised products will remain valid for marketing products in Northern Ireland.

For existing centrally authorised products the Licence Holder should inform the European Medicines Agency (EMA), in conjunction with DMRC, if the medicinal product has been manufactured or distributed in the UK. Subsequent action may be delegated to the DMRC or progressed by the EMA. If the Licence Holder is unsure, the DMRC should be the first point of contact for all issues.

Recalling Defective Medicinal Products: The Responsibilities of Distributors

To accord with the requirements of the Human Medicines Regulations 2012 [SI 2012/1916] the holder of a wholesale dealers licence must comply with the guidelines on Good Distribution Practice. In the case of a Licence Holder in Great Britain, these guidelines would be published under, or that apply by virtue of regulation C17, or in the case of a Licence Holder in Northern Ireland, published by the European Commission in accordance with Article 84 of the 2001 Directive. The holder must maintain an emergency plan to ensure effective implementation of the recall from the market of a medicinal product where recall is either ordered by the licensing authority (or by the competent authority of any European Economic Area (EEA) State in the case of Northern Ireland), or carried out in cooperation with the manufacturer of, or the holder of the marketing authorisation of, the product. The holder must also keep documents relating to the sale or supply of medicinal products under the licence that may facilitate the withdrawal or recall from sale of medicinal products in accordance with their emergency plan (Regulation 43(7) of the Human Medicines Regulations 2012 [SI 2012/1916]).

The holder of the wholesale dealer's licence should have in place detailed procedures that describe the action to be taken when a recall notice is received and must take appropriate steps to inform all customers who may have received stock of the batch(es) and medicinal product(s) that are affected by a recall.

Wholesalers should be aware that not all recalls will be accompanied by a Medicines Recall Notification issued by the MHRA and may be instituted at the request of a manufacturer or Licence Holder. In all cases the MHRA should have been notified of a recall in advance.

If a wholesaler has any doubts about a recall, they should contact the DMRC for advice.

Where a wholesaler receives a complaint regarding a suspected defective medicinal product, it should be referred to the relevant Licence Holder, manufacturer and/or the DMRC.

Note: Manufacturers Licence Holders are, by their nature, carrying out wholesale distribution activities and must comply with the guidelines on good distribution practice in the case of a Licence Holder in Great Britain, published under, or that apply by virtue of regulation C17, or in the case of a Licence Holder in Northern Ireland, published by the European Commission in accordance with Article 84 of the 2001 Directive, as if the Licence Holder were the holder of a wholesale dealer's licence (Regulation 39(8) of the Human Medicines Regulation 2012 [SI 2012/1916]). These guidelines also support the process of medicinal product recalls.

Importing Unlicensed Medicines: Import Notifications

Under regulation 46 of the Human Medicines Regulations 2012 [SI 2012/1916] a medicine must have a marketing authorisation (which includes Product Licences) unless exempt. One of these exemptions, which is in regulation 167 of these regulations, is for the supply of unlicensed medicinal products for the special clinical needs of individual patients. Prospective importers must hold a relevant licence and must notify the MHRA of their intention to import:

- for import from a country on the approved country for import list (currently EU and EEA members) or within the EEA for Northern Ireland, a Wholesale Dealer's Licence valid for import and handling of unlicensed medicinal products;
- for import from a country outside the approved country for import list (currently non-EU and non-EEA members) *or for Northern Ireland outside the EEA*, a Manufacturer's 'Specials' Licence valid for import.

Notifications of the intent to import are processed by the Import Notification System (INS). The MHRA enters the information into the system and issues the Acknowledgement letters. The Pharmaceutical Assessment team assesses the notification taking into account the special need identified, the target population, the product and the manufacturer. The pharmaceutical assessor issues a letter objecting or not to the importation.

Criminal Enforcement Unit

Medicines legislation contains statutory provisions to enforce the requirements of the Human Medicines Regulations 2012 [SI 2012/1916] and the remaining provisions of the 1968 Medicines Act.

This enforcement role is carried out by the MHRA's Criminal Enforcement Unit, which comprises of Criminal Enforcement Intelligence and Criminal Enforcement Investigation sections.

The legislation confers certain powers, including rights of entry, powers of inspection, seizure, sampling and production of documents. Duly authorised Investigation Officers investigate cases using these powers and, where appropriate, criminal prosecutions are brought by the Crown Prosecution Service (CPS). MHRA investigators also investigate offences under other legislation such as the Fraud Act, Trademarks Act and Offences Against the Person Act.

All reported breaches of medicines legislation are investigated. Reports are processed and risk assessed before a course of action is agreed in line with our published Enforcement Strategy.

The aim of the Intelligence Unit is to drive forward the implementation of intelligence-led enforcement and enable a more proactive approach to the acquisition and development of information. The Unit acts as a coordination point for all information-gathering activities and works in conjunction with a wide network of public and professional bodies and trade associations, e.g. UK Border Force, Customs, the Department of Health and Social Care, Trading Standards and Port Health Authorities, the Police Service, and professional organisations such as the General Pharmaceutical Council (GPhC), the General Medical Council and the Association of the British Pharmaceutical Industry (ABPI). Additionally, there is a network of other regulatory agencies and law enforcement bodies within the European Community and in other countries through which the Criminal Enforcement Unit can exchange information and follow trends in crime involving medicines and medical devices.

The Criminal Enforcement Unit coordinates initiatives to counteract and disrupt criminal activity involving the regulated and illegal supply chains. There is a protocol for dealing with falsified medicines infiltrating the licensed medicines supply chain.

Compliance Management and Inspection Action Group

Compliance Management Process

Compliance management is a non-statutory process providing oversight and monitoring of ongoing corrective action plans in response to poor compliance that does not yet meet the threshold for consideration of adverse regulatory action. The process is managed via the Compliance Management Team (CMT) — a non-statutory group of senior GMDP inspectors, selected on the basis of their experience, who coordinate and advise on compliance management activities arising from chronic or significant GMP deficiencies.

Chronic GMP non-compliance: Where major deficiencies are identified over a series of inspection cycles, which the company has not effec-

tively addressed. There is no immediate potential for patient harm but requires attention to avoid adverse regulatory action.

Significant GMP non-compliance: *Where multiple major deficiencies are found at inspection, with no immediate potential for patient harm, which cannot be managed through the Risk Based Inspection (RBI) process but require quick attention to avoid adverse regulatory action.*

The main aim of the compliance management process is to refocus companies towards a state of compliance, thus avoiding the need for regulatory action and potential adverse impacts on patient health through lack of availability of medicines as a result of action against an authorisation, as well as ensuring risk-based decision making and efficient use of inspectorate resources.

The specific Compliance inspection case issues are considered by the CMT, who make decisions in conjunction with the inspector regarding the proportionate inspection and non-inspection compliance management actions required. This may include making recommendations on close monitoring of compliance improvements, recommendations for additional internal or external support or resources required, reductions in capacity to facilitate compliance actions, ensuring that the compliance action plan remains on track, communicating with company senior management, alerting them to any additional compliance concerns, and clearly outlining the consequences of continued non-compliance.

Chronic or significant GMP non-compliance are firstly identified at the inspection and communicated to the CMT, which will collectively decide on an appropriate course of action based on the Inspectors, recommendations. Decisions on compliance-management actions are communicated to the company, following consideration of any written responses to a post- inspection letter, if relevant. The site inspector(s) and CMT will continue to monitor the effectiveness of these actions. The CMT process may also be initiated by the Inspection Action Group (IAG) following referral for significant or serious GMP deficiencies. In cases where consideration of adverse licensing action is no longer required due to improvements or mitigating actions, the IAG may close their case referral and request that the CMT maintain compliance-management oversight until completion of the remediation plans. Upon satisfactory conclusion of the remediation work, the company will be returned to the routine RBI programme; however, referral for consideration of regulatory action may still occur if the required improvements are not achieved in a timely manner.

Conversely, failure to address GMP non-compliance issues when a company is at CMT may result in an upward referral to the IAG so that formal actions against the licence, personnel named on the licence or the marketing authorisation holder can be taken.

MHRA: LICENSING, INSPECTION AND ENFORCEMENT

Referral to the Inspection Action Group (IAG)

Critical findings at inspection are routinely referred to the MHRA's Inspection Action Group (IAG). The group considers referrals involving serious/critical GMP deficiencies.

Serious GMP non-compliance: where regulatory actions should be considered to remove a potential or actual risk to public health or patients/participants in a clinical trial.

The primary objective of the IAG is to protect public health by ensuring that licensable activities meet the required regulatory standards.

The IAG is a non-statutory, multidisciplinary group constituted to advise the Chief Healthcare, Quality and Access Officer on any recommendation for regulatory or adverse licensing action appropriate to the relevant good practice Division. There are two distinct groups:

- IAG1 considers issues related to Good Manufacturing Practice, Good Distribution Practice and Blood Establishment Authorisations (GMP/GDP/BEA) and has 24 scheduled meetings per year, usually the first and third Tuesdays of each month;
- IAG2 considers issues related to Good Clinical and Good Pharmacovigilance Practices (GCP/GPvP) and has 12 scheduled meetings per year, usually the fourth Tuesday of each month.

Where an urgent issue arises, an emergency *ad hoc* meeting can be held. The following attend both IAG1 and IAG2 meetings:

- the nominated Chair;
- at least one MHRA medical assessor;
- at least one MHRA pharmaceutical assessor;
- a solicitor from the Government Legal Services;
- at least one member of the IAG Secretariat;
- any inspector making a referral to the IAG;
- a representative from MHRA Criminal Enforcement Unit (if required);
- members of MHRA staff who may also attend for training purposes.

In addition, the following will attend IAG1:

- an expert/lead senior/senior GMP inspector;
- an expert/lead senior/senior GDP inspector;
- if required, a representative from the Veterinary Medicines Directorate https://www.gov.uk/government/organisations/veterinary-medicines-directorate;
- an expert in blood and blood products (if required).

In addition, the following will attend IAG2:

- an expert/senior GCP inspector;
- an expert/senior GPvP inspector;

- the Clinical Trials Unit manager or deputy;
- the Pharmacovigilance Risk Management Group manager or deputy.

REASONS FOR REFERRAL

This will usually happen if, during the inspection process, the inspector has identified one or more critical "deficiencies" as a result of a Good Practice Standards inspection. However, a referral may also be made as a result of a licence variation, the failure to contact an organisation, the refusal of an organisation to accept an inspection, the outcome of enforcement activity, the outcome of a product recall or a person named on the licence as Production/QC/Qualified Person not fulfilling their legal responsibilities. The company will normally be informed during the closing meeting at inspection that a referral to the IAG will be made. This will be further confirmed in the post-inspection letter and from that point onwards, correspondence from the company should be directed to the IAG Secretariat, copying in the site inspector.

How the process works:

- An inspection reveals serious (critical) deficiencies and the company is told it will be referred to the IAG.
- A post-inspection letter is issued to the company signed by a senior Inspector accredited in that area or a responsible operations manager/lead inspector.
- The IAG discusses the case at its next available meeting (if necessary, an emergency meeting can be called).
- The IAG discusses any proposed action.
- The referred company is informed of any IAG actions and next steps.
- Actions are followed up at subsequent meetings until the situation is resolved.
- The matter is kept on the agenda until the IAG is satisfied that the referral can be closed.

IAG POSSIBLE ACTIONS

IAG1 (GMP/GDP/BEA):

- Refusal to grant a licence or a variation;
- Proposal to suspend the licence for a stated period or vary the licence;
- Notification of immediate suspension of the licence for a stated period (no longer than 3 months);
- Proposal to revoke the licence;
- Notice of suspension, variation or revocation;
- Action to remove a Qualified Person/Responsible Person (QP/RP) from the licence;
- Issue a Cease and Desist order in relation to a Blood Establishment Authorisation (BEA);

- Issue a warning letter to the company/individual;
- Request a written justification for actions of a QP/RP;
- Referral of a QP to their professional body;
- Increased inspection frequency;
- Statement of non-compliance with GMP or GDP;
- Restricted GMP and GDP certificates;
- Impose a production capacity restriction;
- Require engagement of external support for the remediation plan:
- Request the company/individual attend a meeting at the Agency;
- Refer to the Criminal Enforcement Unit for further consideration.

IAG2 (GCP/GPvP):

- Issue an infringement notice in relation to a clinical trial;
- Suspend or revoke a clinical trial authorisation;
- Further follow-up inspections, or triggered inspections at related organ-isations (e.g. issues in GCP may trigger a GMP inspection);
- Referral to Committee for Medicinal Products for Human Use (CHMP) for consideration for or against a marketing authorisation (e.g. sus-pended, varied or revoked);
- Liaison and coordinated action with the European Medicines Agency (EMA) and other Member States regarding concerns;
- Refer the case to the EMA for consideration of the use of the EU Infringe-ment Regulation (which could result in a fine);
- Request a written justification for action of a QPPV (Qualified Person responsible for pharmacovigilance);
- Request the company/individual attend a meeting at the Agency;
- Refer to MHRA Criminal Enforcement Unit for further consideration.

In the case of inspections in third countries:

- a refusal to name a site on a marketing authorisation;
- a recommendation that a site be removed from a marketing authorisation;
- the issuing of a GMP non-compliance statement;
- in the case of an adverse (voluntary or triggered) active pharmaceutical ingredients (API) inspection, this could result in the removal of the API site from the marketing authorisation;
- in the case of an adverse (voluntary or triggered) investigational medic-inal products (IMP) inspection, this could result in the suspension of a clinical trial.

In all cases, an action could result in the withdrawal of product (API, IMP, etc.) from the market. However, this specific action is handled by the Defective Medicines Reporting Centre (DMRC) rather than directly by the IAG.

CRITICAL PRODUCTS

The possible actions that the IAG may take involves consideration of the risks and benefits to patients, and the supply situation where critical medicines are involved following consultation with the Department of Health and Social Care (DHSC) and for overseas products potentially with other national competent authorities.

A critical medicine is defined as one where there is no therapeutic alternative available or where other manufacturers do not have the available capacity to replace the demand when there is disruption to the existing supply chain.

LEGAL BASIS FOR THIS ACTION

The legal basis for licensing action is contained in:

- The Human Medicines Regulations 2012 [SI 2012/1916];
- The Medicines for Human Use (Clinical Trials) Regulations 2004 [SI 2004/1031];
- The Blood Safety and Quality Regulations 2005 [SI 2005/50].

WHAT A LICENCE HOLDER SHOULD DO IF REFERRED TO THE IAG

In the first instance, a referral should be treated as a requirement to correct immediately the deficiencies identified during the inspection and report completed actions to the IAG Secretariat/Inspectorate as soon as possible.

If, due to safety concerns, the referral results in an immediate suspension of a manufacturing/wholesale dealer's licence this will be for a duration of 3 months, and during this time a company should be focused on correcting the inspection deficiencies.

If the referral results in a proposed suspension, variation or revocation of a licence, a company will have the following appeal options prior to a decision being made:

- may make written representations to the licensing authority (MHRA);
- may appear before and be heard by a person appointed for the purpose by the licensing authority (a fee of £10,000 will be charged for a person-appointed request).

If a company submits written representations within the specified time period, the licensing authority shall take those representations into account before determining the matter. In practice, this means that any proposed action will not be progressed until the written representations have been reviewed and considered by the IAG and a recommendation made to the Divisional Director on whether to proceed with the action or not.

If a company submits a request for a Person Appointed Hearing, this will be taken forward by the MHRA Panel Secretariat. Any proposed action will not be progressed until the Person Appointed Hearing has taken place.

It should be noted that a Person Appointed Hearing will only offer its opinion into whether a licence condition has been contravened. A final decision on whether to suspend or revoke a licence will still rest with the licensing authority, who will take the report of the Person Appointed Hearing into account.

Follow-up actions that may be taken:

- a re-inspection to ensure corrective actions implemented;
- request for regular updates on the corrective action plan;
- the issue of a short-dated GMP certificate;
- recommended increase of inspection frequency;
- continued monitoring of the company by IAG via inspectorate updates;
- if serious and persistent non-compliance continues, referral for consideration of criminal prosecution.

Contact for further information: IAGSecretariat@mhra.gov.uk or IAG2Secretariat@mhra.gov.uk

CHARGING FOR COMPLIANCE MANAGEMENT COSTS

The Medicines (Products for Human Use) (Fees) Regulations 2016 section 30(b)(i) permits the MHRA to charge for the additional cost of inspectors' time to review reports, CAPA and responses for companies that have been referred to CMT or IAG. See Compliance Teams blog "It pays to be compliant" for more details: https://mhrainspectorate.blog.gov.uk/2019/01/11/it-pays-to-be-compliant/

Advice

MHRA publishes a series of Guidance Notes relating to its statutory functions. Those of particular interest to manufacturers and wholesale dealers include:

GN 5   Notes for applicants and holders of a manufacturer's licence;
GN 6   Notes for applicants and holders of a wholesale dealer's licence (WDA(H)) or broker registration;
GN 8   A guide to what is a medicinal product;
GN 14   The supply of unlicensed medicinal products "Specials".

Contact details are as follows:

Address:
Customer Services, Medicines and Healthcare products Regulatory Agency, 10 South Colonnade, Canary Wharf, London, E14 4PU, UK
Telephone: +44 (0)20 3080 6000 (weekdays 09:00–17:00)
Fax: +44 (0)20 3118 9803
E-mail: info@mhra.gov.uk
Website: https://www.gov.uk/government/organisations/medicines-and-healthcare-products-regulatory-agency

MHRA: LICENSING, INSPECTION AND ENFORCEMENT

Wholesale Distribution of Medicines

UK Legislation on Wholesale Distribution

Contents

The Human Medicines Regulations 2012 [SI 2012/1916]

Editor's note	These extracts from the Regulations and Standard Provisions of the Human Medicines Regulations 2012 [SI 2012/1916] are presented for the reader's convenience. Reproduction is with the permission of HMSO and the Queen's Printer for Scotland. For any definitive information reference must be made to the original Regulations. The numbering and content within this section corresponds to the regulations set out in the published Statutory Instrument [SI 2012/1916].

Citation and commencement

1 (1) These Regulations may be cited as the Human Medicines Regulations 2012.

(2) These Regulations come into force on 14th August 2012.

Medicinal products

2 (1) In these Regulations "medicinal product" means:

(a) any substance or combination of substances presented as having properties of preventing or treating disease in human beings; or

(b) any substance or combination of substances that may be used by or administered to human beings with a view to:

(i) restoring, correcting or modifying a physiological function by exerting a pharmacological, immunological or metabolic action, or

(ii) making a medical diagnosis.

(2) These Regulations do not apply to:

(a) whole human blood; or

(b) any human blood component, other than plasma, prepared by a method involving an industrial process.

Definition of advanced therapy medicinal product etc.

2A (1) In these Regulations, in their application to products for sale or supply in Great Britain only, "advanced therapy medicinal product" means any of the following products:

(a) a gene therapy medicinal product;

(b) a somatic cell therapy medicinal product; or

(c) a tissue-engineered product.

(2) A "gene therapy medicinal product" is a biological medicinal product which has the following characteristics:

(a) it contains an active substance which contains or consists of a recombinant nucleic acid used in or administered to human beings with a view to regulating, repairing, replacing, adding or deleting a genetic sequence; and

(b) its therapeutic, prophylactic or diagnostic effect relates directly to the recombinant nucleic acid sequence it contains, or to the product of genetic expression of this sequence.

(3) A vaccine against infectious diseases is not to be treated as a gene therapy medicinal product.

(4) A "somatic cell medicinal product" is a medicinal product which has the following characteristics:

(a) it contains or consists of cells or tissues that:

     (i) have been subject to substantial manipulation so that biological characteristics, physiological functions or structural properties relevant for the intended clinical use have been altered; or

     (ii) are not intended to be used for the same essential function in the recipient as in the donor; and

    (b) it is presented as having properties for, or is used in or administered to human beings with a view to, treating, preventing or diagnosing a disease through the pharmacological, immunological or metabolic action of its cells or tissues.

(5) A "tissue-engineered product" is a medicinal product which:

    (a) contains or consists of engineered cells or tissues; and

    (b) is presented as having properties for, or is used in or administered to human beings with a view to, regenerating, repairing or replacing a human tissue.

(6) A tissue-engineered product may contain:

    (a) cells or tissues of human or animal origin;

    (b) viable or non-viable cells or tissues; and

    (c) additional substances, including cellular products, biomolecules, biomaterials, chemical substances, scaffolds or matrices.

(7) A product is not a tissue engineered product if it:

    (a) contains or consists exclusively of non-viable human or animal cells or tissues;

    (b) does not contain any viable cells or tissues; and

    (c) does not act principally by pharmacological, immunological or metabolic actions.

(8) Cells or tissues are engineered if they:

    (a) have been subject to substantial manipulation, so that biological characteristics, physiological functions or structural properties relevant for the intended regeneration, repair or replacement are achieved; or

    (b) are not intended to be used for the same essential function in the recipient as in the donor.

(9) The following manipulations are not substantial manipulations for the purposes of paragraphs (4)(a) and (8)(a):

    (a) cutting;

    (b) grinding;

    (c) shaping;

    (d) centrifugation;

    (e) soaking in antibiotic or antimicrobial solutions;

    (f) sterilisation;

    (g) irradiation;

    (h) cell separation, concentration or purification;

    (i) filtering;

(j) lyophilisation;

(k) freezing;

(l) cryopreservation; and

(m) vitrification.

(10) In these Regulations, in their application to products for sale or supply in Great Britain only, "combined advanced therapy medicinal product" means an advanced therapy medicinal product:

(a) which incorporates, as an integral part of the product, one or more medical devices or one or more active implantable medical devices;

(b) the cellular part of which:

(i) contains viable cells or tissues; or

(ii) contains non-viable cells or tissues which are liable to act upon the human body with an action that can be considered as primary to that of the medical devices.

(11) Where an advanced therapy medicinal product contains viable cells or tissues, the pharmacological, immunological or metabolic action of those cells or tissues is to be treated as the principal mode of action of the product.

(12) An advanced therapy medicinal product containing both autologous and allogeneic cells or tissues is to be treated as being for allogeneic use.

(13) A product which falls within the definition of a tissue-engineered product and within the definition of a somatic cell therapy medicinal product is to be treated as a tissue-engineered product.

(14) A product which falls within the definition of:

(a) a somatic cell therapy medicinal product or a tissue-engineered product;

(b) a gene therapy medicinal product,

is to be treated as a gene therapy medicinal product.

General interpretation

8 (1) In these Regulations (unless the context otherwise requires):

"the 2001 Directive" means Directive 2001/83/EC of the European Parliament and of the Council on the Community Code relating to medicinal products for human use;

"the 2018 Regulations" means the Health Service Products (Provision and Disclosure of Information) Regulations 2018;

"advanced therapy medicinal product" means, in the case of a medicinal product for sale or supply by the holder of a UKMA(NI) or UKMA(UK), a medicinal product described in Article 2(1)(a) of Regulation (EC) No 1394/2007;

"approved country for import list" means the list published by the licensing authority under regulation 18A (approved country for import) and "approved country for import" means a country included in that list;

"Article 126a authorisation" means an authorisation granted by the licensing authority under Part 8 of these Regulations;

"brokering" means all activities in relation to the sale or purchase of medicinal products, except for wholesale distribution, that do not include physical handling and that consist of negotiating independently and on behalf of another legal or natural person;

"EU marketing authorisation" means a marketing authorisation granted or renewed by the European Commission under Regulation (EC) No 726/2004;

"European Economic Area" or "EEA" means the European Economic Area created by the EEA agreement;

"exempt advanced therapy medicinal product" has the meaning given in regulation 171;

"export" means export, or attempt to export, from the United Kingdom, whether by land, sea or air;

"falsified medicinal product" means any medicinal product with a false representation of:

(a) its identity, including its packaging and labelling, its name or its composition (other than any unintentional quality defect) as regards any of its ingredients, including excipients and the strength of those ingredients;

(b) its source, including its manufacturer, its country of manufacturing, its country of origin or its marketing authorisation holder; or

(c) its history, including the records and documents relating to the distribution channels used.

"herbal medicinal product" means a medicinal product whose only active ingredients are herbal substances or herbal preparations (or both);

"homoeopathic medicinal product" means a medicinal product prepared from homoeopathic stocks in accordance with a homoeopathic manufacturing procedure described by:

(a) the European Pharmacopoeia; or

(b) in the absence of such a description in the European Pharmacopoeia,

(i) in relation to a certificate of registration or marketing authorisation for a national homoeopathic product in force in Great Britain only, the British Pharmacopoeia, or in an pharmacopoeia used officially in an country that is included in a list published by the licensing authority for this purpose;

(ii) in relation to a certificate of registration or marketing authorisation for a national homoeopathic product in force in the whole United Kingdom or in Northern Ireland only, in the British Pharmacopoeia or in any pharmacopoeia used officially in an EEA State;

"import" means import, or attempt to import, into the UK, whether by land, sea or air (and "imported" is to be construed accordingly);

"inspector" means a person authorised in writing by an enforcement authority for the purposes of Part 16 (enforcement) (and references to "the enforcement authority", in relation to an inspector, are to the enforcement authority by whom the inspector is so authorised);

"the licensing authority" has the meaning given by regulation 6(2);

"listed NIMAR product" means a product included in a list maintained in accordance with regulation 167B on the date it is dispatched from Great Britain to Northern Ireland;

"manufacturer's licence" has the meaning given by regulation 17(1);

"marketing authorisation" means:

(a) a UK marketing authorisation; or

(b) an EU marketing authorisation;

"medicinal product subject to general sale" has the meaning given in regulation 5(1) (classification of medicinal products);

"the relevant EU provisions" means the provisions of legislation of the European Union relating to medicinal products for human use, except to the extent that any other enactment provides for any function in relation to any such provision to be exercised otherwise than by the licensing authority;

"NIMAR" means Northern Ireland MHRA authorised route;

"relevant European State" means an EEA State or Switzerland;

"relevant medicinal product" has the meaning given by regulation 48;

"special medicinal product" means a product within the meaning of regulation 167 or any equivalent legislation in a country other than the UK;

"traditional herbal medicinal product" means a herbal medicinal product to which regulation 125 applies;

"traditional herbal registration" means a traditional herbal registration granted by the licensing authority under these Regulations and:

(a) "THR(UK)" means such a registration in force in the whole United Kingdom;

(b) "THR(GB)" means such a registration in force in Great Britain only;

(c) "THR(NI)" means such a registration in force in Northern Ireland only.

"UK marketing authorisation" means a marketing authorisation granted by the licensing authority under Part 5 of these Regulations or Chapter 4 of Title III to the 2001 Directive (mutual recognition and decentralised procedure) and:

(a) "UKMA(UK)" means such an authorisation in force in the whole United Kingdom;

(b) "UKMA(GB)" means such an authorisation in force in Great Britain only;

(c) "UKMA(NI)" means such an authorisation in force in Northern Ireland only.

"wholesale dealer's licence" has the meaning given by regulation 18(1).
- In these Regulations, references to distribution of a product by way of wholesale dealing are to be construed in accordance with regulation 18(4) and (5).
- In these Regulations, references to selling by retail, or to retail sale, are references to selling a product to a person who buys it otherwise than for a purpose specified in regulation 18(5).
- In these Regulations, references to supplying anything in circumstances corresponding to retail sale are references to supplying it, otherwise than by way of sale, to a person who receives it otherwise than for a purpose specified in regulation 18(5).

Wholesale dealing in medicinal products

18 (1) A person may not except in accordance with a licence (a "wholesale dealer's licence"):

(a) distribute a medicinal product by way of wholesale dealing; or

(b) possess a medicinal product for the purpose of such [distribution; or]

(c) import a medicinal product from an approved country for import into Great Britain for either purpose; or

(d) supply a listed NIMAR product from Great Britain to Northern Ireland.

(2) Paragraph (1):

(a) does not apply:

(i) to anything done in relation to a medicinal product by the holder of a manufacturer's licence in respect of that product;

(ii) where the product concerned is an investigational medicinal product; or

(iii) if the product is a radiopharmaceutical in which the radionuclide is in the form of a sealed source; and

(b) is subject to regulation 19.

(2A) Paragraph (1)(c) does not apply to imports into Great Britain from an EEA State of medicinal products that have been released for sale, supply or distribution in an EEA State or the United Kingdom before IP completion day.

(2B) For the purposes of paragraph (2A) a medicinal product has been released for sale, supply or distribution where, after the stage of manufacturing has taken place, the product is the subject matter of a written or verbal agreement between two or more persons for the transfer of ownership, any other property right, or possession concerning the product, or where the product is the subject matter of an offer to a person to conclude such an agreement.

(3) Distribution of a medicinal product by way of wholesale dealing, or possession for the purpose of such distribution, is not to be taken to be in accordance with a wholesale dealer's licence unless the distribu-

tion is carried on, or as the case may be the product held, at premises located in the UK and specified in the licence.

(4) In these Regulations a reference to distributing a product by way of wholesale dealing is a reference to:

(a) selling or supplying it; or

(b) procuring or holding it or exporting it for the purposes of sale or supply, to a person who receives it for a purpose within paragraph (5).

(5) Those purposes are:

(a) selling or supplying the product; or

(b) administering it or causing it to be administered to one or more human beings, in the course of a business carried on by that person.

(6) A wholesale dealer's licence does not authorise the distribution of a medicinal product by way of wholesale dealing, or possession of a medicinal product for the purpose of such distribution, unless:

(a) in the case of a product for sale or supply in Great Britain, a UKMA(GB) or UKMA(UK), certificate of registration or traditional herbal registration is in force in respect of the product, or

(b) in the case of a product for sale or supply in Northern Ireland, a UKMA(NI) or UKMA(UK), EU marketing authorisation, Article 126a authorisation, certificate of registration or traditional herbal registration is in force in respect of the product, or

(c) in the case of a listed NIMAR product, a UKMA(GB) or UKMA(UK) is in force in respect of the product,

but this is subject to the exceptions in regulation 43(6).

(7) In paragraph (6)(b), "marketing authorisation" means:

(a) a marketing authorisation issued by a competent authority of a member State in accordance with the 2001 Directive; or

(b) an EU marketing authorisation.

Approved country for import

18A (1) The licensing authority must:

(a) publish a list of countries from which medicinal products may be imported under a wholesale dealing licence ("approved country for import list"); and

(b) only include in that list a country which is included in the approved country for batch testing list.

(2) In order to determine whether a country should be included in the approved country for import list, the licensing authority may, in particular, take into account

(a) the country's system for ensuring that each batch of a medicinal product has been manufactured and checked in accordance with the requirements of its legislation and any authorisation in respect of that product;

(b) the country's rules for good distribution practice;

(c) the regularity of inspections to verify compliance with good distribution practice;

(d) the effectiveness of enforcement of good distribution practice;

(e) the regularity and rapidity of information provided by that country relating to non-compliant manufacturers and distributers of medicinal products;

(f) any on-site review of that country's regulatory system undertaken by the licensing authority;

(g) any on-site inspection of a manufacturing site in that country observed by the licensing authority; and

(h) any other relevant documentation available to the licensing authority.

(3) The licensing authority must:

(a) remove a country from the approved country for import list if that country is removed from the approved country for batch testing list;

(b) in any event review the countries it has included in the approved country for import list to determine if it is still satisfied that the country should remain on that list, and if it is not so satisfied, remove that country from the list; and

(c) undertake that review at least every three years beginning with the date on which that country is included in that list.

Exemptions from requirement for wholesale dealer's licence

19 (1) Regulation 18 does not apply to the sale or offer for sale of a medicinal product by way of wholesale dealing, or possession for the purpose of such sale or offer, where paragraph (2) applies and the person selling or offering the product for sale is:

(a) the holder of:

(i) in the case of a product for sale or supply in Great Britain (including a listed NIMAR product for sale or supply from Great Britain to Northern Ireland) a UKMA(GB), a UKMA(UK), a COR(GB), a COR(UK), a THR(GB) or a THR(UK) (an "authorisation") which relates to the product, or

(ii) in the case of a product for sale or supply in Northern Ireland, a UKMA(NI), a UKMA(UK), a COR(NI), a COR(UK), a THR(NI), a THR(UK), an EU marketing authorisation or an Article 126a authorisation (an "authorisation") which relates to the product, including a holder of an authorisation who manufactured or assembled the product; or

(b) a person who is not the holder of an authorisation in relation to the product but manufactured or assembled the product in the United Kingdom to the order of a person who is the holder of an authorisation relating to the product.

(2) This paragraph applies if:
  (a) until the sale, the medicinal product has been kept on the premises of the person who manufactured or assembled the product (in this regulation referred to as "authorised premises"); and
  (b) those premises are premises authorised for use for manufacture or assembly by that person's manufacturer's licence.
(3) For the purposes of this regulation, a medicinal product is regarded as having been kept on authorised premises at a time when:
  (a) it was being moved from one set of authorised premises to another, or from one part of authorised premises to another part; or
  (b) it was being moved from authorised premises by way of delivery to a purchaser.
(4) Regulation 18 does not apply to a person who in connection with the importation of a medicinal product:
  (a) provides facilities solely for transporting the product; or
  (b) acting as an import agent, handles the product where the product is imported solely to the order of another person who intends to sell the product or offer it for sale by way of wholesale dealing or to distribute it in any other way.
(4A) Regulation 18 does not apply in connection with the distribution by way of wholesale dealing of a medicinal product to be used for vaccination or immunisation against coronavirus or influenza virus, where the person distributing the medicinal product:
  (a) was supplied with the medicinal product for the purposes of the administration of it under relevant arrangements;
  (b) is supplying the medicinal product for the purposes of the administration of it by the person to whom it is being supplied (or by a person employed or engaged by them) under relevant arrangements; and
  (c) is authorised by the body making the arrangements to supply the medicinal product as mentioned in subparagraph (b) under the relevant arrangements.
(4B) Regulation 18 does not apply in connection with the distribution by way of wholesale dealing of a medicinal product to be supplied or administered in accordance with a protocol of the type mentioned in regulation 247, where the person distributing the medicinal product:
  (a) was supplied with the medicinal product for the purposes of the supply or administration of it to a patient under relevant arrangements;
  (b) is supplying the medicinal product for the purposes of the supply or administration of it to a patient by the person to whom it is being supplied (or by a person employed or engaged by them) under relevant arrangements; and
  (c) is authorised by the body making the arrangements to supply the medicinal product as mentioned in sub-paragraph (b) under the relevant arrangements.

(4C) In this regulation, "relevant arrangements" means:
  (a) arrangements for the provision of services as part of:
    (i) in England, the health service as defined by section 275(1) of the National Health Service Act 2006,
    (ii) in Scotland, the health service as defined by section 108(1) of the National Health Service (Scotland) Act 1978(8),
    (iii) in Wales, the health service as defined by section 206(1) of the National Health Service (Wales) Act 2006(9), and
    (iv) in Northern Ireland, the system of health and social care promoted undersection 2(1) of the Health and Social Care (Reform) Act (Northern Ireland)2009(10); or
  (b) arrangements for the provision of services (otherwise than as mentioned in sub-paragraph (a)) as part of the medical services of Her Majesty's Forces.
(4D) Paragraphs (4A) to (4C) cease to have effect on 1st April 2022.
(5) . . .
(6) Regulation 18 does not apply to a person ("P") who imports a medicinal product into Great Britain from an approved country for import for administration to P or to any other person who is a member of P's household.

Application for manufacturer's or wholesale dealer's licence

21 (1) An application for a grant of a licence under this Part must:
  (a) be made to the licensing authority;
  (b) be made in the way and form specified in Schedule 3; and
  (c) contain or be accompanied by the information, documents, samples and other material specified in that Schedule.
  (2) An application must indicate the descriptions of medicinal products in respect of which the licence is required, either by specifying the descriptions of medicinal products in question or by way of an appropriate general classification.

Factors relevant to determination of application for manufacturer's or wholesale dealer's licence

22 (1) In dealing with an application for a manufacturer's licence the licensing authority must, in particular, take into consideration:
  (a) the operations proposed to be carried out under the licence;
  (b) the premises in which those operations are to be carried out;
  (c) the equipment which is or will be available on those premises for carrying out those operations;
  (d) the qualifications of the persons under whose supervision the operations will be carried out; and

    (e) the arrangements made or to be made for securing the safekeeping, and the maintenance, of adequate records in respect of medicinal products manufactured or assembled in pursuance of the licence.

(2) In dealing with an application for a wholesale dealer's licence the licensing authority must in particular take into consideration:

    (a) the premises on which medicinal products of the descriptions to which the application relates will be stored;

    (b) the equipment which is or will be available for storing medicinal products on those premises;

    (c) the equipment and facilities which are or will be available for distributing medicinal products from those premises; and

    (d) the arrangements made or to be made for securing the safekeeping of, and the maintenance of adequate records in respect of, medicinal products stored on or distributed from those premises.

Grant or refusal of licence

23 (1) Subject to the following provisions of these Regulations, on an application to the licensing authority for a licence under this Part the licensing authority may:

    (a) grant a licence containing such provisions as it considers appropriate; or

    (b) refuse to grant a licence if having regard to the provisions of these Regulations and any European Union obligation it considers it necessary or appropriate to do so.

(2) The licensing authority must grant or refuse an application for a licence under this Part within the period of 90 days beginning immediately after the day on which it receives the application.

(3) Paragraph (2) applies to an application only if the requirements of Schedule 3 have been met.

(4) If a notice under regulation 30 requires the applicant to provide the licensing authority with information, the information period is not to be counted for the purposes of paragraph (2).

(5) In paragraph (4), the "information period" means the period:

    (a) beginning with the day on which the notice is given, and

    (b) ending with the day on which the licensing authority receives the information or the applicant shows to the licensing authority's satisfaction that the applicant is unable to provide it.

(6) The licensing authority must give the applicant a notice stating the reasons for its decision in any case where:

    (a) the licensing authority refuses to grant an application for a licence; or

    (b) the licensing authority grants a licence otherwise than in accordance with the application and the applicant requests a statement of its reasons.

Standard provisions of licences

24 (1) The standard provisions set out in Schedule 4 may be incorporated by the licensing authority in a licence under this Part granted on or after the date on which these Regulations come into force.

(2) The standard provisions may be incorporated in a licence with or without modifications and either generally or in relation to medicinal products of a particular class.

(3) In Schedule 4, in relation to a licence holder in Great Britain, references to the principles and guidelines set out in the Good Manufacturing Practice Directive are to those principles and guidelines as they apply under or by virtue of regulation B17.

Duration of licence

25 A licence granted under this Part remains in force until:

(a) the licence is revoked by the licensing authority; or

(b) the licence is surrendered by the holder.

Conditions for wholesale dealer's licence

42 (1) Regulations 43 to 45 (not including regulation 43ZA) (in the case of a wholesale dealer's licence held in Northern Ireland) or regulations 43 to 45AA (including regulation 43ZA) (in the case of a wholesale dealer's licence held in Great Britain) apply to the holder of a wholesale dealer's licence (referred to in those regulations as "the licence holder") and have effect as if they were provisions of the licence (but the provisions specified in paragraph (2) do not apply to the holder of a wholesale dealer's licence insofar as the licence relates to exempt advanced therapy medicinal products).

(2) Those provisions are regulations 43(2) and (8) and 44.

(3) The requirements in Part 2 of Schedule 6 apply to the holder of a wholesale dealer's licence insofar as the licence relates to exempt advanced therapy medicinal products, and have effect as if they were provisions of the licence.

(4) Where a wholesale dealer's licence relates to wholesale dealings in Northern Ireland, the requirements and obligations contained in a provision of Commission Regulation 2016/161 listed in paragraph (5) have effect as if they were provisions of that under this Part.

(5) The provisions mentioned in paragraph (4) are:

(a) Article 10 (verification of the safety features) insofar as it relates to wholesalers;

(b) Article 11 (verification of the authenticity of the unique identifier) insofar as it relates to wholesalers;

(c) Article 12 (unique identifiers which have been decommissioned);

(d) Article 13 (reversing the status of a decommissioned unique identifier) insofar as it relates to wholesalers;

(e) Article 20 (verification of the authenticity of the unique identifier), subject to the exemption contained in Article 21 (derogations from Article 20(b));

(f) Article 22 (decommissioning of unique identifiers); and

(g) Article 24 (actions to be taken in case of tampering or suspected falsification).

(6) Paragraph (4) does not apply in relation to listed NIMAR products in Northern Ireland.

Obligations of licence holder

43 (1) The licence holder must comply with the guidelines on good distribution practice:

(a) in the case of a licence holder in Great Britain, published under, or that apply by virtue of, regulation C17;

(b) in the case of a licence holder in Northern Ireland, published by the European Commission in accordance with Article 84 of the 2001 Directive.

(2) The licence holder must ensure, within the limits of the holder's responsibility, the continued supply of medicinal products to pharmacies, and other persons who may lawfully sell medicinal products by retail or supply them in circumstances corresponding to retail sale, so that the needs of patients in the United Kingdom are met.

(3) The licence holder must provide and maintain such staff, premises, equipment and facilities for the handling, storage and distribution of medicinal products under the licence as are necessary:

(a) to maintain the quality of the products; and

(b) to ensure their proper distribution.

(4) The licence holder must inform the licensing authority of any proposed structural alteration to, or discontinuance of use of, premises to which the licence relates or which have otherwise been approved by the licensing authority.

(5) Subject to paragraph (6), the licence holder must not sell or supply a medicinal product, or offer it for sale or supply, unless:

(a) in the case of a product for sale or supply:

(i) in Great Britain, there is a UKMA(GB), UKMA(UK), a COR(GB), a COR(UK), a THR(GB) or a THR(UK) (an "authorisation"), or

(ii) in Northern Ireland, there is a UKMA(NI), UKMA(UK), a COR(NI), a COR(UK), a THR(NI), a THR(UK), and EU marketing authorisation or an Article 126a authorisation (an "authorisation"),

in force in relation to the product; and

(b) the sale or supply, or offer for sale or supply, is in accordance with the authorisation.

(6) The restriction in paragraph (5) does not apply to:

(a) the sale or supply, or offer for sale or supply, of a special medicinal product in the United Kingdom;

(b) the export from Northern Ireland to an EEA State, or supply for the purposes of such export, of a medicinal product which may be placed on the market in that State without a marketing authorisation, Article 126a authorisation, certificate of registration or traditional herbal registration by virtue of legislation adopted by that State under Article 5(1) of the 2001 Directive;

(ba) the export from Great Britain to an approved country for import, or supply for the purposes of such export, of a medicinal product which may be placed on the market in that country without:

(i) a marketing authorisation, certificate of registration or traditional herbal registration within the meaning of the 2001 Directive, by virtue of legislation adopted by that country under Article 5(1) of that Directive, where the approved country for import is an EEA State, or

(ii) such equivalent authorisation, certificate or registration in the approved country for import, under legislation in that country that makes provision that is equivalent to Article 5(1) of the 2001 Directive, where the approved country for import is not an EEA State;]

(c) the sale or supply, or offer for sale or supply, of an unauthorised medicinal product where the Secretary of State has temporarily authorised the distribution of the product under regulation 174; or

(d) the wholesale distribution of medicinal products:

(i) from Northern Ireland to a person in a country other than Great Britain or a country other than an EEA State; or

(ii) from Great Britain to a person in a country other than Northern Ireland or a country other than an approved country for import.

(7) The licence holder must:

(a) keep documents relating to the sale or supply of medicinal products under the licence which may facilitate the withdrawal or recall from sale of medicinal products in accordance with paragraph (b);

(b) maintain an emergency plan to ensure effective implementation of the recall from the market of a medicinal product where recall is:

(i) ordered by the licensing authority or:

(aa) in the case of a licence holder in Great Britain, by an appropriate authority for the licensing of medicinal products in an approved country for import;

(bb) in the case of a licence holder in Northern Ireland, by the competent authority of any EEA State, or

      (ii) carried out in cooperation with the manufacturer of, or the holder of:

        (aa) in the case of a product for sale or supply in Great Britain, the UKMA(GB) or UKMA(UK), certificate of registration or traditional herbal registration, or

        (bb) in the case of a product for sale or supply in Northern Ireland, the UKMA(NI) or UKMA(UK), EU marketing authorisation, Article 126a authorisation, certificate of registration or traditional herbal registration,

      for, the product; and

    (c) keep records in relation to the receipt, dispatch or brokering of medicinal products, of:

      (i) the date of receipt,

      (ii) the date of despatch,

      (iii) the date of brokering,

      (iv) the name of the medicinal product,

      (v) the quantity of the product received, dispatched or brokered,

      (vi) the name and address of the person from whom the products were received or to whom they are dispatched,

      (vii) where the receipt, dispatch or brokering of medicinal products takes place in Northern Ireland, the batch number of medicinal products bearing safety features referred to in point (o) of Article 54[1] of the 2001 Directive.

(8) A licence holder ("L") in Northern Ireland who imports from another EEA State a medicinal product in relation to which L is not the holder of a marketing authorisation, Article 126a authorisation, certificate of registration or a traditional herbal registration shall:

    (a) notify the intention to import that product to the holder of the authorisation and:

      (i) in the case of a product which has been granted a marketing authorisation under Regulation (EC) No 726/2004, to the EMA; or

      (ii) in any other case, the licensing authority; and

    (b) pay a fee to the EMA in accordance with Article 76(4)[2] of the 2001 Directive or the licensing authority as the case may be, in accordance with the Fees Regulations,

but this paragraph does not apply in relation to the wholesale distribution of medicinal products to a person in a country other than an EEA State.

(8A) Paragraph (8B) applies to a person ("P") who:

    (a) imports into Great Britain a medicinal product, other than for the sole purpose of wholesale distribution of that product to a person in a country other than the United Kingdom; but

---

[1] Point (o) of Article 54a was inserted by Directive 2011/62/EU of the European Parliament and of the Council (OJ No L 174, 1.7.2011, p74).

[2] Article 76(4) was inserted by Directive 2011/62/EU of the European Parliament and of the Council (OJ No L 174, 1.7.2011, p74).

(b) is not the holder of a UK marketing authorisation, certificate of registration or traditional herbal registration in respect of that product.

(8B) Where this paragraph applies, P must:

(a) notify:

(i) the holder of any authorisation, certificate or registration, granted by an authority in the country from which the product is exported, to sell or supply that product in that country, and

(ii) the licensing authority,

of the intention to import that product; and

(b) pay a fee to the licensing authority in accordance with the Fees Regulations.

(9) For the purposes of enabling the licensing authority to determine whether there are grounds for suspending, revoking or varying the licence, the licence holder must permit a person authorised in writing by the licensing authority, on production of identification, to carry out any inspection, or to take any samples or copies, which an inspector could carry out or take under Part 16 (enforcement).

(10) The holder of a licence permitting wholesale dealings in Northern Ireland ("L") must verify in accordance with paragraph (11) that any medicinal products received by L that are required by Article 54a[3] of the Directive to bear safety features are not falsified but this paragraph does not apply in relation to the distribution of medicinal products received from a third country by a person to a person in a third country.

(11) Verification under this paragraph is carried out by checking the safety features on the outer packaging, in accordance with the requirements laid down in the delegated acts adopted under Article 54a(2) of the 2001 Directive.

(12) The licence holder must maintain a quality system setting out responsibilities, processes and risk management measures in relation to their activities.

(13) The licence holder must immediately inform the licensing authority and, where applicable, the UK marketing authorisation holder or EU marketing authorisation holder, of medicinal products which the licence holder receives or is offered which the licence holder:

(a) knows or suspects; or

(b) has reasonable grounds for knowing or suspecting, to be falsified.

(14) Where the medicinal product is obtained through brokering:

(a) a licence holder in Great Britain must verify that the broker involved fulfils the requirements set out in regulation 45A(1)(b);

(b) a licence holder in Northern Ireland must verify that the broker involved is validly registered with the licensing authority or the competent authority of an EEA State.

---

[3] Article 54a was inserted by Directive 2011/62/EU of the European Parliament and of the Council (OJ No L 174, 1.7.2011, p74).

(15) In this regulation, as it applies in the case of a product for sale or supply in Northern Ireland "marketing authorisation" means:

(a) a marketing authorisation issued by a competent authority in accordance with the 2001 Directive; or

(b) an EU marketing authorisation.

Obligations of licence holder in Great Britain supplying listed NIMAR products to Northern Ireland

43ZA (1) This regulation applies only to licence holders in Great Britain supplying listed NIMAR products to Northern Ireland.

(2) A licence holder must comply with the guidelines on good distribution practice, published under, or that apply by virtue of, regulation C17.

(3) So that the needs of patients in Northern Ireland are met, the licence holder must ensure, within the limits of the holder's responsibility, the continued supply of listed NIMAR products to—

(a) registered pharmacies in Northern Ireland;

(b) any person who may lawfully sell those products by retail sale or may lawfully supply them in circumstances corresponding to retail sale in Northern Ireland;

(c) any person who may lawfully administer prescription only medicines in Northern Ireland.

(4) The licence holder must provide and maintain such staff, premises, equipment and facilities for the handling, storage and distribution of listed NIMAR products under the licence as are necessary—

(a) to maintain the quality of the products; and

(b) to ensure their proper distribution.

(5) The licence holder must inform the licensing authority of any proposed structural alteration to, or discontinuance of use of, premises to which the licence relates or which have otherwise been approved by the licensing authority.

(6) The licence holder must not sell or supply, or offer for sale or supply, listed NIMAR products to a person in Northern Ireland, unless—

(a) there is a UKMA(UK) or UKMA(GB) in force in relation to that product; and

(b) the sale or supply is in accordance with that authorisation (except for the fact the product will be in Northern Ireland).

(7) The licence holder must—

(a) keep documents relating to the sale or supply of listed NIMAR products under the licence which may facilitate the withdrawal or recall from sale of such products in accordance with paragraph (b);

(b) maintain an emergency plan to ensure effective implementation of the recall from the market of a listed NIMAR product where recall is—

(i) ordered by the licensing authority; or

    (ii) carried out in co-operation with the manufacturer of, or the holder of the corresponding UKMA(GB) or UKMA(UK) for the product; and

  (c) keep records in relation to the receipt, dispatch or brokering of listed NIMAR products, of—

    (i) the date of receipt,

    (ii) the date of despatch,

    (iii) the date of brokering,

    (iv) the name of the listed NIMAR product,

    (v) the quantity of the product received, dispatched or brokered,

    (vi) the name and address of the person from whom the products were received or to whom they are dispatched; and

  (d) provide the records in sub-paragraph (c) to the licensing authority on request.

(8) For the purposes of enabling the licensing authority to determine whether there are grounds for suspending, revoking or varying the licence, the licence holder must permit a person authorised in writing by the licensing authority, on production of identification, to carry out any inspection, or to take any samples or copies, which an inspector could carry out or take under Part 16 (enforcement).

(9) The licence holder must maintain a quality system setting out responsibilities, processes and risk management measures in relation to their activities.

(10) The licence holder must immediately inform the licensing authority of medicinal products which the licence holder receives or is offered which the licence holder—

  (a) knows or suspects; or

  (b) has reasonable grounds for knowing or suspecting,

to be falsified.

(11) Where the listed NIMAR product is obtained through brokering, a licence holder must verify that the broker involved fulfils the requirements set out in regulation 45A(1)(b).

Requirement for wholesale dealers to decommission the unique identifier

43A (1) This regulation applies only to medicinal products that are required to bear safety features pursuant to Article 54a of the 2001 Directive.

(2) Before supplying a medicinal product to a person in Northern Ireland who falls within one of the classes specified in paragraph (3), the licence holder must verify the safety features and decommission the unique identifier of that medicinal product in accordance with the requirements laid down in Commission Regulation 2016/161.

(3) The classes of person mentioned in paragraph (2) are:

  (a) persons authorised or entitled to supply medicinal products to the public who do not operate within a healthcare institution or within a pharmacy;

(b) persons who receive the product for the purpose of selling, supplying or administering it as a veterinary medicinal product;

(c) dentists;

(d) registered optometrists or registered dispensing opticians;

(e) registered paramedics;

(f) persons who are members of Her Majesty's armed forces;

(g) the Police Service of Northern Ireland;

(h) government institutions maintaining stocks of medicinal products for the purposes of civil protection or disaster control;

(i) universities or other institutions concerned with higher education or research, other than healthcare institutions;

(j) a prison service;

(k) persons carrying on the business of a school;

(l) nursing homes;

(m) hospices.

Requirement that wholesale dealers to deal only with specified persons

44 (1) ...

(2) The licence holder must not obtain supplies of medicinal products from anyone except:

(a) the holder of a manufacturer's licence or wholesale dealer's licence in relation to products of that description;

(b) the person who holds an authorisation granted by an approved country for import (in the case of a licence holder in Great Britain) or by an EEA State (in the case of a licence holder in Northern Ireland) [or]

(c) where the medicinal product is directly received:

(i) in the case of a licence holder in Great Britain, from a country that is not an approved country for import ("A"), for export to a country that is not an approved country for import ("B"), and

(ii) in the case of a licence holder in Northern Ireland, from a state other than an EEA State ("A") for export to another state other than an EEA State ("B"),

the supplier of the medicinal product in country A is a person who is authorised or entitled to supply such medicinal products in accordance with the legal and administrative provisions in country A.

(d) ...

(3) Where a medicinal product is obtained in accordance with paragraph (2)(a) or (b), the licence holder must verify that:

(a) the wholesale dealer who supplies the product complies with the principles and guidelines of good distribution practices; or

(b) the manufacturer or importer who supplies the product holds a manufacturing authorisation.

(4) ...

(5) The licence holder may distribute medicinal products by way of wholesale dealing only to:

(a) the holder of a wholesale dealer's licence relating to those products;

(b) the holder of an authorisation granted by:

   (i)   in the case of a licence holder in Great Britain, the appropriate authority of an approved country for import;

   (ii) in the case of a licence holder in Northern Ireland, the competent authority of another EEA State,

that is responsible for authorising the supply of those products by way of wholesale dealing;

(c) a person who may lawfully sell those products by retail or may lawfully supply them in circumstances corresponding to retail sale;

(d) a person who may lawfully administer those products; or

(e) in relation to supply:

   (i)   in the case of a licence holder in Great Britain to persons in countries other than approved countries for import, a person who is authorised or entitled to receive medicinal products for wholesale distribution or supply to the public in accordance with the applicable legal and administrative provisions of the country to which the product is supplied;

   (ii) in the case of a licence holder in Northern Ireland to persons in a state other than an EEA State, a person who is authorised or entitled to receive medicinal products for wholesale distribution or supply to the public in accordance with the applicable legal and administrative provisions of the state other than an EEA State concerned.

(6) Where a medicinal product is supplied to a person who is authorised or entitled to supply medicinal products to the public in accordance with paragraph (5)(c) or (e), the licence holder must enclose with the product a document stating the:

(a) date on which the supply took place;

(b) name and pharmaceutical form of the product supplied;

(c) quantity of product supplied;

(d) name and address of the licence holder; and

(e) batch number of the medicinal products bearing the safety features referred to in point (o) of Article 54 of the 2001 Directive, in the case of a licence holder in Northern Ireland.

(7) The licence holder must:

(a) keep a record of information supplied in accordance with paragraph (6) for at least five years beginning immediately after the date on which the information is supplied; and

(b) ensure that the record is available to the licensing authority for inspection.

(8) A licence holder in Great Britain may only obtain a medicinal product in respect of which a UKMA(GB) was granted under the unfettered access route if the product satisfies the definition of qualifying Northern Ireland goods.

(9) Paragraph (2)(c) does not apply to:

(a) in the case of a licence holder in Great Britain, products received from Northern Ireland, and

(b) in the case of a licence holder in Northern Ireland, products received from Great Britain.

(10) Paragraph (5)(e) does not apply to:

(a) in the case of a licence holder in Great Britain, products supplied to Northern Ireland, and

(b) in the case of a licence holder in Northern Ireland, products supplied to Great Britain.

Requirement as to responsible persons

45 (1) Subject to regulation 45AA, the licence holder must ensure that there is available at all times at least one person (referred to in this regulation as the "responsible person") who in the opinion of the licensing authority:

(a) has knowledge of the activities to be carried out and of the procedures to be performed under the licence which is adequate to carry out the functions mentioned in paragraph (2); and

(b) has adequate experience relating to those activities and procedures.

(1A) In respect of licence holder in Great Britain, paragraph (1) is subject to regulation 45AA.

(2) Those functions are:

(a) ensuring that the conditions under which the licence was granted have been, and are being, complied with; and

(b) ensuring that the quality of medicinal products handled by the licence holder is being maintained in accordance with the requirements of:

(i) in the case of a licence holder in Great Britain, the UK marketing authorisations, certificates of registration or traditional herbal registrations, and

(ii) in the case of a licence holder in Northern Ireland, the marketing authorisations, requirements of regulation 167A, Article 126a authorisations, certificates of registration or traditional herbal registrations,

applicable to those products.

(3) The licence holder must notify the licensing authority of:

(a) any change to the responsible person; and

(b) the name, address, qualifications and experience of the responsible person.

(4) The licence holder must not permit any person to act as a responsible person other than the person named in the licence or another person notified to the licensing authority under paragraph (3).

(5) Paragraph (6) applies if, after giving the licence holder and a person acting as a responsible person the opportunity to make representations (orally or in writing), the licensing authority thinks that the person:

(a) does not satisfy the requirements of paragraph (1) in relation to qualifications or experience; or

(b) is failing to carry out the functions referred to in paragraph (2) adequately or at all.

(6) Where this paragraph applies, the licensing authority must notify the licence holder in writing that the person is not permitted to act as a responsible person.

Requirement as to responsible persons where licence holder imports from an approved country for import

45AA (1) Subject to paragraph (2), this regulation applies to a licence holder in Great Britain where the licence holder imports a medicinal product from an approved country for import under a wholesale dealer's licence.

(2) The requirements of this regulation do not apply where an unlicensed medicinal product falling under paragraph (1) is imported:

(a) from an approved country for import for the sole purpose of distribution by way of wholesale dealing as a special medicinal product; or

(b) for the sole purpose of wholesale distribution of that product to a person in a country other than an approved country for import.

(3) The licence holder must ensure that there is available at all times at least one person (referred to in this regulation as the "responsible person (import)") whose name is included in the register established under regulation 45AB.

(4) A responsible person (import) must:

(a) carry out the functions under regulation 45(2), unless a responsible person under regulation 45 is performing those functions in respect of the licence; and

(b) ensure that there is appropriate evidence to confirm that each production batch of a medicine imported from an approved country for import under the licence has been certified as provided for in Article 51 of the 2001 Directive, or such equivalent certification procedure as applies in the approved country for import; and

(c) ensure that each production batch of a medicinal product that is subject to the batch testing condition and that is imported into Great Britain from an approved country for import has been certified as being in conformity with the approved specifications in the UK marketing authorisation by:

(i) the appropriate authority, or

(ii) where the batch testing exemption applies, a laboratory in a country that has an agreement with the United Kingdom to the effect that the appropriate authority will recognise that certificate in place of the appropriate authority's own examination.

(5) The licensing authority must publish guidance on the documentation that it considers to be appropriate evidence for the purposes of paragraph (4)(b).

(6) Guidance published under paragraph (5) may be taken into account by the licensing authority in determining whether it considers there has been a failure to comply with this regulation.

(7) The licence holder must apply to vary the licence if a change is proposed to the responsible person (import).

(8) The licence holder must not permit any person to act as a responsible person (import) other than the person named in the licence.

(9) Paragraph (10) applies if:

    (a) the person acting as responsible person (import) in respect of the licence is no longer included in the register under 45AB;

    (b) the licensing authority thinks, after giving the licence holder and a person acting as a responsible person (import) the opportunity to make representations (orally or in writing), that the responsible person (import) is failing to carry out the functions referred to in paragraph (4) adequately or at all.

(10) Where this paragraph applies the licensing authority:

    (a) must notify the licence holder in writing that the person is not permitted to act as a responsible person (import) in respect of that licence; and

    (b) may, subject to regulation 45AB(3)(b), remove that person's name from the register under regulation 45AB.

(11) In this regulation, "unlicensed medicinal product" means a medicinal product in respect of which:

    (a) there is no marketing authorisation, within the meaning of the 2001 Directive, in any EEA State in respect of that product, where the product is imported from an approved country for import that is an EEA State; or

    (b) there is no licence or authorisation in respect of that product as regards its sale or supply in the approved country for import, where the product is imported from an approved country for import that is not an EEA State.

Register for responsible persons (import)

45AB (1) The licensing authority must maintain a register of persons ("the responsible person (import) register") who may carry out the role of responsible person (import) under regulation 45AA.

(2) The licensing authority may only include a person's name in the responsible person (import) register if that person:

    (a) holds:

        (i) a diploma, certificate or other evidence of formal qualifications awarded on completion of a university or other higher education course of study in pharmacy, chemistry, medicine, biology or a related life science, or

        (ii) such other qualification as the licensing authority is satisfied is equivalent;

    (b) is a member of:

        (i) the Royal Society of Biology,

        (ii) the Royal Pharmaceutical Society,

(iii) the Pharmaceutical Society of Northern Ireland,

(iv) the Royal Society of Chemistry, or

(v) such other body as may be specified by the licensing authority for the purpose of this paragraph; and

(c) has a minimum of 2 years' experience in performing the functions of a responsible person under regulation 45, or in performing such other functions that appear to the licensing authority to be equivalent.

(3) The licensing authority:

(a) may remove a person's name from the responsible person (import) register if it no longer considers that the person satisfies the requirements of paragraph (2); but

(b) it may not exercise that power unless it has given that person the opportunity to make representations to it (orally or in writing).

Schedule 4 Standard provisions of licences

PART 4 WHOLESALE DEALER'S LICENCE

All wholesale dealer's licences

28   The provisions of this Part are standard provisions of a wholesale dealer's licence.

29   The licence holder must not use any premises for the handling, storage or distribution of medicinal products other than those specified in the licence or notified to the licensing authority from time to time and approved by the licensing authority.

30   The licence holder must provide such information as may be requested by the licensing authority concerning the type and quantity of medicinal products which the licence holder handles, stores or distributes.

31   The licence holder must take all reasonable precautions and exercise all due diligence to ensure that any information provided by the licence holder to the licensing authority which is relevant to an evaluation of the safety, quality or efficacy of a medicinal product which the licence holder handles, stores or distributes is not false or misleading.

Wholesale dealer's licence relating to special medicinal products

32   The provisions of paragraphs 33 to 42 are incorporated as additional standard provisions of a wholesale dealer's licence relating to special medicinal products.

33   Where and in so far as the licence relates to special medicinal products, the licence holder may only import such products from in the case of an import into Great Britain, an approved country for import and in the case of an import into Northern Ireland, an EEA State:

(a) in response to an order which satisfies the requirements of regulation 167, and

(b) where the conditions set out in paragraphs 34 to 41 are complied with.

34 No later than 28 days prior to each importation of a special medicinal product, the licence holder must give written notice to the licensing authority stating the intention to import the product and stating the following particulars:

   (a) the brand name, common name or scientific name of the medicinal product and (if different) any name under which the medicinal product is to be sold or supplied in the United Kingdom;
   (b) any trademark or the name of the manufacturer of the medicinal product;
   (c) in respect of each active constituent of the medicinal product, any international non-proprietary name or the British approved name or the monograph name, or where that constituent does not have any of those, the accepted scientific name or any other name descriptive of the true nature of the constituent;
   (d) the quantity of medicinal product to be imported, which must not exceed the quantity specified in paragraph 38; and
   (e) the name and address of the manufacturer or assembler of the medicinal product in the form in which it is to be imported and, if the person who will supply the medicinal product for importation is not the manufacturer or assembler, the name and address of the supplier.

35 The licence holder may not import the special medicinal product if, before the end of 28 days beginning immediately after the date on which the licensing authority sends or gives the licence holder an acknowledgement in writing by the licensing authority that it has received the notice referred to in paragraph 34, the licensing authority has notified the licence holder in writing that the product should not be imported.

36 The licence holder may import the special medicinal product referred to in the notice where the licence holder has been notified in writing by the licensing authority, before the end of the 28-day period referred to in paragraph 35, that the product may be imported.

37 Where the licence holder sells or supplies special medicinal products, the licence holder must, in addition to any other records which are required by the provisions of the licence, make and maintain written records relating to:

   (a) the batch number of the batch of the product from which the sale or supply was made; and
   (b) details of any adverse reaction to the product sold or supplied of which the licence holder becomes aware.

38 The licence holder must not, on any one occasion, import more than such amount as is sufficient for 25 single administrations, or for 25 courses of treatment where the amount imported is sufficient for a maximum of 3 months' treatment, and must not, on any one occasion, import more than the quantity notified to the licensing authority under paragraph 34(d).

39   The licence holder must inform the licensing authority immediately of any matter coming to the licence holder's attention which might reasonably cause the licensing authority to believe that a special medicinal product imported in accordance with this paragraph can no longer be regarded as a product which can safely be administered to human beings or as a product which is of satisfactory quality for such administration.

40   The licence holder must not publish any advertisement, catalogue or circular relating to a special medicinal product or make any representations in respect of that product.

41   The licence holder must cease importing or supplying a special medicinal product if the licence holder receives a notice in writing from the licensing authority directing that, from a date specified in the notice, a particular product or class of products may no longer be imported or supplied.

41A   A licence holder:

   (a) in Great Britain may only supply a special medicinal product to a person in Northern Ireland, and
   (b) in Northern Ireland may only supply a special medicinal product to a person in Great Britain,
   in response to an order which satisfies the requirements of regulation 167.

42   In this Part:

   - "British approved name" means the name which appears in the current edition of the list prepared by the British Pharmacopoeia Commission under regulation 318 (British Pharmacopoeia- lists of names);
   - "international non-proprietary name" means a name which has been selected by the World Health Organisation as a recommended international non-proprietary name and in respect of which the Director-General of the World Health Organisation has given notice to that effect in the World Health Organisation Chronicle; and
   - "monograph name" means the name or approved synonym which appears at the head of a monograph in the current edition of the British Pharmacopoeia, the European Pharmacopoeia or a foreign or international compendium of standards, and "current" in this definition means current at the time the notice is sent to the licensing authority.

Wholesale dealer's licence relating to exempt advanced therapy medicinal products

43   The provisions of paragraph 44 are incorporated as additional standard provisions of a wholesale dealer's licence relating to exempt advanced therapy medicinal products.

44   The licence holder shall keep the data referred to in paragraph 16 of Schedule 6 for such period, being a period of longer than 30 years, as may be specified by the licensing authority.

UK LEGISLATION ON WHOLESALE DISTRIBUTION

Schedule 6 Manufacturer's and wholesale dealer's licences for exempt advanced therapy medicinal products

PART 2 WHOLESALE DEALER'S LICENCES

13   The requirements in paragraphs 14 to 20 apply to a wholesale dealer's licence in so far as it relates to exempt advanced therapy medicinal products.

14   The licence holder must obtain supplies of exempt advanced therapy medicinal products only from:

(a) the holder of a manufacturer's licence in respect of those products; or
(b) the holder of a wholesale dealer's licence in respect of those products.

15   The licence holder must distribute an exempt advanced therapy medicinal product by way of wholesale dealing only to:

(a) the holder of a wholesale dealer's licence in respect of those products; or
(b) a person who:
    (i)   may lawfully administer those products, and
    (ii) solicited the product for an individual patient.

16   The licence holder must establish and maintain a system ensuring that the exempt advanced therapy medicinal product and its starting and raw materials, including all substances coming into contact with the cells or tissues it may contain, can be traced through the sourcing, manufacturing, packaging, storage, transport and delivery to the establishment where the product is used.

17   The licence holder must inform the licensing authority of any adverse reaction to any exempt advanced therapy medicinal product supplied by the holder of the wholesale dealer's licence of which the holder is aware.

18   The licence holder must, subject to paragraph 44 of Schedule 4, keep the data referred to in paragraph 16 for a minimum of 30 years after the expiry date of the exempt advanced therapy medicinal product.

19   The licence holder must secure that the data referred to in paragraph 16 will, in the event that:

(a) the licence is suspended, revoked or withdrawn; or
(b) the licence holder becomes bankrupt or insolvent,

be held available to the licensing authority by the holder of a wholesale dealer's licence for the period described in paragraph 18 or such longer period as may be required pursuant to paragraph 44 of Schedule 4.

20   The licence holder must not import or export any exempt advanced therapy medicinal product.

EU Guidelines on GDP and UK Guidance on Wholesale Distribution

Contents

Introduction

Wholesale distribution of medicinal products is defined as all activities consisting of procuring, holding, supplying or exporting medicinal products, apart from supplying medicinal products to the public. To ensure the reliability of the supply chain, the Human Medicines Regulations 2012 regulates wholesale distributors. This also includes virtual operations where no physical handling of the products takes place.

Wholesalers of medicines must comply with Chapters 1–9 of the European Commission's Guidelines on Good Distribution Practice of medicinal products for human use. This chapter sets out the guidelines alongside the expectations for UK wholesalers.

Chapter 1 Quality Management

1.1 Principle

Wholesale distributors must maintain a quality system setting out responsibilities, processes and risk-management principles in relation to their activities[1]. All distribution activities should be clearly defined and systematically reviewed. All critical steps of distribution processes and significant changes should be justified and, where relevant, validated. The quality system is the responsibility of the organisation's management and requires their leadership and active participation, and should be supported by staff commitment.

1.2 Quality system

The system for managing quality should encompass the organisational structure, procedures, processes and resources, as well as activities, necessary to ensure confidence that the product delivered maintains its quality and integrity and remains within the legal supply chain during storage and/or transportation.

The quality system should be fully documented and its effectiveness monitored. All quality system-related activities should be defined and documented. A quality manual or equivalent documentation approach should be established.

A Responsible Person should be appointed by the management, who should have clearly specified authority and responsibility for ensuring that a quality system is implemented and maintained.

The management of the distributor should ensure that all parts of the quality system are adequately resourced with competent personnel, and suitable and sufficient premises, equipment and facilities.

---

[1] Article 80(h) of Directive 2001/83/EC.

The size, structure and complexity of a distributor's activities should be taken into consideration when developing or modifying the quality system.

A change control system should be in place. This system should incorporate quality risk-management principles, and be proportionate and effective.

The quality system should ensure that:

(i) medicinal products are procured, held, supplied or exported in a way that is compliant with the requirements of Good Distribution Practice (GDP);

(ii) management responsibilities are clearly specified;

(iii) products are delivered to the right recipients within a satisfactory time period;

(iv) records are made contemporaneously;

(v) deviations from established procedures are documented and investigated;

(vi) appropriate corrective and preventive actions (commonly known as "CAPA") are taken to correct deviations and prevent them in line with the principles of quality risk management.

1.3 Management of outsourced activities

The quality system should extend to the control and review of any outsourced activities related to the procurement, holding, supply or export of medicinal products. These processes should incorporate quality risk management and include:

(i) assessing the suitability and competence of the contract acceptor to carry out the activity and checking authorisation status, if required;

(ii) defining the responsibilities and communication processes for the quality-related activities of the parties involved;

(iii) monitoring and review of the performance of the contract acceptor, and the identification and implementation of any required improvements on a regular basis.

1.4 Management review and monitoring

The management should have a formal process for reviewing the quality system on a periodic basis. The review should include:

(i) measurement of the achievement of quality system objectives;

(ii) assessment of performance indicators that can be used to monitor the effectiveness of processes within the quality system, such as complaints, deviations, CAPA, changes to processes; feedback on outsourced activities; self-assessment processes, including risk assessments and audits; and external assessments such as inspections, findings and customer audits;

(iii)   emerging regulations, guidance and quality issues that can impact the quality management system;

(iv)   innovations that might enhance the quality system;

(v)   changes in business environment and objectives.

The outcome of each management review of the quality system should be documented in a timely manner and effectively communicated internally.

1.5   Quality risk management

Quality risk management is a systematic process for the assessment, control, communication and review of risks to the quality of medicinal products. It can be applied both proactively and retrospectively.

Quality risk management should ensure that the evaluation of the risk to quality is based on scientific knowledge, experience with the process and ultimately links to the protection of the patient. The level of effort, formality and documentation of the process should be commensurate with the level of risk. Examples of the processes and applications of quality risk management can be found in guideline Q9 of the International Conference on Harmonisation ("ICH").

UK Guidance on Chapter 1 Quality Management

Introduction

A consistent focus on quality is of prime importance for all wholesale distributors in order to maintain an effective and efficient business that meets customer needs and ensures product quality is maintained.

Quality management is as much a mindset as an activity in itself, with the aim of achieving quality processes that permeate throughout all distribution activities, with the ultimate goal of ensuring patient safety.

Quality management system and quality system

A quality system is the sum of all aspects of a system that implements quality policy and ensures that quality objectives are met. This is managed through a quality management system (QMS) which is the system for managing quality and should encompass the organisational structure, procedures, processes and resources, as well as activities necessary to ensure that the product distributed maintains its quality and integrity, and remains within the legal supply chain during all wholesale operations.

Examples of QMS application include:

- quality management review;
- establishment of organisational structure, responsibilities matrix and lines of reporting;
- quality planning and strategy.

The quality system is the vehicle by which quality management is delivered and should encompass all GDP operations. The quality system size and complexity should be proportionate to the distribution activities being undertaken and appropriate for the type of organisation. The GDP Guidelines give a detailed breakdown of the areas that should be covered. Additionally, ICH harmonised guideline ICH Q10 may provide useful information for those designing a quality system.

Good Distribution Practice quality systems should include the following elements:

- quality risk management;
- change management;
- deviation management;
- management of controlled documentation;
- self-inspection;
- control of outsourced activity.

To be fully effective, individual elements of the quality system need to fully integrate both within the organisation's quality system, as well as with any integrated third-party systems such as parent companies or subcontractors. To illustrate this, mitigating risk of medicine theft is provided as an example at the end of this section (example 1).

Quality risk management

Quality risk management (QRM) is the identification and control of risks to product quality through the evaluation of the activities that are being performed. Underpinning this is that the evaluation of the risk is based on knowledge and experience of the process and ultimately links to the protection of the patient. The level of effort, formality and documentation of the process should be commensurate with the level of risk. Where a lack of knowledge is associated with an activity, such as a new process, then the lack of knowledge should be incorporated into the risk evaluation.

Good Distribution Practice guidelines refer to ICH Q9 as a useful guidance document on QRM. This includes the principles and concepts of QRM, with Annex I and II identifying various tools and techniques. Deficiency data indicate that QRM has been poorly understood or implemented, so two examples of application are provided at the end of this section (examples 2 and 3). These illustrate two approaches to show the principles of QRM and will not be suitable for all distributors and circumstances. Common weaknesses seen with GDP QRM include:

- the criticality of risk directly correlates with the degree of urgency rather than the appropriate time to address the risk;
- risk assessments are not reviewed;
- QRM is used as an excuse to avoid developing appropriate mitigation;
- QRM is not understood by managers.

Indications of effective QRM include:

- full integration of QRM principles throughout the quality system;
- QRM is actively used to drive continuous improvement, reduce risks and deviations, and improve understanding of risks;
- the QRM processes are easy to understand and apply.

Change management, corrective and preventative actions

Change management is a formal process that ensures control is maintained while changes that potentially impact on product quality, patient safety or regulatory compliance are carried out. For small- or medium-sized wholesalers, change management and change control are often viewed as the same. Companies with more extensive structure or operations may manage these separately, with change management incorporating changes in addition to quality or operational change controls. These could include IT system change management (including software updates), management of changes incorporated within validation studies or changes to commercial terms.

Extensive operational or quality changes may be managed as a project following the same underlying principles of change management, and be supported by individual activities associated with specific change controls.

There should be a clear distinction between what constitutes the use of change control processes and changes that are managed by other means (e.g. a temporary "planned" deviation from established processes).

Change control

Change control is a formal process whereby changes to a process, key personnel, premises or other changes that potentially impact on product quality, patient safety or regulatory compliance, are identified, monitored and managed in a controlled way. Changes managed by change control may be permanent or temporary. For temporary changes, these could be managed as a temporary change control or temporary deviation dependent on the design of organisations' quality system.

The level of recorded detail should be in line with principles of QRM and in accordance with data integrity, and be proportionate to the extent of the change. A register of change controls will enable traceability of all changes and should include both implemented and rejected changes. Change documentation should be raised at the point that a change is first considered, even if the change is not then implemented.

A typical change control process may consist of several stages:

- Submission of a documented change control request to management.
- Assessment of the request by management. This assessment should consider if there is an overall benefit to the organisation. It should include an impact assessment to record associated areas affected by the change together with identification of potential risks. The assessment should not only evaluate the impact and management following completion of the change (final state), but also how risks are to be managed during the implementation phase of the change.
- Implementation of the change. Monitoring of the implementation stages of the change should be carried out and essential stages recorded. Any deviation from the original implementation plan should be documented.
- Review of the change. A review should take place of the effectiveness of the change, including identification of any new risks, and opportunities for improvement in either the specific change or change implementation. This should be recorded.

Deviation management, corrective and preventative actions

Deviation management is the means by which all deviation types are managed. Many wholesalers apply a deviation process to deviations from procedures, with independent processes to address other deviation types such as temperature excursions, service level complaints, complaints relating to outsourced operations, self-inspection observations or validation excursions. It is important that management and the Responsible Person have oversight of all deviation types.

The term "deviation" is most commonly used by wholesalers to refer to an unplanned event not in compliance with their standard operating processes. Deviations can also refer to authorised departure outside the standard operating procedure or normal way of working (but within regulatory requirements) as a temporary measure.

Deviations require a formal process for reporting and assessment. Those deviations that are unplanned also require investigation. The level of severity is expected to be reflected in the extent of immediate mitigation, documentation, assessment and investigation. Deviations other than very minor ones are likely to be associated with corrective actions and preventive actions, often referred to as CAPA.

Corrective actions are remedial measures taken to address the specific failure. Preventive actions are measures to avoid re-occurrence of the specific failure and, additionally, actions to address existent occurrences of the same failure elsewhere.

The establishment of preventative measures should be a priority where an unplanned event may have a significant impact on public health. The greater the potential impact, the more investigation into root causative effects is required to ensure a robust preventive action plan is created. A variety of tools can be used to ascertain potential root causes depending on the failure type, and a general description of some of these is available in ICH Q9.

Management of controlled documentation

Good documentation practices, including the management of controlled documents, are an essential element of the quality system and are described in chapter 4 – documentation below.

Self-inspection

Self-inspections are the means by which management monitor performance of the quality system and identify opportunities for improvement and deficiencies. It is described in chapter 8 – self inspections below.

Control of outsourced activity

The quality system should extend to the control and review of any outsourced activities related to the procurement, holding, supply or export of medicinal products. The relationship between the organisation or person providing activity on behalf of the wholesaler should be described in an agreement as described in chapter 7 – outsourced activities below. Control measures should incorporate QRM and include:

- assessing the suitability and competence of the contract acceptor to carry out the activity and include confirmation of authorisation status if required;
- defining the responsibilities and communication processes for the quality-related activities of the parties involved;
- monitoring and review of the performance of the contract acceptor, and the identification and implementation of any required improvements on a regular basis.

Management should monitor the performance of the service provider by means of audit. An audit schedule should be maintained outlining the service provider, service provided, audit scope and frequency, and audit format. The audit should be carried out by competent personnel, and where these are specifically contracted, a vendor assessment of the auditor should be carried out to provide assurance of the competency of the auditor. This is especially important where the activity being audited may not be within the full level of understanding of the wholesaler, for example outsourced maintenance of computerised systems may be audited by a contracted auditor with strong experience and knowledge of GDP and computer systems.

Management review and monitoring

Regular review should take place to ensure effectiveness and continual improvement of the QMS.

This review should actively involve company management and key personnel such as the Responsible Person.

The review should incorporate key performance indicators, examples of which include pick accuracy or delivery performance. Performance indicators should be objective and relevant to the organisations activities, alongside driving continuous improvement.

In very small organisations the process of review may require taking a step back and objectively reviewing the operational activities and supporting procedures.

Questions to be considered during the management review may include:

- is the quality system effective, does it reflect the current business model?
- has the recall test or test of the business contingency plan identified weaknesses or opportunities, and have they been followed up?
- are activities being carried out in accordance with the principles of QRM, or are there opportunities for improvement with some processes requiring modification?
- has legislation been amended or guidance published that requires that activities need to be reviewed?
- is the business operating effectively? Are the right products getting to the right customers at the right time?
- are improvements needed to address customer complaints?
- are third parties contracted to provide services, and are they complying with their contractual obligations?
- have there been any unforeseen problems or events, and has effective CAPA been implemented?
- have planned changes been effective?
- are there staff training issues?

The outcome of each management review should be documented, result in a CAPA plan where necessary and should be effectively communicated to staff.

Example 1: Integration of quality and operational processes to mitigation of risk of theft or diversion of medicine

Whether pilfered for personal use or stolen in bulk for diversion, opportunistic or planned, the theft of medicines and diversion of medicines has a broad impact that increases risk to public health and risks the integrity of the medicine supply chain. The potential impact of theft is widespread and includes:

- diversion into the authorised supply chain of medicines damaged by handling in inadequate conditions;
- delay of essential medicine supply to a patient;
- diversion of medicines to unauthorised consumers;
- loss of good reputation of distributors;
- traumatic for staff.

Considering the amount of UK medicines distributed, the proportion of theft is low; however, the potential risk to an individual patient consuming a stolen medicine is potentially high. Without proper safeguards, distributors may either have medicines stolen or unwittingly procure previously stolen stock. Integration of the quality system and operational practices can mitigate the risk of theft or procurement of stolen medicines. Some measures for consideration are listed below.

Quality management: monitoring of unusual sales patterns, monitoring changes in risk profiles for products supplied and evidence of theft or near-misses within deviation reports. Quality risk management incorporates security risks evaluation embedded throughout the quality system.

Personnel: security pre-employment checks, training of drivers in security, development of an open culture that supports reporting and whistleblowing, restricted personnel access to high risk areas and policies in place for management of visitors, control of security passes. Where security awareness within the organisation is low, or where a significant theft has taken place, specialised security consultants may be used, in which case appropriate vetting of these should take place.

Facility and equipment design and maintenance: security measures are built into the design, including restriction of vehicular access to loading bay areas, location of high-risk stock within the warehouse, maintenance repair and servicing of buildings, perimeter fences and equipment, including shutters and CCTV.

Documentation: stock records safeguarded from unauthorised alteration, including both hard copy and computerised records, stock discrepancies addressed at an appropriate level, records enable clear visibility of discrepancies including under-picked stock, mislaid stock, under-delivered stock and evidence of destroyed stock, including stock for destruction supplied to third-countries. Procedures describe how to report medicine theft to the MHRA.

Operations: procurement controls include robust authentication of suppliers and customers, incentivisation of purchasing or sales staff does not conflict with increasing risk of distributing diverted medicines and witness checking for high-risk operations, including picking controlled drugs. Control of access and use of security seals.

Complaint management: trending of under-delivered or lost stock.

Returned medicines: control of courier used for reverse logistics, and verification that returned stock is genuine and is supported by appropriate documentation.

Falsified medicines: clear understanding in all areas of the organisation for standards of operations and how to report suspect medicines and transactions.

Outsourced activities: integration with couriers through written agreements including immediate reporting to the contract giver of anomalies, assurance of a chain of custody, risk profiling of contractors, monitoring contractor and control of additional subcontracting by the contractor.

Transportation: security features identified as part of user-requirement specification, security profiling for high-risk consignments and driver trained in security practices.

Example 2: Application of quality risk management to GDP transportation risks

This example illustrates some of the QRM considerations and GDP expectations, as it applies to transportation, which remains a significant weakness for many wholesalers, especially those that do not own their own fleet.

Distribution of medicines has inherent risks, and by applying QRM it is possible to identify and define the risks, possibly remove some and create the means to improve detection of risk events and thereby reduce their impact. It can also help identify what is an acceptable level of risk.

A summary of inherent risks and their criticality assists managers in being mindful of risks in different areas of their organisation thereby showing consequential change in risk caused by an action, and can also provide a benchmark of current risk level.

Apart from the summary of inherent risks, individual quality risk assessments also feed into risk management. These can be both subject-based assessments, such as evaluation of risks associated with transportation, or incorporated into quality system processes, such as part of evaluation of a change control or a deviation. The latter helps to reduce total risk rather than resolve one issue but create a larger risk elsewhere. Quality risk assessments can include the following stages:

- risk assessment;
- risk control;
- risk communication;
- risk review.

RISK ASSESSMENT

An assessment of the transport chain should help identify which parts are associated with greater risk. This can be performed either as a single approach for a route, or by grouping similar routes and transport modes into different transport lanes. For example, one lane may consist of ambient products by air freight to mainland Europe; the next lane might include cold chain air freight to Europe; the next lane may describe road freight to Europe using own transport; and a fourth might describe road transport to Europe using a courier. Each of these lanes will have risk profiles common to all shipments within it but distinct from the other lanes. Separate types of risk should be identified, e.g. high and low product temperature excursions, security breach, damage in transit and failure to deliver in full and on time.

If high temperature excursion is identified as a potential significant risk, the probability of the excursion, impact of the excursion and the likelihood of detection will be predicted. Probability will be affected by factors such as geographical differences. Initially, the estimate of probability may by subjective based only on experience and knowledge within the organisation. As the model develops and temperature data are accumulated, the objectivity and quality of the estimate of probability will improve. Early subjective probability therefore requires a safety factor to be included in order to mitigate against initial weakness of data and knowledge.

The next stage is to assess the impact of the temperature excursion both on the shipment and also on specific products or product groups.

It is rare to find sound scientific justification for acceptance of a load subject to an excursion, and, in the uncommon instances where a supplier or customer contacts the marketing authorisation holder for stability information, it is often not directly comparable to the excursion experienced. The most common presented reason for accepting a consignment with a temperature excursion is purely commercial, which may put patients at risk and undermines any risk management carried out by the company. In some cases, attempts are made to inappropriately apply mean kinetic temperature to underestimate impact rather than develop good control and preventive measures.

Increasing the likelihood of detection provides for earlier excursion warning, may help prevent an excursion and gives greater assurance that temperature conditions have been maintained. In circumstances where each shipment is not monitored for temperature, a very robust validation is required with clearly defined limits of validation, and where these are breached then the whole load is compromised. In practical terms it is normally easier to monitor temperature throughout the load or as monitoring combined with vehicle temperature mapping. Technological advances have provided easy and inexpensive means to relay temperature at receipt or as live data. It is important to ensure appropriate alerts are set in order to highlight potential excursions.

RISK CONTROL

The control of risk involves accepting levels of risk or reducing it to an acceptable level based on sound scientific reasoning. Approaches taken may include the avoidance of distributing medicines to specific territories outside the capability of the distributor or outsourcing shipping to couriers better suited for controlled temperature transport. With any risk control measure, the company needs to ensure potential new risks are identified and any related risk assessment is re-evaluated.

RISK COMMUNICATION

This includes communication of risk information within and outside of the organisation. In our transportation example, staff in Customer Services or Finance should not select use of a courier based purely on low price, but should draw from approved couriers where there has been formal quality risk assessment. A written agreement between the supplier and third-party courier provides a route of communication between both parties and can incorporate risk-mitigation measures such as restriction on uncontrolled further subcontracting, minimum specification of vehicles and drivers used, and prohibition of high risk activity such as cross-docking in an unauthorised manner.

Where new fleet is being selected, user requirement specification should incorporate areas of risk such as design criteria and functionality. Good specification design documents support risk communication between different departments, e.g. Finance, Transportation Department, Warehousing, Quality, Fleet Supplier.

RISK REVIEW

Quality risk management is dynamic and should adapt as circumstances within or external to the company change. It should be reviewed routinely and after any significant event or deviation.

Example 3: Application of quality risk management to development of a business continuity plan

The QMS should ensure that business activity is maintained and minimise the impact of unforeseen events. In these circumstances, a disaster contingency or business continuity plan may safeguard the organisation from service disruption as a consequence of internal or external factors. Examples of these factors may include:

- systems failure due to hacking of essential IT system;
- severe weather affecting the distribution chain locally or remotely;
- lack of availability of key personnel, including the Responsible Person or a subject-matter expert;
- supply disruption from a sole supplier;
- liquidation of 3PL warehouse holding stock;
- changes in operations due to exit from the EEA.

The global COVID-19 pandemic was an example of an external factor with wide-reaching impacts on wholesalers, who experienced a range of issues. These included:

- cost escalation of operations due to the implementation of new processes for hygiene and less efficient processes due to separation of shifts and distancing requirements;
- cost fluctuations of medicines due to changes in product availability and increased demand of some lines;
- operational impact due to reduced product flow through the supply chain as a consequence of customers not releasing products or not collecting products due to shielding;
- increased cost to customers;
- uncertainty of financial forecasting;
- staff management, including management of furloughs, staff isolating, introduction of homeworking and use of agency contingency staff.

The business continuity plan should be developed and tested in line with QRM principles. The level of detail of the plan may be correlated with the size of organisation, complexity of operations and complexity of the event the contingency is targeted at. For wholesalers that distribute medicines that provide an immediate risk to patients if the supply from the wholesaler is interrupted, then the plan should be used to protect continued supply and is likely to be extensive.

A good business continuity plan not only identifies risks, but also assists resource planning if the event occurs and assists the robustness of processes. It can facilitate implementation of approved alternative arrangements of non-critical activities, e.g. temporary homeworking arrangement for office staff, while streamlining core critical operations. Business continuity plans provide clear responsibilities and communication channels for all concerned and provides confidence to third parties where they have an involvement in operations.

Where a continuity plan is effective, it may provide competitive advantage to the wholesaler when compared to similar organisations that have not adequately prepared. During the development of the business continuity plan, consideration should be made of those processes critical to public health, e.g. the ability to maintain effectiveness of medicinal product recalls alongside the incident.

The continuity plan should be assessed following closure of the incident, following testing or as a periodic review in order to ascertain effectiveness.

Chapter 2 Personnel

2.1 Principle

The correct distribution of medicinal products relies upon people. For this reason, there must be sufficient competent personnel to carry out all the tasks for which the wholesale distributor is responsible. Individual responsibilities should be clearly understood by the staff and be recorded.

2.2 Responsible Person

The wholesale distributor must designate a person as responsible person. The responsible person should meet the qualifications and all conditions provided for by the legislation of the Member State concerned[2]. A degree in pharmacy is desirable. The responsible person should have appropriate competence and experience, as well as knowledge of and training in GDP.

The responsible person should fulfil their responsibilities personally and should be continuously contactable. The responsible person may delegate duties but not responsibilities.

The written job description of the responsible person should define their authority to take decisions with regard to their responsibilities. The wholesale distributor should give the responsible person the defined authority, resources and responsibility needed to fulfil their duties.

The responsible person should carry out their duties in such a way as to ensure that the wholesale distributor can demonstrate GDP compliance and that public service obligations are met.

The responsibilities of the responsible person include:

(i)   ensuring that a quality management system is implemented and maintained;
(ii)   focusing on the management of authorised activities and the accuracy and quality of records;
(iii) ensuring that initial and continuous training programmes are implemented and maintained;

---

[2] Article 79(b) of Directive 2001/83/EC.

(iv) coordinating and promptly performing any recall operations for medicinal products;

(v) ensuring that relevant customer complaints are dealt with effectively;

(vi) ensuring that suppliers and customers are approved;

(vii) approving any subcontracted activities which may impact on GDP;

(viii) ensuring that self-inspections are performed at appropriate regular intervals following a prearranged programme and necessary corrective measures are put in place;

(ix) keeping appropriate records of any delegated duties;

(x) deciding on the final disposition of returned, rejected, recalled or falsified products;

(xi) approving any returns to saleable stock;

(xii) ensuring that any additional requirements imposed on certain products by national law are adhered to[3].

2.3 Other personnel

There should be an adequate number of competent personnel involved in all stages of the wholesale distribution activities of medicinal products. The number of personnel required will depend on the volume and scope of activities.

The organisational structure of the wholesale distributor should be set out in an organisation chart. The role, responsibilities and inter-relationships of all personnel should be clearly indicated.

The role and responsibilities of employees working in key positions should be set out in written job descriptions, along with any arrangements for deputising.

2.4 Training

All personnel involved in wholesale distribution activities should be trained on the requirements of GDP. They should have the appropriate competence and experience prior to commencing their tasks.

Personnel should receive initial and continuing training relevant to their role, based on written procedures and in accordance with a written training programme. The Responsible Person should also maintain their competence in GDP through regular training.

In addition, training should include aspects of product identification and avoidance of falsified medicines entering the supply chain.

---

[3] Article 83 of Directive 2001/83/EC.

Personnel dealing with any products which require more stringent handling conditions should receive specific training. Examples of such products include hazardous products, radioactive materials, products presenting special risks of abuse (including narcotic and psychotropic substances) and temperature-sensitive products.

A record of all training should be kept, and the effectiveness of training should be periodically assessed and documented.

2.5 Hygiene

Appropriate procedures relating to personnel hygiene, relevant to the activities being carried out, should be established and observed. Such procedures should cover health, hygiene and clothing.

UK Guidance on Chapter 2 Personnel

Responsible Person

Regulation 45 of the Human Medicines Regulations 2012, as amended, requires that all licensed wholesale dealers should have at their disposal at least one person available as the Responsible Person (RP). The Responsible Person should have appropriate competence and experience, as well as knowledge of and training in Good Distribution Practice (GDP).

The points below set out the MHRA requirements and expectations for the RP, and are designed to help companies and RPs when nominating an RP.

Eligibility requirements

The experience of the RP is expected to be closely aligned to the wholesale distribution activities carried out by the company for which they are nominated. An RP with experience in one type of wholesale business is not automatically eligible to be nominated as an RP on another more complex licence and where there is a significant change in a business model, an RP may not necessarily remain suitable for that organisation.

Responsibilities of an RP

The RP is responsible for ensuring that the conditions under which the licence was granted have been, and are being, complied with; and ensuring that the quality of medicinal products handled by the licence holder is being maintained in accordance with the requirements of the marketing authorisations applicable to those products. The responsibilities of an RP include:

(i)   ensuring that a quality management system is implemented and maintained;

(ii)   focusing on the management of authorised activities and the accuracy and quality of records;

(iii)   ensuring that initial and continuous training programmes are implemented and maintained;

(iv)   coordinating and promptly performing any recall operations for medicinal products;

(v)   ensuring that relevant customer complaints are dealt with effectively;

(vi)   ensuring that suppliers and customers are approved;

(vii)   approving any subcontracted activities that may impact on GDP;

(viii) ensuring that self-inspections are performed at appropriate regular intervals following a prearranged programme and necessary corrective measures are put in place;

(ix)   keeping appropriate records of any delegated duties;

(x)   deciding on the final disposition of returned, rejected, recalled, or falsified products;

(xi)   approving any returns to saleable stock;

(xii)   ensuring that any additional requirements imposed on certain products by national law are adhered to.

The Responsible Person should fulfil their responsibilities personally and should be continuously contactable. The RP should be resident in the UK and proof of identity and address is required as part of the application process.

Where there is more than one RP named on the licence, each is expected to take full responsibility for the role, within the scope of their responsibilities as defined in their job description and agreed with the licence holder. It should be clear within the quality system which of the RPs is primarily accountable for the responsibilities described in GDP; responsibilities may be allocated either by function (e.g. oversight of the training programme) or where a company operates more than one site it may be possible to allocate responsibilities by site, providing full oversight of activities at a particular site or sites.

Contract RPs

The RP does not have to be an employee of the licence holder but must be continuously contactable. Where the RP is not an employee, there should be a written contract between the licence holder and the RP specifying responsibilities, duties, authority and time on site. Where a contract RP provides services from within a contracting company, the contract should be with the specific RP and not the contracting company.

When contracting an RP, the licence holder should carefully consider the competence and knowledge of the RP in relation to the proposed licensed activity. For example, if the primary plan is to export medicines the contract RP must have experience and knowledge of that area of wholesale distribution. As with any outsourced activity the licence holder should monitor and review the performance of the contract RP.

The contracted RP should also ensure they have adequate knowledge and experience to carry out the role. The RP must fully understand and have knowledge of the activities being carried out at a site. The RP should conduct a thorough review of operations before committing to a contract to act as RP to assure themselves that GDP will be complied with at the contracted site and any companies that are closely linked to it.

Contracting to be an RP for a company is a serious commitment requiring a high degree of vigilance to ensure that the company has an appropriate awareness of their obligation to comply with GDP and the Human Medicines Regulations.

The contract RP is expected to ensure they do not over extend themselves and apply to act as RPs or consultants for too many companies.

Obligations of the Licence Holder

The Human Medicines Regulations 43 to 45 set out the obligations of the licence holder in relation to holding a wholesale dealer's licence. The licence holder is the company to which the licence is issued. The licence holder is ultimately responsible for complying with GDP and the Human Medicines Regulations 2012 through persons employed by the company. The licence holder must have training and awareness of GDP and the Human Medicines Regulations.

It is for the licence holder to appoint a suitable RP that provides it with reassurance that:

- the conditions under which the licence was granted have been, and are being, complied with; and
- ensuring that the quality of medicinal products handled by the licence holder is being maintained in accordance with the requirements of the marketing authorisations applicable to those products.

The licence holder is also responsible for informing the Licensing Authority of any changes in the RP. Any changes must be advised immediately, and no person may act as RP other than those named on the licence or notified to the Licensing Authority.

The licence holder should ensure that there is a process for receiving advice and comment from the RP and recording the consequent action taken as may be necessary.

Knowledge requirements

The RP should have access to relevant pharmaceutical and technical knowledge and advice when it is required, and have personal knowledge of:

- the relevant provisions of the Human Medicines Regulations 2012 and amendments;
- the relevant legislation in the intended market the organisation is supplying to;
- the Guidelines on Good Distribution Practice;
- the conditions of the Wholesale Dealer's Licence for which nominated;
- the products traded under the licence and the conditions necessary for their safe storage and distribution;
- the categories of persons to whom products may be distributed.

The RP should also maintain their competence in GDP through regular training and keep records as evidence.

Experience requirements

The RP must demonstrate they have at least 1 year's practical experience of the activities authorised on the licence, i.e. procuring, holding, supplying or exporting. The RP must have obtained the technical knowledge of how to qualify suppliers, identify medicinal products, understand storage conditions and temperature control, qualify customers and how to transport medicinal products.

The RP should have at least 1 year's experience in maintaining a quality management system appropriate to the licence for which nominated.

The RP should be able to demonstrate they have completed relevant training in GDP.

Assessment of RP knowledge and experience

The knowledge and experience of an RP may be assessed by an inspector:

- when a variation is submitted to name them on a wholesale dealer's licence;
- during an inspection;
- on an ad hoc basis if non-compliance is established.

If the RP cannot demonstrate the required experience and knowledge or is not adequately carrying out those duties, the Licensing Authority may compulsorily vary the licence to remove the RP or refuse acceptance of the RP on that licence application. These actions may be extended to any other licence on which the RP is named.

Reporting arrangements

To carry out their responsibilities, the RP should:

- have a clear reporting line to the licence holder;
- have the defined authority, resources and responsibility needed to fulfil their duties;
- have access to all areas, sites, stores, staff and records relating to the licensable activities being carried out;
- demonstrate regular review and monitoring of all such areas, sites and staff, etc.;
- have delegated arrangements whereby the RP receives written reports that such delegated actions have been carried out on behalf of the RP in compliance with standard operating procedures and GDP. The RP remains responsible and should have demonstrable oversight of delegated duties;
- focus on the management of licensable activities, the accuracy and quality of records, compliance with standard operating procedures and GDP, the quality of handling and storage equipment and facilities, and the standards achieved;
- keep appropriate records relating to the discharge of the RP responsibilities.

The delegation of RP duties

Where the licence covers a number of sites, the RP may have a nominated deputy with appropriate reporting and delegating arrangements. However, the RP should be able to demonstrate to the Licensing Authority that the necessary controls and checks are in place. The term "Deputy RP" is not legally recognised but is often used. Only the Responsible Person(s) named on a wholesale dealer's licence have legal responsibility for the organisation's compliance and remain responsible for any duties that have been delegated.

Dispute resolution

Should it prove impossible to resolve a disagreement between the licence holder and the RP, the Licensing Authority should be consulted.

While a joint referral is clearly to be preferred, either party may approach the Licensing Authority independently. If an RP finds difficulty in performing statutory responsibilities or the activities being carried out under the licence, the Licensing Authority should be consulted in strict confidence.

The Responsible Person Gold Standard

The Human Medicines Regulations 2012 require holders of a wholesale dealer's licence to designate and ensure that there is available at all times at least one person, referred to in the regulations as the "Responsible Person", who, in the opinion of the licensing authority:

(a) has knowledge of the activities to be carried out and of the procedures to be performed under the licence; and

(b) has adequate experience relating to those activities and procedures.

Guidance on the role and responsibilities of the RP is set out in Chapter 2 of the GDP guidelines and these remain the same irrespective of whether the RP is a permanent employee of a company or is an external party working under the terms of a contract.

The RP plays a vital part in ensuring the quality and the integrity of medicinal products are maintained throughout the distribution chain and it is essential that they have the right knowledge, demonstrate competence and deploy the right skills so that patients and healthcare professionals have the confidence and trust to use medicines.

In order to facilitate this and to standardise the requirements for individuals operating as, or aspiring to be, a RP, Cogent (the national skills body for the science industries) has, following extensive discussion with pharmaceutical companies and the MHRA, published a "Gold Standard" role profile for the RP.

This sets out an industry-agreed framework that identifies the skills required in four competency areas and includes not only traditional qualifications and technical requirements, but also the behavioural skills necessary to do the job to a high standard. The Gold Standard is a competency framework, or role profile, and should be used by:

- the Licence Holder to assist in selection and induction of the RP;
- the RP in identifying the extent to which he/she fulfils the role and in compiling a training programme;
- the prospective RP in planning their learning and experience to prepare for a future role.

Responsible Person
Medicinal Products

The Human Medicines Regulations require a distributor to designate a Responsible Person(s), named on the applicable licence. Regulation 45 and the EU GDP Guide set out the requirements and the responsibilities.

Where the RP is contracted to a company, the duties remain the same as for those of the permanently employed RP. The responsibilities should be covered in a contract.

Compliance	**The Gold Standard** Job Role skills, knowledge and behaviours
	the individual should understand: • *the role of MHRA in the licensing of medicines and as the competent authority including the risk-based inspection process, the role of the enforcement group, the Inspection Action Group (IAG), and resulting actions that can be taken due to non-compliance* • *the UK regulations in relation to Wholesale Distribution* • *the European Pharmaceutical Directive related to Wholesale Distribution of Medicinal Products* • *Good Distribution Practice (GDP)* • *the importance of a clear reporting line to the wholesale distribution authorisation holder, senior manager and/or CEO* *the individual shall:* • *employ due diligence in the discharge of their duties, maintaining full compliance to procedures and appropriate regulations* • *report to senior management, the Marketing Authorisation holder and the MHRA any suspicious events of which they become aware* *in addition, the individual also has knowledge of:* • *the role of the professional bodies and organisations that regulate those supplying medicinal products to the public e.g. GPhC* • *the role of the Home Office in relation to the handling of Controlled Drugs* • *the role of the Veterinary Medicines Directorate (VMD) in relation to veterinary medicines* • *the role of the European Medicines Agency (EMA) and use of EUDRAGMDP* • *the Falsified Medicines Directive* • *the Principles and Guidelines of Good Manufacturing Practice and how the principles of GDP maintain product quality throughout the distribution chain*
Knowledge	**The Gold Standard** Job Role skills, knowledge and behaviours
	the individual should have: • *the prior relevant knowledge and experience related to the distribution of medicinal products* • *access to pharmaceutical knowledge and advice when it is required* • *knowledge of the products traded under the licence* • *if not a pharmacist or QP, one year's relevant practical and managerial experience of medicinal products*

 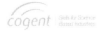

Responsible Person
Medicinal Products

Technical Competence	The Gold Standard Job Role skills, knowledge and behaviours

	the individual is able to perform duties including:
	
	Quality Management
	the individual shall ensure that a quality management system proportionate to the distributor's activities is implemented and maintained including:
	  • *Quality Risk Management*
	  • *Corrective and Preventative Actions (CAPA) to address deviations*
	  • *Change Control*
	  • *Measurement of performance indicators and management review*
	
	Personnel
	The Responsible Person is required to:
	  • *understand their own responsibilities*
	  • *carry out all duties in such a way as to ensure that the wholesale distributor can demonstrate GDP compliance*
	  • *define personal and staff roles, responsibilities and accountabilities and record all delegated duties*
	  • *ensure that initial and continuous training programmes are implemented and maintained*
	  • *ensure all personnel are trained in GDP, their own duties, product identification, the risks of falsified medicines and specific training for products requiring more stringent handling*
	  • *maintain training records for self and others and ensure training is periodically assessed*
	
	Premises & Equipment
	  • *ensure that appropriate standards of GDP are maintained for own premises and contracted storage premises*
	  • *identify medicinal products, legal categories, storage conditions and different Marketing Authorisation types*
	  • *maintain the safety and security of medicinal products within the appropriate environments, including product integrity and product storage*
	  • *use the appropriate systems to segregate, store and distribute medicinal products*
	  • *maintain records for the repair, maintenance, calibration and validation of equipment including computerised systems*
	  • *ensure storage areas are temperature mapped, qualified and validated*
	
	Documentation
	The individual shall focus on:
	  • *the accuracy and quality of records*
	  • *contemporaneous records*
	  • *records storage*
	  • *maintaining comprehensive written procedures that are understood and followed*
	  • *ensure procedures are valid and version controlled*

 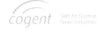

Responsible Person
Medicinal Products

	Operations • carry out due diligence checks and ensure that suppliers and customers are qualified • ensure all necessary checks are carried out and that medicinal products are authorised for sale • manage authorised activities to ensure operations do not compromise the quality of medicines and can demonstrate compliance with GDP • demonstrate the application of activities and provisions in accordance with the wholesale distribution authorisation and of company processes and procedures • ensure that any additional requirements imposed on certain products by national law are adhered to e.g. specials, unlicensed imports & Controlled Drugs **Complaints, returns, suspected falsified medicinal products and medicinal product recalls** • ensure relevant customer complaints are dealt with effectively, informing the manufacturer and/or marketing authorisation holder of any product quality/product defect issues • decide on the final disposition of returned, rejected, recalled or falsified products • approve any returns to saleable stock • coordinate and promptly perform any recall operations for medicinal products • co-operate with marketing authorisation holders and national competent authorities in the event of recalls • have an awareness of the issues surrounding falsified medicines **Outsourced Activities** • approve any subcontracted activities which may impact on GDP **Self-Inspection** • ensure that self-inspections are performed at appropriate regular intervals following a prearranged programme and necessary corrective measures are put in place **Transportation** • apply the appropriate transport requirements and methods for cold chain, ambient and hazardous product • ensure all transport equipment is appropriately qualified **Brokers** • ensure that transactions are only made with brokers who are registered • ensure that any broker activities performed are registered
Business Improvement	**The Gold Standard** Job Role skills, knowledge and behaviours
	the individual should: • practise continuous improvement practices and utilise appropriate tools and techniques to solve problems

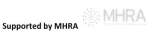

Supported by MHRA

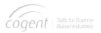

Responsible Person
Medicinal Products

Functional & Behavioural	**The Gold Standard** Job Role skills, knowledge and behaviours

	the individual has:
	 • *relevant skills in:*
	      ○ *English (level 2)*
	      ○ *Mathematics (level 2)*
	      ○ *ICT*
	
	 the individual can demonstrate relevant personal qualities in:
	     Autonomy
	      ○ *take responsibility for planning and developing courses of action, including responsibility for the work of others*
	      ○ *exercise autonomy and judgement within broad but generally well-defined parameters*
	 • *Management & Leadership*
	      ○ *develop and implement operational plans for their area of responsibility*
	      ○ *manage diversity & discrimination issues*
	      ○ *provide leadership for their team*
	
	 • *Working with others*
	      ○ *ensure effective delegation whilst retaining ownership of the outcome*
	      ○ *develop and maintain productive working relationships with colleagues and stakeholders*
	      ○ *monitor the progress and quality of work within their area of responsibility*
	
	 • *Personal development*
	      ○ *manage their professional development by setting targets and planning how they will be met*
	      ○ *review progress towards targets and establish evidence of achievements*
	
	 • *Communication*
	      ○ *put across ideas in clear and concise manner and present a well-structured case*
	      ○ *communicate complex information to others*
	
	 • *Business*
	      ○ *understands the business environment in which the company operates*
	      ○ *has an appreciation of the industry sector and competitors*
	
	 • *Customers*
	      ○ *understands the customer base and is aware of customer requirements*

For more information on how to achieve the Gold Standard contact us on 01325 740900	
Version 2 July 2014	

 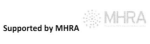

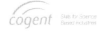

EU GUIDELINES ON GDP AND UK GUIDANCE ON WHOLESALE DISTRIBUTION

The licence holder is required to provide an RP with adequate knowledge and experience. Learning "on the job" is usual in this industry, but experiential training can only provide for some elements of the full package. There is a place for good-quality external training and this should be considered by all licence holders. Before arranging any external training, the licence holder and RP should be fully aware of the collaborative work on the Responsible Person Gold Standard between the GDP Inspectorate and Cogent Skills.

There is, effectively, a hierarchy of RP training provision in the UK. The following shows the range of external training and the extent to which they are recognised by MHRA.

- Any training provider may offer RP training. Current offerings range from extremely generic courses to targeted courses delivered in the work place. The buyer must verify the content is accurate and suited to their needs.
- A training provider may align their training with the Responsible Person Gold Standard but without recognition from the MHRA. Once again, there is a range in quality, and the buyer must be wary.
- A list of RP training providers recognised by MHRA/Cogent Skills is available on the Cogent Skills website[4].

RPs may demonstrate their suitability to the licence holder and the inspector as follows:

- knowledge of GDP and the relevant regulations, and application of that knowledge to the organisation's operations;
- industry experience – relevant GDP experience;
- familiarity with the business operations of the licence holder – this can be particularly challenging in a large or complex organisation;
- induction/primary training – role familiarity;
- role definition and place within the organisation – sufficient seniority and influence;
- delegation and training others – the RP is responsible for all GDP activities, even those delegated;
- training records – RP, licence holder and staff;
- continuing development for the RP – as the supply chain continually presents new challenges.

There is no real substitute for reading and re-reading the GDP Guidelines and relevant regulations. Many licence holders include the GDP

---

[4] Responsible Person in Good Distribution Practice – Consultancy & Courses (cogentskills.solutions).

Guidelines within their quality system, which sends the right message to all staff. Reading and understanding the Guidelines should be seen as a clear learning activity and should form part of the RP's training record. Further sources of information are inspectorate blogs, and information published on the GOV.UK website.

INDUSTRY EXPERIENCE

It is essential that the RP can demonstrate practical industry experience related to the authorised activities on the licence and GDP. For example, conducting an effective recall by ensuring sufficient staff, storage space and written procedures are in place and clearly understood by those involved.

FAMILIARITY WITH THE GDP OPERATIONS OF THE LICENCE HOLDER

The RP should familiarise themselves with all aspects of the GDP operations and company structure. Where the RP lacks sufficient oversight or knowledge of the day-to-day operational activities, non-compliance issues can occur. For instance, the licence holder may be conducting GDP activities from an unlicensed site which the RP is unaware of.

INDUCTION/PRIMARY TRAINING

The induction process is essential when onboarding a new RP. The licence holder must ensure that the nominated RP has the appropriate knowledge and experience to carry out their duties and provide adequate time at the induction stage.

The nominated RP must ensure they are fully conversant with all aspects of GDP and associated regulations; it may take several years before an RP is fully coherent with the roles and responsibilities.

ROLE DEFINITION AND PLACE WITHIN THE ORGANISATION

There should be a clear reporting line to the licence holder and the RP should have adequate resource available to ensure the organisation's compliance. Respective responsibilities between the RP and the licence holder should be clearly defined and understood. In the larger organisation, the RP is frequently in the Quality Department. The position of the RP should always allow sufficient oversight of activities such as the warehouse management system, staff rosters, transport, etc.

DELEGATION AND TRAINING OTHERS

GDP clearly sets out that all staff should be trained in their role, in GDP, in the identification of medicines and in the avoidance of falsified medicines entering the supply chain. There should be a clear training programme describing these. The RP must ensure that initial and continuous training programmes are implemented and maintained; and, although the RP need not conduct all the training themselves, the RP should have sufficient oversight to demonstrate the trainers, training materials and records are suitable. Licence holders are also expected to undergo training.

TRAINING RECORDS

Training records can be paper-based or electronic and should include a wide range of learning activities from SOP reading and external training to ad hoc learning such as shadowing staff. Records should cover all staff; this includes the RP and licence holder. The GDP Inspectorate considers an RP's suitability based on a range of evidence – this would include how they perform their role, as well as the range of training they have undertaken.

CONTINUING DEVELOPMENT FOR THE RP

Continuing professional development (CPD) is a natural progression from initial training. Some professions will require that ongoing learning is recorded in the form of CPD, e.g. pharmacists and pharmacy technicians registered with the General Pharmaceutical Council (GPhC). These records can be used as the RP's training record so long as the CPD covers the scope of the role and the records are made available on inspection. Many make use of external training courses – many of these are of a high standard and cover a specific area within GDP. Other external courses are intended to be generally applicable to all RPs and these can still be of use in continuing development.

The Responsible Person (Import)

A wholesale dealer in Great Britain may only import Qualified Person (QP) certified medicines from the European Economic Area (EEA) if certain checks are made by the "Responsible Person (import) (RPi)". Great Britain is England, Wales and Scotland.

Products that do not require RPi oversight

Medicinal products sourced from Northern Ireland for wholesale purposes are out of scope of this guidance. This is permitted under the supervision of a Responsible Person (RP).

Products with a UK or Great Britain marketing authorisation that are imported into Great Britain from outside the UK without QP certification from a country on the list will require QP certification under a UK manufacturing and import authorisation before being placed on the market.

Products without a marketing authorisation in the UK, Northern Ireland, Great Britain or a listed country are outside the scope of this guidance. Importation of such products is permitted under the supervision of a Responsible Person (RP), with notification to the MHRA of each importation that is for supply to the Great Britain market.

Introduction

The RPi is responsible for implementing a system to confirm for products that have been imported into Great Britain from countries on an approved country for import list (initially, this will be countries in the EEA):

- that the required QP certification has taken place;
- that the required independent batch release certificate is available for biological products (described on a wholesale dealer's licence as "immunologicals and blood products").

The RPi may delegate the activity of checking this certification has taken place but remains responsible for ensuring the effectiveness of these checks.

The RPi is required to implement a system for confirming QP certification and independent batch release certification (for biological products) has taken place when importing into Great Britain the following products from a listed country:

- a UK or Great Britain licensed medicine for use in Great Britain;
- a UK or Great Britain licensed medicine for supply to another third country;
- a Northern Ireland or approved country licensed medicine for supply to fulfil special clinical needs;
- a Northern Ireland or approved country licensed medicine imported as an introduced medicine for supply to another third country;
- a Northern Ireland or approved country licensed medicine for use as a parallel import.

What evidence can be used for QP certification

The RPi should ensure that written evidence is available to demonstrate that each batch of product has been QP certified as required in Article 51 of Directive 2001/83/EC.

Not all options listed below may be suitable for different supply chain relationships; however, just one of these pieces of evidence is sufficient to satisfy the requirements of regulation 45AA of the Human Medicines Regulations 2012. Other evidence may be acceptable provided it confirms that QP certification has taken place for the batch in question.

EVIDENCE FOR GREAT BRITAIN WHOLESALE DEALERS LICENCE (WDA(H)) HOLDERS IMPORTING A UK, NORTHERN IRELAND, GREAT BRITAIN OR EEA LICENSED MEDICINE FROM A LISTED COUNTRY

Batch certification by a QP may be confirmed using evidence such as:

- batch certificate confirming QP certification in accordance with Article 51 of Directive 2001/83/EC);

- a copy of the 'control report' (Appendix II to EU Good Manufacturing Practice Annex 16);
- statement of certification (ad hoc, confirming certification in accordance with Article 51 of Directive 2001/83/EC);
- reference to company internal systems (e.g. global Enterprise Resource Planning system) that shows batch certification;
- confirmation that the final manufacturing step (other than batch certification) of an authorised medicine has been performed by a Manufacturing and Import Authorisation holder in a listed country. A copy of the Marketing Authorisation and technical agreement with the manufacturer should be available to place reliance on this supply chain control;
- for medicines authorised in a listed country, batch certification may be verified by confirming that the medicine has been purchased from an authorised wholesaler after it has been "placed on the market" in the listed country.

A blanket document from your supplier declaring that all the medicines they supply have been QP certified and sourced from authorised wholesalers after they have been placed on the market is not considered suitable evidence.

WHAT EVIDENCE CAN BE USED FOR INDEPENDENT BATCH RELEASE CERTIFICATION?

Biological products requiring independent batch release certification are listed on the European Directorate for Quality of Medicines website. (https://www.edqm.eu/en/human-ocabr-guidelines).

Independent batch release may be confirmed using evidence such as:

- a statement from the marketing authorisation holder confirming that a batch certificate has been issued by NIBSC or a Mutual Recognition Agreement partner;
- a copy of the batch certificate issued by NIBSC or a Mutual Recognition Agreement partner;
- confirmation from NIBSC that a batch certificate has been issued. Enquiries should be sent to CPB@nibsc.org.

Batches of QP certified biological medicines that require independent batch release should not be sold or supplied by the importing wholesale dealer in Great Britain until independent batch release certification is also confirmed.

Additional guidance

SUPPLY CHAIN SECURITY

Checks on products imported from a listed country should also ensure that the product is not the subject of a recall or reported as stolen and is available on the market within the listed country's licensed supply chain. Good Distribution Practice (GDP) requirements for supplier qualification set out in GDP 5.2 must be maintained. The MHRA's supplier verification blog provides additional information. Products that have been certified by a QP but have been diverted to countries not within a listed country or Northern Ireland must be imported by the holder of an MIA and recertified by a QP.

PRODUCTS IMPORTED FOR PARALLEL IMPORT OR SPECIAL NEED

From 1 January 2022, the RPi should implement a process to confirm the status of the unique identifier for Prescription Only Medicines, if wholesale dealers are importing products:

- for parallel import;
- for use for special clinical need or introduction.

This is required by the EU's Falsified Medicine Directive. Confirmation of decommissioning may be provided by using evidence such as National Medicines Verification System records from the supplier.

From 1 January 2022, products that are supplied as decommissioned must be decommissioned by the final EEA supplier and not at any other point in the supply chain.

GREAT BRITAIN WDA(H) HOLDERS ACTING AS OR ON BEHALF OF THE UK MARKETING AUTHORISATION HOLDER (MAH)

For Great Britain WDA(H) holders acting as or on behalf of the UK or Great Britain MAH, the expectation is that products have been certified prior to importation. Shipment to Great Britain under pre-certification quarantine is not acceptable for the WDA(H) importation model.

If supply chains require shipment under quarantine prior to QP certification for technical reasons (e.g. products with very short shelf life) the MAH should seek further advice from MHRA by e-mail to GDP. Inspectorate@mhra.gov.uk

Working as an RPi

If you are named as an RPi on a WDA(H) you have an important role in ensuring the safe control of medicines. You have training and an understanding of the industry in order to qualify for the role, where you have the legal responsibility to ensure that batches of authorised medicines imported from countries on a list have been appropriately certified prior to being placed on the Great Britain market.

You will take responsibility for implementing a system for the WDA(H) as a whole. There is no requirement for each site on the WDA(H) to name its own RPi. You do not have to be an employee of the licence holder, but you must be continuously contactable. Where you are not an employee, there should be a written contract between the licence holder and the RPi specifying responsibilities, duties, authority and time on site.

If you are a contract RPi then you are expected to ensure you do not over-extend yourself and apply to act as RPi for too many companies.

Becoming an RPi

There are several stages to becoming named as an RPi.

You must first demonstrate that you are eligible to act as an RPi. This is through a combination of relevant qualifications and experience. It is also expected that you will be a full member of a professional body with a published code of conduct. Once eligibility has been assessed and accepted by the MHRA, you can be named on a register; the register will be maintained by the MHRA and will include all persons eligible to be named as an RPi.

The regulations set out expectations for qualifications, experience and membership of professional bodies.

Acceptable qualifications are a diploma, certificate or other evidence of formal qualifications awarded on completion of a university or other higher education course of study in:

- pharmacy;
- chemistry;
- medicine;
- biology;
- a related life science.

Equivalent qualifications acceptable for RPi candidates include:

- level 5 qualifications from Chartered Institute of Logistics and Transport;
- a Quality Management System Lead Auditor or Pharmaceutical GMP Lead Auditor qualification awarded by Chartered Quality Institute.

Other qualifications may also be acceptable. These will be checked during the application process. You can check the suitability of your qualifications by e-mail to GDP.Inspectorate@mhra.gov.uk

You must be able to demonstrate, e.g. by providing a curriculum vitae (CV), that you have a minimum of 2 years' experience in performing the functions of a Responsible Person on a WDA(H). Evidence of performing other functions, e.g. a quality assurance role for a pharmaceutical manufacturer, may also be considered equivalent.

Acceptable professional body memberships are:

- Royal Society of Biology;
- Royal Pharmaceutical Society;
- Pharmaceutical Society of Northern Ireland;
- Royal Society of Chemistry.

Additional bodies that the licensing authority considers to be equivalent for RPi candidates include:

- the Chartered Institute of Logistics and Transport;
- the Chartered Quality Institute.
- the Organisation for Professionals in Regulatory Affairs
- Association of Pharmacy Technicians UK (APTUK)

Other professional associations may be acceptable. These will be checked during the application process. You can check the suitability of your professional body membership by e-mail to GDP.Inspectorate@mhra.gov.uk

You will need to be a "full member" rather than an affiliate or student member of a professional body corresponding to your qualifications and experience. Affiliate membership of a professional body where you do not have a related qualification is not acceptable. You will need to demonstrate continual professional development and comply with the professional code of conduct expected by the professional body.

QUALIFIED PERSONS ACTING AS RPi

If you are a person named on the Qualified Persons register you will also be eligible to act as an RPi. You must still apply to be named on the RPi register. As an alternative to providing evidence of your qualifications and membership of a professional body you may provide evidence of your QP registration.

SUITABILITY

You must also demonstrate suitability to be named on a specific WDA(H) licence. At the time of application, the MHRA will confirm whether you are named on the register, and check whether your experience is suitable for the proposed licence activity. For example, an eligible RPi without prior experience in parallel importation might not be considered suitable to be named on WDA(H) where the company is importing licensed products for parallel trade.

APPLYING TO BE NAMED AS A RPi

RPi applications may be submitted through the MHRA Portal from 1 January 2021.

The Responsible Person (import) (RPi) is described in regulations 45AA and 45AB of the Human Medicines Regulations 2012 (as amended).

The RPi should be a UK resident. You will need to provide proof of address and identity when you apply.

Chapter 3 Premises and Equipment

3.1 Principle

Wholesale distributors must have suitable and adequate premises, installations and equipment[5], so as to ensure proper storage and distribution of

---

[5] Article 79(a) of Directive 2001/83/EC.

medicinal products. In particular, the premises should be clean, dry and maintained within acceptable temperature limits.

3.2 Premises

The premises should be designed or adapted to ensure that the required storage conditions are maintained. They should be suitably secure, structurally sound and of sufficient capacity to allow safe storage and handling of the medicinal products. Storage areas should be provided with adequate lighting to enable all operations to be carried out accurately and safely.

Where premises are not directly operated by the wholesale distributor, a contract should be in place. The contracted premises should be covered by a separate wholesale distribution authorisation.

Medicinal products should be stored in segregated areas which are clearly marked and have access restricted to authorised personnel. Any system replacing physical segregation, such as electronic segregation based on a computerised system, should provide equivalent security and should be validated.

Products pending a decision as to their disposition or products that have been removed from saleable stock should be segregated either physically or through an equivalent electronic system. This includes, e.g., any product suspected of falsification and returned products. Medicinal products received from a third country but not intended for the Union market should also be physically segregated. Any falsified medicinal products, expired products, recalled products and rejected products found in the supply chain should be immediately physically segregated and stored in a dedicated area away from all other medicinal products. The appropriate degree of security should be applied in these areas to ensure that such items remain separate from saleable stock. These areas should be clearly identified.

Special attention should be paid to the storage of products with specific handling instructions as specified in national law. Special storage conditions (and special authorisations) may be required for such products (e.g. narcotics and psychotropic substances).

Radioactive materials and other hazardous products, as well as products presenting special safety risks of fire or explosion (e.g. medicinal gases, combustibles, flammable liquids and solids), should be stored in one or more dedicated areas subject to local legislation and appropriate safety and security measures.

Receiving and dispatch bays should protect products from prevailing weather conditions. There should be adequate separation between the receipt and dispatch and storage areas. Procedures should be in place to maintain control of inbound/outbound goods. Reception areas where deliveries are examined following receipt should be designated and suitably equipped.

Unauthorised access to all areas of the authorised premises should be prevented. Prevention measures would usually include a monitored intruder alarm system and appropriate access control. Visitors should be accompanied.

Premises and storage facilities should be clean and free from litter and dust. Cleaning programmes, instructions and records should be in place. Appropriate cleaning equipment and cleaning agents should be chosen and used so as not to present a source of contamination.

Premises should be designed and equipped so as to afford protection against the entry of insects, rodents or other animals. A preventive pest-control programme should be in place.

Rest, wash and refreshment rooms for employees should be adequately separated from the storage areas. The presence of food, drink, smoking material or medicinal products for personal use should be prohibited in the storage areas.

3.2.1 TEMPERATURE AND ENVIRONMENT CONTROL

Suitable equipment and procedures should be in place to check the environment where medicinal products are stored. Environmental factors to be considered include temperature, light, humidity and the cleanliness of the premises.

An initial temperature mapping exercise should be carried out on the storage area before use, under representative conditions. Temperature monitoring equipment should be located according to the results of the mapping exercise, ensuring that monitoring devices are positioned in the areas that experience the extremes of fluctuations. The mapping exercise should be repeated according to the results of a risk assessment exercise or whenever significant modifications are made to the facility or the temperature controlling equipment. For small premises of a few square meters which are at room temperature, an assessment of potential risks (e.g. heaters) should be conducted and temperature monitors placed accordingly.

3.3 Equipment

All equipment impacting on the storage and distribution of medicinal products should be designed, located and maintained to a standard which suits its intended purpose. Planned maintenance should be in place for key equipment vital to the functionality of the operation.

Equipment used to control or to monitor the environment where the medicinal products are stored should be calibrated at defined intervals based on a risk and reliability assessment.

Calibration of equipment should be traceable to a national or international measurement standard. Appropriate alarm systems should be in place to provide alerts when there are excursions from predefined storage conditions. Alarm levels should be appropriately set and alarms should be regularly tested to ensure adequate functionality.

Equipment repair, maintenance and calibration operations should be carried out in such a way that the integrity of the medicinal products is not compromised.

Adequate records of repair, maintenance and calibration activities for key equipment should be made and the results should be retained. Key equipment would include, e.g. cold stores, monitored intruder alarm and access-control systems, refrigerators, thermo-hygrometers, or other temperature and humidity recording devices, air handling units and any equipment used in conjunction with the onward supply chain.

3.3.1 COMPUTERISED SYSTEMS

Before a computerised system is brought into use, it should be demonstrated, through appropriate validation or verification studies, that the system is capable of achieving the desired results accurately, consistently and reproducibly.

A written, detailed description of the system should be available (including diagrams where appropriate). This should be kept up to date. The document should describe principles, objectives, security measures, system scope and main features, how the computerised system is used and the way it interacts with other systems.

Data should only be entered into the computerised system or amended by persons authorised to do so.

Data should be secured by physical or electronic means and protected against accidental or unauthorised modifications. Stored data should be checked periodically for accessibility. Data should be protected by backing up at regular intervals. Back-up data should be retained for the period stated in national legislation but at least 5 years at a separate and secure location.

Procedures to be followed if the system fails or breaks down should be defined. This should include systems for the restoration of data.

3.3.2 QUALIFICATION AND VALIDATION

Wholesale distributors should identify what key equipment qualification and/or key process validation is necessary to ensure correct installation and operation. The scope and extent of such qualification and/or validation activities (such as storage, pick and pack processes) should be determined using a documented risk assessment approach.

Equipment and processes should be respectively qualified and/or validated before commencing use and after any significant changes, e.g. repair or maintenance.

Validation and qualification reports should be prepared summarising the results obtained and commenting on any observed deviations. Deviations from established procedures should be documented and further actions decided to correct deviations and avoid their re-occurrence (corrective and preventive actions). The principles of CAPA should be applied where necessary. Evidence of satisfactory validation and acceptance of a process or piece of equipment should be produced and approved by appropriate personnel.

UK Guidance on Chapter 3 Premises and Equipment

Qualification and validation of equipment, including computerised systems

The main GDP expectation for qualification and validation of equipment is that the company has identified what equipment is critical to their operations, and they have a proportionate approach to qualification during installation or following repair or modification in line with quality risk-management principles.

A wholesaler may, for example, consider qualification of an uninterrupted power supply generator to power a cold room as being critical and likely to include a high degree of input from external engineers with high impact if it fails, so testing of the system is likely to be extensive to ensure the unit will operate reliably. Less critical equipment, such as a thermometer may be considered by the wholesaler to require less extensive qualification, especially where they are of simple design, and multiple thermometers enable some continuous monitoring.

Examples of equipment often deemed most critical include uninterrupted power supply generators, cooling system for cold rooms and electronic staff access systems.

Computerised systems cover a wide range of functions, and, as with other equipment, the company should be aware of the most critical systems, as well as inherent risks. Factors that may contribute to risk related to software include:

- application (WMS, inventory management, product scanning, premises security);
- design (off-the-shelf, customisable off-the-shelf, bespoke);
- connectivity (customer access portals, networking across company sites, compatibility with other software systems, including on-site and with field force);
- maintenance and stability;
- management (in-house, outsourced);
- criticality of data (corruption prevention, protection against unauthorised changes, back-up and restoration functions, archiving).

The extent of qualification or validation for computerised systems should challenge the weakest parts of the systems and take account of the greatest risk of system non-compliance or potential failure, rather than simply relying on validation or qualification of the most robust parts of any system.

Temperature control and monitoring

Manufacturers subject their products to stability studies that are used to determine appropriate storage conditions, including those for temperature. These conditions are therefore specific for each product, and a licensed wholesale dealer should refer to manufacturers' information when deciding the storage conditions to use.

Following manufacture, some medicinal products can be stored and transported at ambient temperature, while others may require lower than ambient temperatures to assure their quality and efficacy.

These are often referred to as "cold chain products" or "fridge lines", and wholesale dealers are expected to store and distribute them in strict accordance with the product labelling requirements as stated in the GDP Guidelines: Chapters 5.5 (Storage) and 9.2 (Transportation) give more information.

Medicinal products experiencing an adverse temperature may undergo physical, chemical or microbiological degradation. In the most serious of cases this may lead to conversion of the medicine into ineffective or harmful forms. The ability to detect these changes may not appear until the medicine is consumed, and it is therefore essential that appropriate temperature conditions are controlled and monitored throughout each step of the supply chain. This section concerns temperature mapping and the ongoing temperature monitoring and control required throughout the wholesale supply chain.

Temperature mapping

Chapter 3.2.1 of the GDP Guidelines states:

"An initial temperature mapping exercise should be carried out on the storage area before use, under representative conditions.

Temperature monitoring equipment should be located according to the results of the mapping exercise, ensuring that monitoring devices are positioned in the areas that experience the extremes of fluctuations.

The mapping exercise should be repeated according to the results of a risk assessment exercise or whenever significant modifications are made to the facility or the temperature controlling equipment.

For small premises of a few square meters which are at room temperature, an assessment of potential risks (e.g. heaters) should be conducted and temperature monitors placed accordingly."

While the guidelines say that mapping should take place, this should be specific and relevant to your own storage area. The duration of a mapping exercise should be determined based on the variability of the environment and data recorded rather than a standard set period.

Temperature mapping should be carried out to demonstrate by way of documented evidence that the chosen storage area is suitable for the storage of temperature-sensitive medicinal products. A mapping exercise of the proposed storage area will also ensure that the company understands their storage area and has identified any potential areas therein that may be unsuitable to store medicines. A mapping exercise will also inform as to where permanent thermometers should be located.

Temperature mapping should be carried out, before stock is stored. This might not be possible where a storage area is being reconfigured. In smaller empty storage areas, dummy products could be used to simulate normal operational storage without compromising genuine product, including cold stores and fridges/freezers. In an empty storage area, a mapping exercise should be repeated when fully stocked. Data arising from the exercise should be documented and a risk assessment documented with any hot or cold spots identified. This exercise should then be repeated accounting for seasonal variations.

To temperature map, firstly look at the area to be used for storage and identify the highest point of storage, not the highest shelf or pallet location. Identify any potential problem areas such as heaters, lighting, windows and doors, loading bays or high storage areas such as mezzanine floors. These areas should be covered in the exercise. Areas such as CD rooms, packing areas, returns and quarantine should be included. When deciding on a storage area, it can be difficult to cool storage areas down as well as heat them up. Calibrated monitoring probes should be used in sufficient numbers dependent on the size of the storage area.

Once the initial mapping exercise is complete, the data should be recorded and risk assessed to determine the most appropriate positions for the permanent monitoring probes and should cover the areas that have the widest temperature fluctuations or indicate areas with any hot or cold spots. A risk assessment would also define and justify the regularity of any future mapping exercises and must also be regularly reviewed, perhaps as part of the self-audit process.

The exercise should be repeated to cover seasonal variations or if the storage area is subsequently reconfigured.

The RP should be party to the whole mapping process and should be fully aware of the mapping exercise findings, risk-assessment recommendations and review process. The RP's involvement does not stop at the

EU GUIDELINES ON
GDP AND UK GUIDANCE ON
WHOLESALE DISTRIBUTION

mapping process, however; the RP should also be able to demonstrate supervision and review of subsequent daily minimum/maximum routine temperature monitoring and recording and should be consulted in the event of any temperature excursions.

Refrigerated and ambient medicinal products: receipt, storage and packing

RECEIPT OF REFRIGERATED PRODUCTS

When cold chain products are received, it is important that they are checked-in as a matter of priority and placed in a pharmaceutical refrigerator.

The person responsible for receiving the delivery must also satisfy themselves that the goods have been transported under appropriate conditions (e.g. there has been no direct contact between the products and gel or ice blocks or if the consignment is warm to the touch).

If it cannot be confirmed that the products have been transported under appropriate conditions and there is concern that their quality may have been compromised, the delivery should be quarantined in a suitable refrigerator while enquiries are made with the supplier.

Until the issue has been clarified the products in question should be considered as unsuitable and should not be supplied.

If, following enquiries, there is still doubt as to the quality of the medicines received, the delivery should not be accepted and should be returned to the supplier.

STORAGE OF REFRIGERATED PRODUCTS IN A PHARMACEUTICAL REFRIGERATOR

The equipment used for the storage of refrigerated medicinal products should be demonstrably suitable and fit for purpose. Due to the configuration of domestic refrigerators, they are often found to be unsuitable for the storage of pharmaceutical products.

The air within a pharmaceutical refrigerator is typically circulated by a fan, which provides a uniform temperature profile and a rapid temperature pull down after the door has been opened.

Temperature monitoring is recorded by a calibrated electronic minimum/maximum thermometer, with an accuracy of ±0.5°C, which can be read without opening the refrigerator door.

Additional benefits are that these refrigerators can be locked and some have the option of either an audio or visual alarm system to alert staff in the event of temperature deviations.

Many refrigerators have glass-fronted doors giving greater visibility of stock levels, aiding stock management and also deterring the storage of non-medicinal products.

When purchasing a new refrigerator, factors to consider might also include how long the unit can maintain the required temperatures if the power is turned off and to what extent the temperature is affected by external ambient temperature variation, e.g. in hot spells.

TEMPERATURE MONITORING IN A REFRIGERATOR

As is applicable for transportation, products stored in a refrigerator should be subject to daily temperature monitoring by a minimum and maximum calibrated device with a supporting appropriate calibration certificate.

Temperature records should identify any temperature deviations and give details of corrective actions taken as a result.

For instances where there has been a temperature deviation, best practice would be to take a further reading later the same day, to ensure that it was a transient deviation and show that the temperature was now back within prescribed parameters.

The Responsible Person should be informed of any deviations.

Temperature records are especially important in the event of a problem with a product and may be required as evidence of appropriate storage. With this in mind, they should be free from alterations or corrections and the person responsible for taking the readings each day should have a trained deputy to cover for absences.

The records should be routinely reviewed and signed off by the Responsible Person.

SMALL REFRIGERATORS

Refrigerators used to store pharmaceuticals should be demonstrated to be fit for purpose. In the simplest of cases a new off-the-shelf refrigerator installed according to the manufacturer's instructions and temperature monitored with an appropriate device may be considered appropriately qualified for storing cold chain product that is shown to be unaffected by minor temperature excursions. A refrigerator used for holding more susceptible stock such as biological products will require more extensive qualification.

In addition to temperature mapping and monitoring there should be safeguards to preserve appropriate storage conditions. Some small refrigerators are purported to be medical or pharmaceutical refrigerators, but this on its own does not automatically render them suitable for wholesale use. The refrigerator should be capable of restoring the temperature quickly after the door has been opened and without danger of overshooting to extreme cold. This could be assisted by an internal fan and good shelf design that enables an efficient air flow. There should be no internal ice box and no internal temperature dials capable of being inadvertently knocked and adjusted.

Storage practices for using small refrigerators should include consideration of segregation of stock with different status, e.g. incoming, quarantine, returned and outgoing stock. Sufficient space should be maintained to permit adequate air circulation and product should not be stored in contact with the walls or on the floor of the refrigerator. If the refrigerator is filled to capacity the effect on temperature distribution should be investigated. Where non-refrigerated items are introduced to the refrigerator, such as non-conditioned gel packs, the impact of introducing these items should be assessed regarding the increase in temperature they cause.

LARGE COMMERCIAL REFRIGERATORS AND WALK-IN COLD ROOMS

Large commercial refrigerators and walk-in cold rooms should be of appropriate design, suitably sited and be constructed with appropriate materials. Consideration should be given to protecting entry points from ingress of warm air. The design should ensure general principles of GDP can be maintained, such as segregation of stock. Condensate from chillers should not be collected inside the unit and there should be a capability to carry out routine maintenance and service activities as much as possible from outside the unit. The temperature should be monitored with an electronic temperature-recording device that measures load temperature in one or more locations depending on the size of the unit, and alarms should be fitted to indicate power outages and temperature excursions.

FREEZERS

Most of the problems seen with use of freezers also apply to refrigerators. The same general principles apply to freezers as apply to other cold chain storage units mentioned above. Walk-in freezers pose a significant operator health and safety risk, and the impact of ways of working should be reviewed with consideration of risk to causing temperature excursions.

Design considerations

When buying a new freezer the user should consider what it is to be used for and how they intend on using it. This may appear obvious, but the use of freezers that are not fit for use and unsuitable operating practices are regularly seen.

The most common use of freezers by wholesalers is for storing and conditioning cold packs for inclusion in passive transport containers. There may also be a need to store frozen medicinal products such as some vaccines, although the range of medicines that require to be stored frozen is small.

The intended use will determine the extent to which a particular freezer design meets your needs, or if any special measures need to be put in place. Consideration should be given to what temperature range you require, with a diversity of freezer models being available that maintain a variety of frozen temperatures. Storage conditions for specific medicines may be found by reference to packaging details or the Summary of Product Characteristics available from the manufacturers' medicines regulatory authority or from the manufacturer.

Considerations of use

Prior to use the freezer should be fully qualified in line with GDP qualification requirements and the exercise documented both for small freezers, in which case qualification may be very simple, and large freezers installed by external specialists. Installation of the freezer should include risk assessment of the impact of the installation, e.g. effect of heat generation by the freezer on the surrounding area. Personnel should be instructed on how to use the freezer, and there should be notification to staff who are restricted from using it.

As with all equipment (including freezers and cold packs), do not just rely on qualification data from the marketing brochure or sales representative: make sure the qualification fully meets your needs.

Domestic freezers are unlikely to have adequate power to rapidly freeze cold packs from room temperature and may not be suitable for the storage of frozen pharmaceutical products.

Storage of medicines

The range of medicines that require storage in a freezer is small, and the storage equipment most often seen are small freezers holding a small quantity of medicine. There is often a temptation to use the same freezer for other purposes such as the conditioning of cold packs. This increases risk to the stored medicines, as high temperature excursions are created either by unconditioned cold packs loaded in bulk or by increased access to the freezer to load or remove the cold packs. It is therefore recommended that freezers used for storing medicines are dedicated in use or otherwise demonstrated to be not adversely affected by freezing cold packs. If the volume of frozen medicines is very small then the wholesaler should consider whether it is worth either not holding those lines or outsourcing the holding of cold chain medicines to a wholesaler better suited to storing them.

Some companies compromise by using dual refrigerator/freezer units. Although less expensive and with a smaller footprint than separate units, if one unit becomes non-functional then the both units are compromised. In addition, if both units are served by a single compressor, then the ability of the equipment to maintain temperature in one unit may affect its ability to maintain the other unit. This may be a concern if frozen medicines are stored and the refrigerator is in frequent use, if regular defrosting of the refrigerator occurs or where the thermostat setting for one unit is adjusted.

The majority of frozen medicines require storage in the range of −15°C to −20°C, and the responsibility is on the wholesaler to ensure they know what frozen temperature is required for a particular product and that the freezer used can maintain this. Requirements to temperature monitor and map freezers for storing medicines or conditioning cold packs are the same as for refrigerators.

Not all frozen medicines require storage at the same frozen temperature.

Conditioning of cold packs

In order for cold packs to perform consistently, several points need to be considered. The first is to ensure that the correct type of pack is used as they are designed to maintain different temperatures. This is brought about by the use of different phase change materials, which are materials that change between liquid and solid phases at specific temperatures. One effect of this change in phase is that the pack maintains a stable temperature throughout the change. A pack designed for −15°C may therefore not be suitable for maintaining +5°C.

The packs should be used in accordance with either the manufacturers' instructions or the conditions established through undertaking a qualification exercise. This is because all packs are not the same, for example some packs designed to be conditioned within a refrigerator may not be suitable for conditioning within a freezer, and some types are not suitable for multiple freeze/thaw cycles.

CONTROL AND MONITORING OF STORAGE AREAS

Where medicines that may be required in an emergency are stored then contingency measures should be put in place such as linking essential equipment in a large warehouse to a source of emergency power. These emergency measures should be routinely tested, such as the confirmation of restoration of stored data and settings when emergency power supply is activated and after normal power is resumed. For these products there should be a system in place to ensure that on-call personnel are notified in the event of power failure or temperature alarms being triggered including notification outside of normal working hours.

BEST PRACTICE

Whatever type of refrigerator or cold store is used, once a mapping exercise has taken place, products should be stored in an orderly fashion on shelves – not directly on the floor of the unit – to ensure air circulation, consistent temperatures throughout and to facilitate cleaning.

Calibrated temperature monitoring probes should be sited in a central location within the refrigerator and, preferably, between the products.

Probes should not be placed in the door.

The refrigerator should be cleaned regularly (as part of a general cleaning rota) and serviced at least annually.

If the refrigerator is fitted with an audible or visual alarm, this should be routinely tested to confirm correct operation at specified appropriate temperatures.

The stock within the refrigerator should be subject to effective stock rotation based on first expiry, first out (FEFO).

It should not be assumed that the most recent deliveries will have a longer expiry period.

Refrigerators containing medicinal products must not be used for the storage of food and drink or anything that might contaminate the medicinal products.

Calibration of temperature monitoring devices including ambient

In order to have confidence in temperature readings, monitoring devices should be calibrated to demonstrate they have appropriate accuracy and precision. Temperate storage thermometers should be accurate to ±1°C, and cold chain devices accurate to ±0.5°C. Calibration should extend across the whole of the anticipated working range, so for a temperate storage range of 15°C to 25°C the calibration range may be 10°C to 30°C to allow the thermometer to be used in assessing temperature excursions or to be used in temperature mapping exercises. Results of the calibration exercise should be presented in a report or calibration certificate approved by the calibrator and demonstrated to be appropriate for use by the wholesaler. The certificate should include the following details:

- serial number of the calibrated instrument;
- serial numbers of test instruments;
- traceability to National or International calibration standards;
- calibration test method used;
- ISO or equivalent registration details of calibration laboratory;
- date of calibration;
- calibration results;
- unique certificate number;
- approval of results by calibrator.

Where a temperature monitoring device reads the temperature from a main monitoring unit plus a remote probe it should be clear from the calibration certificate which part of the device the calibration refers to. Calibration should be carried out annually and, where adjustments are made to the equipment as part of calibration, an assessment of accuracy and precision should be made before and after adjustment. On completion a suitable representative from the wholesaler should approve the calibration, indicating its suitability for use.

Short-Term Storage of Ambient and Refrigerated Medicinal Products – Requirements for a Wholesale Dealer's Licence

The GDP Guidelines define wholesale distribution as: "… all activities consisting of procuring, holding, supplying or exporting medicinal products…"

GDP Chapter 9 requires that "provision should be made to minimise the duration of temporary storage while awaiting the next stage of the transportation route."

The Glossary of Terms defines holding as "storing medicinal products". Medicinal products should therefore only be stored on premises that are covered by a wholesale dealer's licence. However, there are certain cases where medicinal products are held for short periods of time during transportation and prior to onward shipment, e.g. in overnight freight depots. In such instances it has been determined that, as a matter of policy, a site is not required to be licensed where:

- ambient products remain for less than 36 hours;
- cold chain products are transported and stored overnight in continuously refrigerated vehicles or in qualified packaging;
- vehicles are in transit and product is not unloaded at the site.

As a matter of policy, a site must be licensed where:

- ambient products are held in excess of 36 hours;
- products requiring refrigeration are placed in a cold store, even when this is for less than 36 hours;
- wholesaling activities other than storage are being carried out. This includes the handling of returned goods and where decisions are made regarding suitability for resale, as well as the usual activities of picking against orders;
- ownership has been transferred.

Where transportation is performed by a third party and they are holding product, then they require a WDA(H) naming the relevant sites. Whether the licensed sites require naming as third parties on the supplying wholesaler's licence will depend on the nature of the commercial and GDP contracts. In general, if the product is "in transit", the transport site is not required to be named as a third party on the supplier's licence.

Chapter 4 Documentation

4.1 Principle

Good documentation constitutes an essential part of the quality system. Written documentation should prevent errors from spoken communication and permits the tracking of relevant operations during the distribution of medicinal products.

4.2 General

Documentation comprises all written procedures, instructions, contracts, records and data, in paper or in electronic form. Documentation should be readily available/retrievable.

With regard to the processing of personal data of employees, complainants or any other natural person, Directive 95/46/EC[6] on the protection of individuals applies to the processing of personal data and to the free movement of such data.

Documentation should be sufficiently comprehensive with respect to the scope of the wholesale distributor's activities and in a language understood by personnel. It should be written in clear, unambiguous language and be free from errors.

Procedure should be approved, signed and dated by the Responsible Person. Documentation should be approved, signed and dated by appropriate authorised persons, as required. It should not be handwritten, although, where it is necessary, sufficient space should be provided for such entries.

Any alteration made in the documentation should be signed and dated; the alteration should permit the reading of the original information. Where appropriate, the reason for the alteration should be recorded.

Documents should be retained for the period stated in national legislation for at least 5 years. Personal data should be deleted or anonymised as soon as their storage is no longer necessary for the purpose of distribution activities.

Each employee should have ready access to all necessary documentation for the tasks executed.

Attention should be paid to using valid and approved procedures. Documents should have unambiguous content; title, nature and purpose should be clearly stated. Documents should be reviewed regularly and kept up to date. Version control should be applied to procedures. After revision of a document a system should exist to prevent inadvertent use of the superseded version. Superseded or obsolete procedures should be removed from workstations and archived.

Records must be kept either in the form of purchase/sales invoices, delivery slips or on a computer or any other form, for any transaction in medicinal products received, supplied or brokered.

Records must include at least the following information: date; name of the medicinal product; quantity received, supplied or brokered; name and

---

[6] OJ L 281, 23.11.1995, p. 31.

address of the supplier, customer, broker or consignee, as appropriate; and batch number at least for medicinal product bearing the safety features[7].

Records should be made at the time each operation is undertaken.

UK Guidance on Chapter 4 Documentation

Document control

Document control encompasses document lifecycle management and is required for control of quality and operational aspects of an organisation. Documentation must be controlled at all times. There are various levels of control that must be applied in line with the principles of quality risk management. For example, copies of procedures may be provided to third parties as uncontrolled copies of the controlled document or just valid on the day of printing. The system of controlling documents and document templates should be described within a procedure.

The document lifecycle

Quality documents need to follow a lifecycle approach in order to ensure adequate control. The basic stages of the lifecycle are as follows:

CREATION

The requirement of the document needs to be clearly identified. Relevant subject matter experts should be involved, which not only ensures it reflects intended use, but also that it is likely to be understood by all users and may assist their buy-in. The use of a standard template helps to ensure all relevant sections are included, and assists the reader in navigation throughout the document.

REVIEW

The created document should be reviewed prior to approval, in order to check technical accuracy, assess its adherence to business objectives and corporate standards for controlled documents, assess any inconsistencies with other documents in the quality system, and to ensure its main objective has been met.

APPROVAL

If the draft document is deemed satisfactory, it should be approved by an appropriate authorised person and entered onto the register of controlled documents.

---

[7] Article 80(e) and Article 82 of Directive 2001/83/EC.

IMPLEMENTATION

The issue date may precede the implementation date to allow time to distribute and train the document, in which it should be clearly stated when the new document takes effect. Documents should be readily accessible to those who are required to use them. All distributed copies should be traceable, including those issued to external parties. It is likely that issuance is aligned with the training programme for major revisions.

USE

The procedure is readily available and in use.

WITHDRAWAL

Notice should be given to all relevant parties when their copy of the document is to be withdrawn. This is likely to align with issuance of a new version. Reconciliation of all circulated copies should take place and followed up where a copy has not been returned.

DESTRUCTION

Documents should be destroyed in line with relevant retention periods. Where more than one retention period exists (e.g. Home Office controlled drug records), the longest required retention period should be adhered to. For GDP records this is generally 5 years; however, exceptions are in place.

Operating procedures

It is vital that procedures are written with the full involvement of the organisation for which they are intended. This not only ensures that procedures are reflective of the organisation, but also enables the organisation to define and develop its own processes. Where procedures intended for other organisations are used, this can often result in inefficiency and non-compliance.

When writing procedures, considerations should be made for all relevant users such as quality personnel, operators and trainers. Documentation should be sufficiently comprehensive with respect to the scope of the wholesale distributor's activities and use a technical level of language understood by personnel. All acronyms and company-specific terms should be clearly defined either within the document or dedicated glossary. Complex processes can be represented by the use of flow charts or visual representations.

Records

The retention and control of records is also an essential aspect of good documentation practice. Records are present in various categories and include:

- financial records, e.g. a purchase order or sales invoice;
- quality records, e.g. deviations and CAPAs;
- employee training and competence records;

- routine monitoring records, i.e. records of equipment maintenance, temperature records and pest control;
- qualification records, i.e. evidence of temperature mapping and transport validation.

Different types of records may need specific considerations to enable full control, e.g.: Sales invoices are often a duplicate form also serving as a delivery note by the supplier. There may be a risk that a copy of this used by the Accounts Department is not maintained as an exact copy with the consequence that they become contradictory, especially where stock adjustments have been made on one copy.

Where controlled forms have different sections that are managed individually, such as a deviation and associated CAPAs, the individually assigned CAPA forms can become separated from the parent deviation. Records can also become inconsistent with closure of the deviation being inconsistent with closure of the associated CAPA.

Training records should be available for all members of staff involved and do not often reflect competence of staff. Records should demonstrate briefing of staff that do not have direct GDP responsibilities but could impact GDP operations by their activities, e.g. where they work in a shared warehouse.

Routine monitoring records: The most commonly reviewed monitoring records are temperature monitoring records. Very often these are only reviewed to confirm temperatures are in range, and not reviewed for trending, which may indicate a system is about to fail. Externally signed maintenance records (e.g. heating, ventilation and air conditioning (HVAC) servicing or pest control) are not always confirmed by the wholesaler, and not always legible or completed to an appropriate standard of recording.

Qualification records are often not correlated with an appropriately defined objective or protocol, which in turn prevents the ability to ascertain if the exercise was successful or not. Reports of externally generated exercises need to be understood by the wholesaler, and approved if appropriate. This is a common problem observed with external calibration of devices.

In order to ensure that records are fully traceable, appropriate logs or registers should be in place. Examples of registers may include a log of procedures, training logs, registers of CAPAs and change control logs. These should be easy to update and maintain in an accurate state.

Restrictions on availability of records

Measures must be in place in order to enable the appropriate control of access to sensitive information, including records and other documents.

For permanent staff, this may include limitation to access documents pertinent to their role. Personnel information should be protected in line with GDPR or other similar requirements. Access to commercially sensitive information may need to be restricted from temporary staff and contractors. Patient-specific information associated with orders needs to be restricted from non-relevant staff. The Responsible Person needs to maintain oversight of such information in order to ensure that these supplies are maintained and measures are in place to prevent supply of medicines against falsified redacted prescriptions.

It is vital that the Responsible Person has adequate oversight of the document control process and access to relevant records in order to fulfil their responsibilities.

Data Integrity

In order to trust GDP records, the data need to be created in line with data integrity (DI) expectations. Data integrity is the extent to which all data are complete, consistent and accurate throughout the data lifecycle. It is essential that this principle of DI is followed in order to ensure traceability of GDP activities and associated records and other documentation. Failure to meet this requirement has been present in all areas of GxP, and, as a result, the MHRA has provided guidance published on the MHRA website. The reader is encouraged to refer to these documents for a complete list of definitions and broader guidance.

Basic concepts

Failure in DI is often caused by weakness in implementation of measures that ensure that DI standards are implemented and maintained, referred to as data governance. The MHRA expects that appropriate measures are taken in respect to DI and data governance, and it should be clear which data are critical to regulatory compliance and product safety, in order to ensure appropriate resource is applied to the more critical data. For data that are not as important, less effort will be expected along with a rationale as to what data are deemed by the company as being not critical.

Criticality of data

Quality risk management lends itself as a useful tool to determine which data and records are critical to operations and therefore require more robust data governance measures. If GDP activity cannot be reconstructed should specific data be lost, then it can be assumed that the data in question is critical. For equipment that generates data the extent of qualification in respect to DI should correlate with data criticality. Quality risk management can also be applied to identify which data and records are not critical such as secondary records and put in place measures to ensure that critical data do not inadvertently end up on the secondary record. An example of a secondary record is of a customer invoice that gets copied on receipt of stock and retained in the warehouse as evidence of delivery while the original is sent to the accountant. If the warehouse copy is subsequently annotated, e.g. to amend stock quantity booked in, then it is no longer a true copy of the original and therefore both need to be considered as master documents.

If data are transcribed from an instrument or hard copy record onto a computerised system and the original record is considered by the company to be non-critical, then consideration must be made as to how the company considers the original record as not being critical. Appropriate measures of review and approval of the transcribed records must be put in place. Any inconsistency in the computerised record would indicate failure not only in the integrity of the data, but also failure of the governance process concerned with the review and approval of transcription, and any other records approved in the same way including records not related to this event would be circumspect.

ALCOA applied to GDP

A ATTRIBUTABLE TO THE PERSON GENERATING THE DATA

Any critical data or information recorded for GDP purposes must be attributed to the originator. For hard copy records, entries should be traceable to the person making the record, with initialling and dating being developed as an unconscious habit. Where computerised systems are in use, individuals are expected to only access systems by a unique password that can be traced to a level of permission. To guarantee this there should be adequate provision of terminals and a culture of logging out when not using shared devices to prevent work-around arrangements from being developed. A person with administrator access must not use this mode for anything other than maintenance operations and should have a separate user account for daily operations.

Where signatures or names relate to personnel outside of the organisation, e.g. engineer, then the name should be printed in addition to signing and they should also print their job role. For regular contacts, e.g. customers, a signature log may be developed and managed as a controlled document. Where shipments are international and parts of the delivery are outsourced, additional control measures should be put in place to maintain the chain of custody for the delivery from the warehouse to the customer.

L   LEGIBLE AND PERMANENT

Hard copy records are often not legible due to poor training of staff, poor form design and poor process design, and lead to errors in reading and transcription. Simple solutions include the provision of clipboards to prevent warehouse and delivery forms being completed on top of non-flat surfaces leading to poor writing, development of forms that accommodate those with large writing, and training staff in how to record errors and how to use traceable footnotes rather than squeeze notes into a small comments box. Replacement of hard copies with electronic records may improve legibility but may pose other problems such as poor accessibility to records.

The trend towards replacing manual systems with computerised ones has not always been met with appropriate assessment of risk, e.g. there may be emphasis placed on data back-up of records but little attention paid to ability to restore records. Where computer systems are updated and previous software or hardware is no longer supported then a quality risk assessment should be carried out and appropriate action undertaken to ensure records can be retrieved.

The versatility and ease of use of electronic spreadsheets has led to them being very common. They lose the ability to retain original data that is overwritten and entries are normally not attributable to the recorder unless strict document control measures are put in place, including access control and versioning. Other approaches to control spreadsheets include printing in hard copy or PDF form, and retaining a log of each approved version.

C   CONTEMPORANEOUS

Records should be traceable to the time the activity is carried out in order to reduce the chance of the record being forgotten or traceability of actions lost. Some events are more time-critical than others, such as execution of a medicine recall or qualification of a transport lane. In these circumstances recording of events must be consistent, especially where activity spans different time zones or different date formats are in use by different organisations that are involved.

O   ORIGINAL RECORD (OR TRUE COPY)

The original record refers to data as originally generated, preserving the integrity (accuracy, completeness, content and meaning) of the record, e.g. original paper record of manual observation, or electronic raw data file from a computerised system.

A true copy refers to a copy of original information that been verified as an exact (accurate and complete) copy having all of the same attributes and information as the original. The copy may be verified by dated signature or by a validated electronic signature.

Where hard copy documents are scanned into electronic format for archiving there needs to be a process of verification that all records are complete and are an accurate representation of the original. Problems can exist where some documents in a bundle are of poor print quality, double-sided or where a highlighter has been used. In these cases the electronic records may not be complete or a true copy of the original.

On occasions where documents are provided from third parties, such as copies of or translations of customer wholesale dealer's licences, the document must be authenticated as a true copy by reference to an appropriate source such as a regulatory authority. Reliance solely on the word of the third party is not acceptable.

Where copies of originals are made they should be clearly able to be differentiated from the original and prevent mix-up. Possible control measures include use of watermarks, embossing or having original documents on coloured paper with restricted access to the paper.

A ACCURATE

Accuracy of data is essential to GDP, and having good processes to manage errors supports this. Deviation management should ensure corrections are traceable and approved, and original incorrect data not lost. Processes and systems should be developed that drive accuracy rather than challenge it and where data are manipulated then there should be defined rules controlling this, e.g. number rounding and conversion of units of measure. A common failure in this respect is in the management of stock adjustments where physical stock count and stock records do not match. Stock records need to be managed in an open and honest manner and adjustments not hidden but corrected with appropriate justification and authorisation.

When formulae are used in electronic spreadsheets they are rarely qualified, in which case errors can be introduced without being noticed. The use of check boxes and formulae that detect nonsense values can help reduce errors.

Data governance

Having good quality data and records is not only essential to GDP, but also a contributory factor in managing an effective and efficient operation. A fundamental requirement is development of a quality culture where all staff are able to identify weaknesses without feeling intimidated and understand the importance of maintaining accurate records and adherence to procedures.

Good training and level of knowledge are also required, especially for staff in quality-assurance roles as they are often responsible for provision of training, design of processes and procedures, evaluation of deviations and creation of quality culture. If they are weak in any of these then the staff required to make accurate records are at a disadvantage. Training can also be provided specifically in relation to DI so, e.g., staff understand the difference between a witness signature and a check signature and the risks to DI associated with a particular process, as well as reviewing records to ensure that data makes sense in addition to confirming all entries are complete.

One of the most common failures in GDP is inadequate control of quality system documents. Where events such as complaints or deviations are recorded in free-vend template forms these are often not reconciled or reconcilable. This may lead to records being lost or incorrect template versions being used. Good system design with consideration of DI provides the means to ensure all records are complete with use of simple solutions, such as use of hard-bound forms or controlled issue of numbered and indexed forms.

Data integrity can be monitored by incorporation into self-inspections or as a single separate horizontal audit to enable best practice to be shared across departments. Monitoring of near misses in addition to full breaches and consideration of opportunities for continuous improvement all add to the data governance tools that can be reviewed during quality management reviews that, in turn, lead to further development of a healthy quality culture.

When reviewing data it is important to consider whether the data can be fully relied upon. For example, in an ambient storage warehouse the thermometer indicates a minimum temperature of 5°C and a maximum of 36°C. Potential root causes may include failed calibration history or damage of the thermometer, or low competence of staff using the device. These reasons could indicate unreliability of the records.

Such outlying data as described in the example are easy to spot, but when faced with data that look within trend, it is less likely to be challenged; however, the integrity of data can be just as unreliable even though it all appears within the expected range.

GDP COMPUTERISED SYSTEMS

The advance of computerised system and application development has enabled operators to carry out activities at an increasingly fast pace, including flash transactions, sometimes without having sight of stock. The intention to use non-trackable software such as WhatsApp for quality-critical event reporting has been proposed by wholesalers – and refused on the grounds of not being capable to comply with DI requirements; however, the use of computerised systems is encouraged providing they are appropriately qualified and controlled, especially if they are bespoke to your organisation. The MHRA GxP Data Integrity guidance provides a lot of information on this topic.

The use of robots and electronic audit trails can lead to a false sense of security in relation to data integrity. The simple act of ensuring that stock is delivered to the right address can fail when an electronic proof-of-delivery signal cannot be picked up either in remote Africa or in mid-Wales, and work-arounds are created. Additional problems of maintaining a full audit trail arises when stock changes from one organisation or department to another, for example delivery of a consignment through a network of third-party couriers leading to an incomplete document audit trail. Also, some couriers only retain their track-and-trace records for a few weeks before destroying them.

Where records are converted from one form to another, e.g. hard-copy supplier invoices converted to PDF, or hard-copy temperature records transcribed into an electronic record, then these should be confirmed as being accurate and complete by a person of appropriate seniority. This process should also be assessed for potential failure modes, e.g. when converting hard-copy supplier invoices to PDF there may be more than one version of the document (same original but with different annotations on it). Both versions may therefore need to be retained. In addition, some double-sided documents may incorrectly be only scanned single-sided. Copying such documents can be tedious and is often delegated to an office junior, but the implications of not having a complete, accurate and legible set of scanned records will mean you will not be able to trace activities and will not comply with regulations.

THE USE OF SPREADSHEETS

Spreadsheets are a useful tool for managing and presenting data due to their versatility and ease of use, which has led to their wide application within GDP. It is important to note, however, that when data within a spreadsheet cannot be reconstructed elsewhere and are essential to GDP activity then data governance measures must be rigorous. Caution should be taken when number-rounding, converting from one unit of measurement to another or from numbers to graphs.

If the spreadsheet has multiple users it may be impossible to ascertain who (Attributable) made an entry, whether entries have been over-written and replaced (permanent), and when the data entries had been made (Contemporaneous). If the spreadsheet is not version-controlled and managed as a controlled document, then there may be different versions in use (Original). Where formulae and other functions are used there is potential for these to be corrupted without being detected (Accurate).

Possible ways of gaining appropriate control include restricting the use of spreadsheets only for non-critical data and locking down cells or sheets within it so write access is restricted. Another potential solution is to use the spreadsheet to create a hard-copy version that is version-controlled, approved and dated, locked down and managed as the controlled version. In this case it is the approved version that needs to be used as the working document, not the unapproved spreadsheet used to create it. This approach can be useful when data are not entered frequently such as a staff training matrix that may only be revised a few times each year or confirmation of supplier or customer authentication carried out every fortnight.

Where Macros or formulae are used within a spreadsheet, these should be defined (e.g. within an operating procedure), tested for accuracy and protected against unauthorised changes. Confirming these are not corrupted should be part of regular data-integrity review.

Some considerations for preparing documentation for a regulatory inspection

Wholesalers have an obligation to ensure that documents are readily available for presentation to a regulatory inspector. Where companies operate over several sites, it may be problematic to have all records available. In these circumstances, the organisation should notify the inspector as soon as possible regarding the notice period for obtaining documents, especially if they are archived off-site.

Where documents are managed electronically, the organisation may need to provide access to the inspector to navigate the documentation system. It may facilitate the inspection to have print facilities for review of electronic documents as hard copies. Some records may be printed prior to the inspection, in which case the inspector should be consulted if they require this. Any printed documents should be clearly legible.

SPECIFIC DOCUMENTATION CONSIDERATIONS: CASE STUDIES

Case study 1: Export to a third country

When exporting to a third country, several considerations need to be made from a documentation and record keeping perspective. These include:

- Procedures and written agreements containing sufficient detail of the export process.
- Evidence of authentication of the customer and their entitlement to receive medicinal products. This may include copies of the customer's licence, assessment of their financial status, and confirmation against the UK embargo lists of persons and companies.
- Approval of the consignment; this includes confirmation against UK medicine export restrictions, confirmation of import restrictions into the third country and import licences from the national competent authority.
- A complete documentation chain of custody for the medicinal products from the point of the suppliers authorised storage location to the authorised premises of the customer. This may include purchase order, instructions to the freight forwarder, Customs declarations, sales orders, sales invoices, bill of lading or airway bill, and temperature monitoring records.
- Clear financial records that are consistent with the physical chain of custody.
- Authenticated translations of documentation.

- A clear protocol detailing the methodology and logic behind the mapping exercise.
- The quality of the records enables conclusions to be drawn.
- Written agreements in place for external mapping contractors.
- All externally generated data are provided to the wholesaler.
- Documentation is managed within the document control system.
- Records should be traceable so that it is clear who created individual records and participated in the exercise.
- Names of any external persons involved should be printed in addition to any signatures.

Chapter 5 Operations

5.1   Principle

All actions taken by wholesale distributors should ensure that the identity of the medicinal product is not lost and that the wholesale distribution of medicinal products is performed according to the information on the outer packaging. The wholesale distributor should use all means available to minimise the risk of falsified medicinal products entering the legal supply chain.

All medicinal products distributed in the EU by a wholesale distributor must be covered by a marketing authorisation granted by the EU or by a Member State[8].

Any distributor, other than the marketing authorisation holder, who imports a medicinal product from another Member State must notify the marketing authorisation holder and the competent authority in the Member State to which the medicinal product will be imported of their intention to import that product[9]. All key operations described below should be fully described in the quality system in appropriate documentation.

5.2   Qualification of suppliers

Wholesale distributors must obtain their supplies of medicinal products only from persons who are themselves in possession of a wholesale distribution authorisation, or who are in possession of a manufacturing authorisation which covers the product in question[10].

---

[8] Articles 76(1) and (2) of Directive 2001/83/EC.
[9] Article 76(3) of Directive 2001/83/EC.
[10] Article 80(b) of Directive 2001/83/EC.

Wholesale distributors receiving medicinal products from third countries for the purpose of importation, i.e. for the purpose of placing these products on the EU market, must hold a manufacturing authorisation[11].

Where medicinal products are obtained from another wholesale distributor the receiving wholesale distributor must verify that the supplier complies with the principles and guidelines of good distribution practices and that they hold an authorisation, for example by using the Union database. If the medicinal product is obtained through brokering, the wholesale distributor must verify that the broker is registered and complies with the requirements in Chapter 10[12].

Appropriate qualification and approval of suppliers should be performed prior to any procurement of medicinal products. This should be controlled by a procedure and the results documented and periodically rechecked.

When entering into a new contract with new suppliers the wholesale distributor should carry out "due diligence" checks in order to assess the suitability, competence and reliability of the other party. Attention should be paid to:

(i)   the reputation or reliability of the supplier;
(ii)   offers of medicinal products more likely to be falsified;
(iii)   large offers of medicinal products which are generally only available in limited quantities; and
(iv)   out-of-range prices.

5.3 Qualification of customers

Wholesale distributors must ensure they supply medicinal products only to persons who are themselves in possession of a wholesale distribution authorisation or who are authorised or entitled to supply medicinal products to the public.

Checks and periodic rechecks may include requesting copies of customer's authorisations according to national law, verifying status on an authority website, requesting evidence of qualifications or entitlement according to national legislation.

Wholesale distributors should monitor their transactions and investigate any irregularity in the sales patterns of narcotics, psychotropic substances or other dangerous substances. Unusual sales patterns that may constitute diversion or misuse of medicinal product should be investigated and reported to competent authorities where necessary. Steps should be taken to ensure fulfilment of any public service obligation imposed upon them.

---

[11] Article 40, third paragraph of Directive 2001/83/EC.
[12] Article 80, fourth paragraph of Directive 2001/83/EC.

5.4   Receipt of medicinal products

The purpose of the receiving function is to ensure that the arriving consignment is correct, that the medicinal products originate from approved suppliers and that they have not been visibly damaged during transport.

Medicinal products requiring special storage or security measures should be prioritised and once appropriate checks have been conducted they should be immediately transferred to appropriate storage facilities.

Batches of medicinal products intended for the EU and EEA countries should not be transferred to saleable stock before assurance has been obtained in accordance with written procedures that they are authorised for sale. For batches coming from another Member State, prior to their transfer to saleable stock, the control report referred to in Article 51(1) of Directive 2001/83/EC or another proof of release to the market in question based on an equivalent system should be carefully checked by appropriately trained personnel.

5.5   Storage

Medicinal products and, if necessary, healthcare products should be stored separately from other products likely to alter them and should be protected from the harmful effects of light, temperature, moisture and other external factors. Particular attention should be paid to products requiring specific storage conditions.

Incoming containers of medicinal products should be cleaned, if necessary, before storage.

Warehousing operations must ensure appropriate storage conditions are maintained and allow for appropriate security of stocks.

Stock should be rotated according to the "first expiry, first out" (FEFO) principle. Exceptions should be documented.

Medicinal products should be handled and stored in such a manner as to prevent spillage, breakage, contamination and mix-ups. Medicinal products should not be stored directly on the floor unless the package is designed to allow such storage (such as for some medicinal gas cylinders).

Medicinal products that are nearing their expiry date/shelf life should be withdrawn immediately from saleable stock either physically or through other equivalent electronic segregation.

Stock inventories should be performed regularly taking into account national legislation requirements. Stock irregularities should be investigated and documented.

5.6   Destruction of obsolete goods

Medicinal products intended for destruction should be appropriately identified, held separately and handled in accordance with a written procedure.

Destruction of medicinal products should be in accordance with national or international requirements for handling, transport and disposal of such products.

Records of all destroyed medicinal products should be retained for a defined period.

5.7 Picking

Controls should be in place to ensure the correct product is picked. The product should have an appropriate remaining shelf life when it is picked.

5.8 Supply

For all supplies, a document (e.g. delivery note) must be enclosed stating the date; name and pharmaceutical form of the medicinal product (batch number at least for products bearing the safety features); quantity supplied; name and address of the supplier; name and delivery address of the consignee[13] (actual physical storage premises, if different); and applicable transport and storage conditions. Records should be kept so that the actual location of the product can be known.

5.9 Export to third countries

The export of medicinal products falls within the definition of "wholesale distribution"[14]. A person exporting medicinal products must hold a wholesale distribution authorisation or a manufacturing authorisation. This is also the case if the exporting wholesale distributor is operating from a free zone.

The rules for wholesale distribution apply in their entirety in the case of export of medicinal products. However, where medicinal products are exported, they do not need to be covered by a marketing authorisation of the Union or a Member State[15]. Wholesalers should take the appropriate measures in order to prevent these medicinal products reaching the Union market. Where wholesale distributors supply medicinal products to persons in third countries, they shall ensure that such supplies are only made to persons who are authorised or entitled to receive medicinal products for wholesale distribution or supply to the public in accordance with the applicable legal and administrative provisions of the country concerned.

---

[13] Article 82 of Directive 2001/83/EC.
[14] Article 1(17) of Directive 2001/83/EC.
[15] Article 85(a) of Directive 2001/83/EC.

UK Guidance on Chapter 5 Operations

Qualification of customers and suppliers

The qualification and re-qualification of suppliers and customers are fundamental pillars of good distribution practice, and one of the highest risk areas of Good Distribution Practice (GDP). The MHRA requires organisations to have qualification and re-qualification procedures implemented within their quality management system.

Before commencing wholesale dealing activities with a supplier or customer (trading partners), licensed wholesale dealers must ensure that their proposed trading partners are entitled to trade with them. Checks must demonstrate that trading partners either hold the required manufacturing and wholesale dealer's licence where necessary or that they are entitled to receive medicines for the purpose of retail supply, to a person who may lawfully administer the products or for use in the course of their business.

Qualification of suppliers

Maintaining the integrity of the supply chain is one of the most important aspects of wholesale distribution. A robust fully documented system to ensure medicines are sourced appropriately must be in place and subjected to regular review. Licensed wholesale dealers must ensure their suppliers are appropriately licensed to supply medicines. The qualification of suppliers requires the following steps to be fully compliant:

- The first step is to verify that supplies of medicinal products only come from persons who are themselves in possession of a wholesale distribution authorisation, or who are in possession of a manufacturing authorisation that covers the product in question.

  Traditionally, copies of licences have been requested from suppliers, but this is no longer required as details of a licence of the supplier can be viewed via the MHRA's register of wholesalers. While the MHRA register is updated regularly it must not be relied on as a sole means of qualifying suppliers' authority to supply. The information should also be verified by using the MHRAGMDP[16] website, as this is updated daily. Currently, the MHRAGMDP website does not contain details of the legal categories of products that can be handled or third-party sites used and must not be relied on as a sole means of qualifying suppliers. When searching for companies use an asterisk (*) on either side of a name or number to broaden the search.

---

[16] https://cms.mhra.gov.uk/

One practical way to demonstrate qualification of suppliers could be a printed copy of the appropriate pages, signed and dated as evidence the checks were made, when and by whom. Evidence held by a company of validation checks should be appropriately traceable to users and include dates of qualification and retained in line with GDP document retention requirements.

Supplies from any other source, such as pharmacies, is not permitted. There remains a persistent misunderstanding that pharmacies can supply a small amount of medicines without a wholesale dealers licence. This is not the case as the exemption that allows this trade was removed in 2013. Where a pharmacy holds a WDA(H), a company should ensure that they are procuring from the correct legal entity.

- The second step requires that wholesalers verify that any wholesale supplier complies with the principles and guidelines of good distribution practices. To establish GDP compliance, the GDP certificate of the wholesaler should be viewed on the MHRAGMDP website. Certificates when issued are valid for up to 5 years. The date of the certificate expiry should be recorded.

The MHRA adds conditioning statements to GDP certificates for new applicants and those companies where the inspection outcome indicated a more frequent inspection schedule is required, limiting certificate expiry to 2 years.

Where certificates have reached expiration dates, further enquiries should be made with those companies to ascertain their compliance status.

- The third step is periodic rechecking of the information obtained and due diligence.

Wholesalers must be aware of issues that could affect their suppliers' continued authority to supply. Qualification processes must ensure that documented checks are made at least twice a month of MHRA's list of suspended licence holders and regular checks on MHRAGMDP or EudraGMDP website for issued GMP and GDP statements of noncompliance. There should be at a minimum an annual full revalidation of the information held on suppliers; however, companies should ensure that re-qualification of suppliers is conducted on a risk basis.

Supporting all of the checks made so far is effective due diligence by the Responsible Person. The MHRA has seen evidence of serious non-compliance pertaining to qualification; quantities of a high-value medicine were stolen and re-introduced to the supply chain. The medicine was sold in an unusually large quantity and purchased by several wholesalers.

After the event, looking at the evidence available to the purchasers, it was apparent that the company selling the stock had a conditioned GDP certificate, a poor financial history and no previous access to such large volumes of high-value stock.

When entering into a new contract with new suppliers, the wholesale distributor should carry out "due diligence" checks in order to assess the suitability, competence and reliability of the other party. Questions that should be considered could include:

- checking the financial status of the supplier, how long have they been trading, and do they have an acceptable credit history?
- has an audit been performed of the supplier, or has anyone in your company visited them? If so what was their impression?
- where is the stock coming from and is the product offered a new product for your company?
- is the product being offered available in quantities or volumes that are unusually high or is the price being offered lower than the usual price?
- how transparent is the supply chain of this transaction?
- what will be the method of transportation?
- is the contact managing the business relationship linked to the company they purport to represent? For example, do web domains, IP addresses and phone numbers support claims being made by persons or organisations?
- has there been a recent, rapid change of senior management, or offering of medicines outside of the usual business practices associated with the supplier?

Due diligence checks should be implemented and documented when dealing with a company or transaction that is outside of an established trading pattern.

Organisations must be aware that criminals actively look for weak spots in the supply chain for gain. The MHRA frequently receives reports that companies with wholesale dealer licences are being "cloned". Here, a company uses the licence and address details of a legitimate company but sets up a fake website and bank account that is similar to the real operation. Typically, this fake company will offer some tempting stock and send information using genuine company details but from a different e-mail account. Observed methodologies have included, e.g., substituting .com for .co.uk, utilising hyphenation, utilising unrelated e-mail domains and closely mimicking a related website name. The bank account information will be for the fake company. Please take extreme care if your supplier advises the bank details have changed and your accounts team should be made aware of this practice. Other methods include the purchase of a company and change of ownership, not detectable by routine licence review, and the subsequent supply of high-value medicines.

Any detection of suspicious activity, near misses or active engagement with suspected dishonest actors in the supply chain should be reported to the Licensing Authority.

For companies that are involved in the sourcing of medicines from a third country for export to third countries then there are different requirements. Companies are obliged to document that checks are made to show that where the medicinal product is directly received from a third country ("A") for export to a third country ("B"), the supplier of the medicinal product in country A is a person who is authorised or entitled to supply such medicinal products in accordance with the legal and administrative provisions in country A. Any licences obtained should have been translated into English and authenticated by a notary with appropriate due diligence carried out.

If there is no GDP certificate available then other evidence of GDP compliance by the wholesale supplier should be obtained, such as a copy of their last inspection close out letter confirming GDP compliance. For suppliers from EEA Member States the same checks should be made on EudraG-MDP and via licences that have been translated. The translated licences should be authenticated as such by a notary.

COMPLIANCE WITH GDP

Licensed wholesale dealers must verify that wholesale suppliers comply with the principles and guidelines of good distribution practices. To establish GDP compliance, the GDP certificate of the wholesaler should be viewed on the relevant website. Certificates when issued are valid for up to 5 years. The date of the certificate expiry should be recorded. The MHRA adds conditioning statements to GDP certificates for new applicants and those companies where the inspection outcome indicated a more frequent inspection schedule is required, limiting certificate expiry to 2 years. If there is no GDP certificate available then other evidence of GDP compliance by the wholesale supplier should be obtained, such as a copy of the inspection close-out letter confirming GDP compliance.

ROUTINE RE-QUALIFICATION

Licensed wholesale dealers must be aware of issues that could affect their suppliers' continued authority to supply. The following should be carried out:

- regular checks at least twice a month of MHRA's list of suspended licence holders;
- regular checks on MHRAGMDP and EudraGMDP websites for issued GMP and GDP statements of non-compliance;
- a risk based re-qualification process, conducted at least annually, including a documented full re-qualification of suppliers.

DUE DILIGENCE

When entering into a new contract with new suppliers, the licensed wholesale dealer should carry out "due diligence" checks in order to assess the suitability, competence and reliability of the other party. Questions that should be considered could include, but are not limited to, the following:

- Checking the financial status of the supplier, how long have they been trading, and do they have an acceptable credit history?
- Has an audit been performed of the supplier, or has anyone in your company visited them? If so what was their impression?
- Where is the stock coming from and is the product offered a new product for your company?
- Is the product being offered available in quantities or volumes that are unusually high or is the price being offered lower than the usual price?
- How transparent is the supply chain of this transaction?
- What will be the method of transportation?
- Is the contact managing the business relationship linked to the company they purport to represent? For example, do web domains, IP addresses and telephone numbers support claims being made by persons or organisations?
- Is the company directorship consistent with supplied documentation?

Due diligence checks should be implemented and documented when dealing with a company or transaction that is outside of an established trading pattern.

PROCUREMENT FROM THIRD COUNTRIES

For companies that are involved in the sourcing of medicines from a third country for supply to third countries, there are different requirements. Companies are obliged to document that checks are made to show that where the medicinal product is directly received from a third country ("A") for export to a third country ("B"), the supplier of the medicinal product in country A is a person who is authorised or entitled to supply such medicinal products in accordance with the legal and administrative provisions in country A. Any licences obtained should have been translated into English and authenticated by a notary with appropriate due diligence carried out.

Customer qualification

Licensed wholesale dealers have a key role in guaranteeing medicines are only supplied to authorised organisations, persons entitle to hold medicines and qualified prescribers. For distribution to a wholesale customer, the checks that must be made are similar to the qualification of suppliers, and application of the principles of due diligence and risk based periodic re-qualification applies.

This should include:

- The first step is to verify that wholesale recipients of medicinal products are themselves in possession of a wholesale distribution authorisation.

Traditionally, copies of licences have been requested from customers, but this is no longer required as details of a licence of a UK customer can be viewed via the MHRA's register of wholesalers. While the MHRA register is updated regularly it must not be relied on as a sole means of qualifying customers' authority to receive medicines. The information should also be verified by using the MHRAGMDP website as this is updated daily. Currently, the MHRAGMDP website does not contain details of third-party sites used and must not be relied on as a sole means of qualifying customers. When searching for companies use an asterisk (*) on either side of a name or number to broaden the search.

One practical way to demonstrate qualification of customers could be a printed copy of the appropriate pages, signed and dated as evidence the checks were made, when and by whom. Evidence held by a company of validation checks should be appropriately traceable to users and include dates of qualification and retained in line with GDP document retention requirements.

- The second step requires that wholesalers should verify that any wholesale customer complies with the principles and guidelines of good distribution practices and are entitled to hold the category of medicine they intend to procure. To establish GDP compliance, the GDP certificate of the wholesaler should be viewed on the MHRAGMDP website. Certificates when issued are valid for up to 5 years. The date of the certificate expiry should be recorded.

The MHRA adds conditioning statements to GDP certificates for new applicants and those companies where the inspection outcome indicated a more frequent inspection schedule is required, limiting certificate expiry to 2 years.

Where certificates have reached expiration dates, further enquiries should be made with those companies to ascertain their compliance status.

- The third step is periodic rechecking of the information obtained and due diligence.

Wholesalers must be aware of issues that could affect their customers' continued authority to supply. Qualification processes must ensure that documented checks are made at least twice a month of the MHRA's list of suspended licence holders and regular checks on the MHRAGMDP or EudraGMDP websites for issued GMP and GDP statements of non-compliance. There should be, at a minimum, an annual full revalidation of the information held on customers; however, companies should ensure that re-qualification of customers is conducted on a risk basis.

Supporting all of the checks made so far is effective due diligence by the Responsible Person. The MHRA has seen evidence of serious non-compliance pertaining to qualification; quantities of a high-value medicine liable for misuse were stolen and re-introduced to the supply chain.

The medicine was sold in an unusually large quantity and purchased by several wholesalers.

After the event, looking at the evidence available to the purchasers, it was apparent that the company selling the stock had a conditioned GDP certificate, a poor financial history and no previous access to such large volumes of high-value stock.

When entering into a new contract with new customers, the wholesale distributor should carry out 'due diligence' checks in order to assess the suitability, competence and reliability of the other party. Questions that should be considered could include:

- Checking the financial status of the customer, how long have they been trading, and do they have an acceptable credit history?
- Has an audit been performed of the customer, or has anyone in your company visited them? If so what was their impression?
- What will be the method of transportation?
- Is the contact managing the business relationship linked to the company they purport to represent? For example, do web domains, IP addresses and telephone numbers support claims being made by persons or organisations?
- Do supplies delivery addresses match details provided on documentation which has been validated?

Due diligence checks should be implemented and documented when dealing with a company or a transaction had been identified that is outside of an established trading pattern.

In relation to wholesale distribution of scheduled controlled medicines to other wholesalers, companies must check their customers hold both a wholesale dealer's licence and a Home Office controlled drugs licence of the appropriate schedule.

For the qualification of a person who may lawfully administer the products then the following registers must be checked prior to supplying:

- Pharmacists and registered pharmacies – General Pharmaceutical Council or Pharmaceutical Society of Northern Ireland website register.
- Doctors – General Medical Council list of registered medical practitioners.
- Dentists – General Dental Council list of registered dental practitioners.
- Paramedics/podiatrists/chiropodists – Health and Care Professions Council (HCPC) website register with listings for prescription-only medication (POM) and local anaesthetic use, if these are the product categories sold.
- Practice nurses – Nursing and Midwifery Council register.
- Hospitals – the Care Quality Commission (CQC) in England or equivalents in Wales, Scotland and Northern Ireland.

See Appendix 3 for further information.

SUPPLY TO THIRD COUNTRIES

Licensed wholesale dealers exporting medicinal products to persons in third countries must ensure that such supplies are only made to persons who are authorised or entitled to receive medicinal products for wholesale distribution or supply to the public in accordance with the applicable legal and administrative provisions of the country concerned. As an example, some companies attempt to export products such as Botox to doctors and clinics in the USA. The US FDA only permits healthcare providers to obtain and use FDA-approved medications purchased directly from the manufacturer or from wholesale distributors licensed in the US. In certain circumstances, the FDA may authorise limited importation of medications that are in short supply. Such medications are imported from approved international sources and distributed in the USA through a controlled network, and would not be sold in direct-to-clinic solicitations. UK-licensed versions of FDA-approved drugs are not treated by FDA as equivalent and must not be sold in the USA to doctors or clinics.

A company must satisfy itself that local legal requirements have been met prior to import. A company should consider and be able to demonstrate knowledge of:

- local legal framework in destination countries;
- any requirements for importation documentation;
- customs, freight or transportation requirements specific to the destination country;
- any paperwork associated with the supply of medicines, including transportation.

Companies should be able to demonstrate delivery to the end location point they had qualified.

The company should retain copies of the above documentation. Any suspicion of diversion or obtaining medicines by false representation should be reported to the Licensing Authority.

DUE DILIGENCE

Licensed wholesale dealers have an obligation in GDP to monitor their transactions and investigate any irregularity in the sales patterns of narcotics, psychotropic or other dangerous substances. This may include medicines which may not appear to be vulnerable as a finished product, such as antihistamine medicines, including but not limited to cetirizine and pseudoephridrine-containing products. Unusual sales patterns that may constitute diversion or misuse of medicinal product should be investigated and reported to Licensing Authorities where necessary.

When conducting due diligence checks, a company should never rely on information solely provided by the trader. The following should be considered:

- conducting independent research into the company, by way of review of wider official sources of information, such as Companies House records;
- ensuring details provided by an organisation match their online presence;
- calling numbers or testing contact details obtained independently;
- validating bank details in line with your expectations from experience;
- ensuring internal training programmes encompass departments that may be approached outside of your direct knowledge, such as finance, and equip staff with mechanisms to report changes to supplier or customer details you may not be aware of;
- what processes and assessments you have in place to confidently establish the identity of a prospective supplier or customer;
- the types, volumes and prices of products being offered and usual availability as a potential risk;
- ensuring commercial activities, such as procurement, sales and marketing teams, have appropriate training and regulatory oversight;
- if your risk-management processes minimise the prospect of falsified medicines entering the supply chain;
- when re-qualifying suppliers, consider if any significant changes in directorship or ownership have occurred;
- how staff and management can be confident that replies are only sent to approved and valid e-mail addresses;
- how reporting mechanisms from goods in processes generate deviations and integrate into the quality management system;
- how new contact details are reviewed by your company;
- how the company manages trade shows or commercial events and any outputs from these.

The MHRA recognises that determined efforts by unauthorised persons or criminals can be convincing. Nonetheless, there is an expectation that licence holders have appropriate systems to safeguard the supply chain. This may include ensuring detailed records of collection and delivery activities are made, to assure organisations that actors involved in your supply chain at every step are legitimate, and that activities have been appropriately reviewed, risk assessed and have oversight.

Instances of falsified GDP certificates and wholesale dealer authorisations have been observed throughout the supply chain and organisations must remain vigilant as to risks to patients when dealing with suppliers, customers and brokers.

The MHRA has become aware that certain medicines subject to abuse, including but not limited to diazepam, nitrazepam, zopiclone, codeine linctus, tramadol zolipdem and pseudoephidrine have been diverted from the regulated supply chain and made available for sale illegitimately. These products are Schedule 4 controlled drugs under the Misuse of Drugs Act. Significant amounts of genuine licensed packs of these products from various manufacturers have been seized and recovered throughout the UK and internationally. Instances of high-value hospital lines being supplied in large quantities represent further risk of diversion and falsification of which organisations should remain vigilant.

Wholesalers are reminded that they have an obligation in GDP to monitor their transactions and investigate any irregularity in the sales patterns of narcotics, psychotropic or other dangerous substances. Unusual sales patterns that may constitute diversion or misuse of medicinal product should be investigated and reported to competent authorities where necessary. Organisations should establish processes to review transactions and trends on a regular basis to identify what within their particular business model is considered unusual or suspicious.

In relation to wholesale distribution of scheduled controlled medicines to other wholesalers, companies must check their customers hold both a wholesale dealer's licence and a Home Office controlled drugs licence of the appropriate schedule.

For distribution to a wholesale customer, the checks that should be made are similar to the qualification of suppliers. A hard copy of the Home Office licence must be obtained from your customers prior to any supply being made and the validity of this assessed by appropriate staff.

For supplies to pharmacies, hospitals and clinics these organisations are not required to have a Home Office licence as their supplies are for patients. It is particularly important that the usage pattern is considered when fulfilling orders and that order volumes are commensurate with the expected demand of an organisation and their intended market. For example, a retail pharmacy without a WDA(H) would not generally require the same volumes of controlled substances as a specialist hospital unit. There should be procedure in place that sets defined limits to the size of routine orders that can be placed by customers that alert the company's Responsible Person to investigate if excessive amounts are ordered.

Other concerns that arise in relation to customer supplies include medical practitioners who request supplies to their home address. The GMC medical register does not include the address of registered doctors so companies should avoid sending products to home addresses. Doctors operating in the independent sector will be working from clinics registered with the CQC in England, Healthcare Inspectorate in Wales, Healthcare Improvement in Scotland and The Regulation and Quality Improvement Authority in Northern Ireland. Medicines should usually be dispatched to these verifiable addresses rather than residential properties. Where medicines are ordered on behalf of a doctor, the medicines should be stored in a verifiable location where those medicines are entitled to be held, or are otherwise licensed by the Home Office.

For wholesale distributors exporting medicinal products to persons in third countries, they must ensure that such supplies are only made to persons who are authorised or entitled to receive medicinal products for wholesale distribution or supply to the public in accordance with the applicable legal and administrative provisions of the country concerned. Wholesalers should be aware that suspicious and unusual transactions may also include export activities and organisations must apply the same vigilance to export orders as to domestic.

The principles pertaining to the qualification of suppliers and customers remains consistent with export customers as with any other customer type, and re-qualification should occur on a risk-defined periodic basis.

If licensed wholesale dealers have any concerns pertaining to the procurement or supply of medicines, including unusual sales patter reporting, in the first instance they should e-mail GDP.Inspectorate@mhra.gov.uk. Details of the company and the name and quantities of products that have been ordered in the last 6 months should be included. This will be dealt with in confidence.

In instances where reporting directly to the Inspectorate may pose a risk to individuals, or you wish to inform the MHRA anonymously of any relevant matters, please contact the whistleblowing section.

E-mail: whistleblower@mhra.gov.uk

Any suspicions of fraudulent activity or attempts to impersonate a licence holder should be reported promptly to the Licensing Authority and your local police. Case Referrals, within our Enforcement Team, is the responsible team at the MHRA and they will be able to provide support if you need to raise a report:

- Case Referral Centre/Fakemeds Hotline
- Telephone (weekdays 09:00–17:00): 020 3080 6330
- Telephone (out-of-hours emergency): 07795 825 727
- E-mail: casereferrals@mhra.gov.uk

Parallel Importation

The Human Medicines Regulations 2012 refers to lists of approved countries for:

- importation of medicines under a wholesale dealer's licence;
- batch testing of medicines;
- manufacturing of active substances with regulatory standards equivalent to the UK.

The list of approved countries will enable UK importers and wholesalers to continue to recognise QP certification and regulatory standards for active substance manufacture performed in certain countries in the same way as before 1 January 2021. The UK's acceptance of batch testing done in EEA countries will be reviewed before 31 December 2022. A 2-year notice period will be given in the case of changes.

The UK Parallel Import Licensing Scheme allows nationally authorised medicinal products from approved countries for authorised human medicines (29) to be marketed in the UK, provided the imported products have no therapeutic difference from the equivalent UK products. It also allows centrally (EMA) authorised products to be imported into Great Britain (England, Wales and Scotland) under the same condition. Parallel importation exists in the absence of price harmonisation of pharmaceutical products between UK/GB and from approved countries, i.e. when there are significant price differences between approved countries; where prices of medicines are not governed by free competition laws, but are generally fixed by local national government.

It involves the transfer of genuine, original branded or generic products, marketed in one approved countries for authorised human medicines at a lower price (the source country) to the UK/GB (the country of destination) by a parallel importer, and placed on the market in competition with a therapeutically identical product already marketed there at a higher price by or under licence from the owner of the brand. The scope of the UK Parallel Import scheme is limited to nationally authorised products, i.e. those medicinal products that have been granted a marketing authorisation by a competent authority of an approved country for authorised human medicines.

For GB only it extends to centrally authorised medicinal products, granted a marketing authorisation by the EMA that is valid in all approved countries. For Northern Ireland only the transfer from approved countries of these products is termed "Parallel Distribution". The EMA administers a Parallel Distribution scheme for these types of products. Further information on the EMA parallel distribution scheme can be found on the EMA website and in the section below titled "Parallel Distribution".

Products that are parallel imported from an approved country for authorised human medicines require a Product Licence for Parallel Import (PLPI) granted by the Licensing Authority, the MHRA, following extensive checks to ensure that the imported drug is therapeutically the same as the domestic version. Further information on the PLPI licensing procedure can be found on the MHRA website.

A company intending to import medicines from approved countries for authorised human medicines must ensure their licence allows for such activity and that an RPi is in post.

Parallel importers operating in the UK require a wholesale dealer's licence.

In addition, parallel importers in the UK involved in re-packaging or re-labelling of product must hold a manufacturer's licence (MIA) authorising product assembly and will be inspected regularly for compliance with GMP. Alternatively, repackaging/relabelling can be contracted out to another company that already holds such a licence.

Parallel importers are required to have effective recall procedures in place. The MHRA has systems in place to receive and investigate reports of packaging and labelling problems with medicines, including parallel imported products.

https://www.gov.uk/guidance/medicines-apply-for-a-parallel-import-licence

Parallel distribution

Centrally authorised medicinal products are medicines that have been granted a marketing authorisation by the EMA that is valid in all approved countries and also in Northern Ireland.

The sourcing of centrally authorised medicines (not in the official language of the destination market) from one approved country to another independent of the Marketing Authorisation Holder is termed Parallel Distribution.

The EMA administers a Parallel Distribution scheme whereby holders of a wholesale dealer's licence wishing to import from EEA markets to Northern Ireland must notify the EMA of their intent to import, re-package and distribute the product and provide the EMA with the latest product information and labelling in the language of the Member State of destination to be checked for compliance with the marketing authorisation and latest EU legislation on medicinal products. This requirement is set out in Article 76 of Directive 2001/83/EC on the Community code relating to medicinal products for human use.

Similarly to parallel importation, a company wishing to act as a parallel distributor must hold a wholesale dealer's licence. In addition, if they intend to carry out the re-packaging/re-labelling themselves, the company will require an MIA or they can contract this activity out to an MIA holder authorised for assembly.

Further information on Parallel Distribution can be found on the EMA website:

http://www.ema.europa.eu/ema/index.jsp?curl=pages/regulation/general/general_content_000067.jspampmid=WC0b01ac0580024594

Products Imported from Countries on a List

Medicinal products sourced from Northern Ireland for wholesale purposes are out of the scope of this guidance. This is permitted under the supervision of a Responsible Person (RP).

Products with a UK or Great Britain marketing authorisation that are imported into Great Britain from outside the UK without QP certification from a country on the list will require QP certification under a

UK manufacturing and import authorisation before being placed on the market.

Products without a marketing authorisation in the UK, Northern Ireland, Great Britain or a listed country are outside the scope of this guidance. Importation of such products is permitted under the supervision of a Responsible Person, with notification to the MHRA of each importation that is for supply to the Great Britain market.

Where a company imports products from a country on a list, a Responsible Person for Import (RPi) must be nominated and mechanisms for ensuring the proper authorisation and release of those medicines in the origin market must be implemented.

The RPi is responsible for implementing a system to confirm for products that have been imported into Great Britain from countries on an approved country for import list:

- that the required QP certification has taken place;
- that the required independent batch release certificate is available for biological products (described on a wholesale dealer's licence as "immunologicals and blood products").

The RPi is required to implement a system for confirming QP certification and independent batch release certification (for biological products) has taken place when importing into Great Britain the following products from a listed country:

- a UK or Great Britain licensed medicine for use in Great Britain;
- a UK or Great Britain licensed medicine for supply to another third country;
- a Northern Ireland or approved country licensed medicine for supply to fulfil special clinical needs;
- a Northern Ireland or approved country licensed medicine imported as an introduced medicine for supply to another third country;
- a Northern Ireland or approved country licensed medicine for use as a parallel import.

Companies must have appropriate batch-specific controls to qualify and ensure:

- that the required QP certification has taken place;
- that the required independent batch release certificate is available for biological products (described on a wholesale dealer's licence as "immunologicals and blood products");
- that where products have originated in the EEA, that they have been decommissioned prior to receipt, or otherwise have systems in place to assess the unique identifier for Prescription Only Medicines, if wholesale dealers are importing products if medicines are being imported for parallel import, unique clinical need or introduction;

- the product is not the subject of a recall or reported as stolen and is available on the market within the listed country's licensed supply chain.

The RPi should ensure that written evidence is available to demonstrate that each batch of product has been QP certified as required in Article 51 of Directive 2001/83/EC. Documentary evidence of this must be kept by a company.

Not all options listed below may be suitable for different supply chain relationships; however, just one of these pieces of evidence is sufficient to satisfy the requirements of regulation 45AA of the Human Medicines Regulations 2012. Other evidence may be acceptable provided it confirms that QP certification has taken place for the batch in question.

- Batch certificate confirming QP certification in accordance with Article 51 of Directive 2001/83/EC).
- A copy of the "control report" (Appendix II to EU Good Manufacturing Practice Annex 16).
- Statement of certification (ad-hoc, confirming certification in accordance with Article 51 of Directive 2001/83/EC).
- Reference to company internal systems (e.g. global Enterprise Resource Planning system) that shows batch certification.
- Confirmation that the final manufacturing step (other than batch certification) of an authorised medicine has been performed by a Manufacturing and Import Authorisation holder in a listed country. A copy of the Marketing Authorisation and technical agreement with the manufacturer should be available to place reliance on this supply chain control.
- For medicines authorised in a listed country, batch certification may be verified by confirming that the medicine has been purchased from an authorised wholesaler after it has been "placed on the market" in the listed country.

What Evidence can be used for Independent Batch Release Certification?

Biological products requiring independent batch release certification are listed on the European Directorate for Quality of Medicines website.

Independent batch release may be confirmed using evidence such as:

- a statement from the marketing authorisation holder confirming that a batch certificate has been issued by NIBSC or a Mutual Recognition Agreement partner;
- a copy of the batch certificate issued by NIBSC or a Mutual Recognition Agreement partner;
- confirmation from NIBSC that a batch certificate has been issued. Enquiries should be sent to CPB@nibsc.org.

Batches of QP-certified biological medicines that require independent batch release should not be sold or supplied by the importing wholesale dealer in Great Britain until independent batch release certification is also confirmed.

Processes should be in place to ensure physical or electronic segregation of stock.

Continued Supply

Under the Human Medicines Regulations 2012, the marketing authorisation holder is required to notify the competent authority (the MHRA in the UK) of the date of actual marketing of the medicinal product, taking account of the various presentations authorised, and to notify the competent authority if the product ceases to be placed on the market either temporarily or permanently. Except in exceptional circumstances, the notification must be made no less than 2 months before the interruption.

Any authorisation which within 3 years of granting is not placed on the market will cease to be valid. In respect of generic medicinal products, the 3-year period will start on the grant of the authorisation, or at the end of the period of market exclusivity or patent protection of the reference product, whichever is the later date. If a product is placed on the market after authorisation, but subsequently ceases to be available on the market in the UK for a period of 3 consecutive years, it will also cease to be valid. In these circumstances the MHRA will, however, when it is aware of the imminent expiry of the 3-year period, notify the marketing authorisation holder in advance that their marketing authorisation will cease to be valid. In exceptional circumstances, and on public health grounds, the MHRA may grant an exemption from the invalidation of the marketing authorisation after 3 years. Whether there are exceptional circumstances and public health grounds for an exemption will be assessed on a case-by-case basis. When assessing such cases, the MHRA will, in particular, consider the implications for patients and public health more generally of a marketing authorisation no longer being valid.

Those provisions are implemented in the UK by Part 5 of the Human Medicines Regulations 2012.

In accordance with the MHRA's interpretation of the expression "placing on the market" the MHRA's view is that a product is "placed on the market" at the first transaction by which the product enters the distribution chain in the UK. The marketing authorisation holder must, therefore, notify the MHRA when a product with a new marketing authorisation is first placed into the distribution chain, rather than the first date it becomes available to individual patients. The MHRA requests that you notify us of this first "placing on the market" within 1 calendar month. In order to ensure that a marketing authorisation continues to be valid, the marketing authorisation holder must ensure that at least one packaging presentation (e.g. bottle or blister pack) of the product, which can include own-label supplies, authorised under that marketing authorisation is present on the market.

The marketing authorisation holder must report all cessations/interruptions to the MHRA. However, the MHRA does not need to be notified of the following:

(a) normal seasonal changes in manufacturing and/or distribution schedules (such as cold and flu remedies);

(b) short-term temporary interruptions in placing on the market that will not affect normal availability to distributors.

If you are in doubt about whether or not you need to notify an interruption in supply, you should err on the side of caution and report it to the MHRA in the normal way. You must notify the MHRA if any of the presentations authorised under a single marketing authorisation cease to be placed on the market either temporarily or permanently, but, as stated above, the absence of availability of one or more presentations – as long as one presentation of the product authorised under the single marketing authorisation remains on the market – will not invalidate the marketing authorisation. Problems relating to manufacturing or assembly should also be discussed with the appropriate GMP Inspector and issues of availability of medicines relating to suspected or confirmed product defects should be directly notified to, and discussed with, the Defective Medicines Reporting Centre (tel.: 020 3080 6574).

The Department of Health and Social Care (DHSC) is responsible for the continuity of supply of medicines, and manufacturers have a legal requirement to inform DHSC of any supply problems. DHSC works closely with the Medicines Healthcare products Regulatory Agency (MHRA), NHSE&I, pharmaceutical companies, the wider NHS, wholesalers and others in the supply chain to ensure consistency of supply of medicines.

Under Part 6 of the Health Service Products (Provision and Disclosure of Information) Regulations 2018, manufacturers are legally required to provide information to the DHSC Medicines Supply Team about availability of UK licensed medicines and about discontinuation or anticipated supply shortages. The regulations were introduced in January 2019, superseding previous voluntary arrangements. These requirements ensure that the DHSC Medicines Supply Team have relevant information from manufacturers at the earliest point to help manage supply shortages and mitigate any potential impacts on patients. Marketing authorisation holders are expected to be fully accountable for their supply chain to the UK market and required to understand the potential impact on UK patients should supplies of their products become unavailable. Any Information submitted by companies as outlined in regulation 29(2) of the Health Service Products (Provision and Disclosure of Information)

Regulations 2018 is commercially confidential information and treated sensitively by DHSC.

The Human Medicines Regulations 2012 (45)(2) under which the marketing authorisation holder and the distributors of a medicinal product actually placed on the market shall, within the limits of their responsibilities, ensure appropriate and continued supplies of that medicinal product to pharmacies and persons authorised to supply medicinal products so that the needs of patients in the UK are covered. Failure by a marketing authorisation holder to comply with this obligation is a criminal offence, unless the marketing authorisation holder took all reasonable precautions and exercised all due diligence to avoid such a failure.

Obtaining medicines for wholesale using prescriptions

The MHRA is aware of a growing use of false NHS and private prescriptions to obtain medicines from Marketing Authorisation Holders (MAH). Prescriptions are requested by the MAH for a variety of reasons, but mainly to provide evidence the product is needed for a patient. Typically, prescriptions are requested for high-cost medicines not usually seen in dispensing pharmacies. Redacted prescriptions are presented by a pharmacy to the MAH, implying there is a patient, the product is supplied, but is then wholesaled and not dispensed to a patient.

MAHs have an obligation to ensure appropriate and continued supplies of medicinal product to pharmacies and persons authorised to supply medicinal products so that the needs of UK patients are met, set out in The Human Medicines Regulations 2012. Some MAHs have decided to manage the distribution of specific products by requesting a redacted prescription to ensure the supply is for a UK patient.

Medicines for wholesale supply cannot under any circumstances be obtained by way of a prescription and doing so is a breach of the conditions of the WDA(H) set out in regulation (43)(2). Companies are reminded that any procurement must be conducted by, and from, holders of WDA(H), and failure to adhere to this is a critical departure from GDP.

Where pharmacies also hold wholesaler authorisations, a clear distinction between pharmacy and wholesale procurement must be maintained.

Storage

Medicinal products and, if necessary, healthcare products should be stored separately from other products likely to alter them and should be protected from the harmful effects of light, temperature, moisture and other external factors. Particular attention should be paid to products requiring specific storage conditions.

Incoming containers of medicinal products should be cleaned, if necessary, before storage.

Warehousing operations must ensure appropriate storage conditions are maintained and allow for appropriate security of stocks. There should be a physical or electronic system of segregation in place between wholesale and retail stock ensuring that products are held within the correct environment in accordance with the labelled conditions.

Stock should be rotated according to the "first expiry, first out" (FEFO) principle. Any exceptions should be confirmed and documented.

Medicinal products should be handled and stored in such a manner as to prevent spillage, breakage, contamination and mix-ups. Medicinal products should not be stored directly on the floor unless the package is designed to allow such storage (such as for some medicinal gas cylinders).

Medicinal products that are nearing their expiry date/shelf life should be withdrawn immediately from saleable stock either physically or through other equivalent electronic segregation.

Stock inventories should be performed regularly accounting for national legislation requirements. Stock irregularities should be investigated and documented.

Where wholesalers conduct retail operations, electronic of physical segregation should be maintained and an audit trail implemented demonstrating the procurement of medicines for each specific mechanism, and the final fate of inventory.

The Responsible Person on a WDA(H) must be able to demonstrate that all medicines have been purchased appropriately and in line with GDP.

Whereas it may be appropriate to transfer wholesale inventory to retail stock in some occasions, it is not permitted to move retail products into wholesale remits.

DHSC have implemented restrictions on goods that can be hoarded. Companies must ensure that processes are implemented to prevent the hoarding and excessive stocking of medicines detailed within a list of medicines published by DHSC.

Companies can continue to withhold medicines as part of stock management arrangements agreed with marketing authorisation holders, which is not considered hoarding.

Companies can also continue to maintain contingency stockpiles built up at the request of the Department of Health and Social Care (DHSC) or Public Health England (PHE).

Destruction of obsolete goods

Medicinal products intended for destruction should be appropriately identified, held separately and handled in accordance with a written procedure.

Destruction of medicinal products should be in accordance with national or international requirements for handling, transport and disposal of such products.

Records of all destroyed medicinal products should be retained for a defined period.

Picking

Controls should be in place to ensure the correct product is picked. The product should have an appropriate remaining shelf life when it is picked.

Stock segregation

There should be a physical or electronic system of segregation in place between wholesale and retail stock ensuring that products are held within the correct environment in accordance with the product labelled conditions.

The Responsible Person on a WDA(H) must be able to demonstrate that all medicines have been purchased appropriately and in line with GDP.

The purchasing of medicines from company to company constitutes wholesale distribution, and any company procuring on behalf of another must hold a WDA(H) and be named on a licence as a third-party site. Written agreements defining responsibilities must be in place to properly control the activity.

It is prohibited for pharmacies to obtain stock using redacted prescriptions for wholesale dealing.

It is a breach of the conditions of the wholesale dealer licence set out in regulation 43(2) of the Human Medicines Regulations by impinging on the ability of the MAH to discharge its obligations that the needs of UK patients are met.

Supply

For all supplies, a document, whether hard or electronic copy, (e.g. delivery note) must be enclosed or recorded stating the date; name and pharmaceutical form of the medicinal product, batch number at least for products bearing the safety features; quantity supplied; name and address of the supplier; name and delivery address of the consignee[17] (actual physical storage premises, if different); and applicable transport and storage conditions. Records should be kept so that the actual location of the product can be verified and is traceable.

---

[17] Article 82 of Directive 2001/83/EC.

Companies should be able to demonstrate where proportionate, by way of risk management, validation and mapping:

- the goods are transported within label conditions and active or passive shipping solutions are suitable to ensure this;
- considerations of extremes of climate;
- the route that medicine will take from despatch to end destination;
- any mitigation strategies employed during transportation to protect the integrity of medicines.

Integration Operational Processes to Mitigation of Risk of Theft or Diversion of Medicine

The theft and diversion of medicines has a broad impact that increases risk to public health and risks the integrity of the medicine supply chain.

Robust operational practices can mitigate the risk of theft or procurement of stolen medicines. Some measures for consideration are listed below.

Operations undertaken by the company should ensure sufficient measures are in place to mitigate the risk of theft of medicines. The company should consider as part of their operations:

Quality management: monitoring of unusual sales patterns, monitoring changes in risk profiles for products supplied and evidence of theft or near-misses within deviation reports. Quality risk management incorporates security risks evaluation embedded throughout the quality system.

Personnel: security pre-employment checks, training of drivers in security, development of an open culture that supports reporting and whistleblowing, restricted personnel access to high-risk areas and policies in place for the management of visitors and control of security passes.

Facility and equipment design and maintenance: security measures are built into the design including restriction of vehicular access to loading bay areas, location of high-risk stock within the warehouse, maintenance repair and servicing of buildings, perimeter fences and equipment, including shutters and CCTV.

Documentation: stock records safeguarded from unauthorised alteration including both hard copy and computerised records, stock discrepancies addressed at an appropriate level, records enable clear visibility of discrepancies including underpicked stock, mislaid stock, under-delivered stock, evidence of destroyed stock, including stock for destruction supplied to third countries. Procedures describe how to report medicine theft to the MHRA.

Operations: procurement controls include robust authentication of suppliers and customers, incentivisation of purchasing or sales staff does not conflict with increasing risk of distributing diverted medicines, witness checking for high-risk operations including picking controlled drugs. Control of access into high risk areas and use of consignment security seals.

Standardised packaging of inventory designed to protect and mitigate risk to products from adulteration or theft

Reporting mechanisms to local police forces and the MHRA.

Complaint management: identifying trends of under-delivered or lost stock.

Returned medicines: control of courier used for reverse logistics, verification that returned stock is genuine and is supported by appropriate documentation.

Falsified medicines: clear understanding in all areas of the organisation for standards of operations and how to report suspect medicines and transactions.

Outsourced activities: integration with couriers through written agreements, including immediate reporting to the contract giver of anomalies, assurance of a chain of custody, risk profiling of contractors, monitoring contractor and control of additional subcontracting by the contractor.

Transportation: security features identified as part of user requirement specification, security profiling for high-risk consignments, driver trained in security practices.

REPORTING STOLEN AND MISSING MEDICINES TO THE MHRA

Theft of medicines that may pose a significant risk to public health should be reported in a timely manner to the MHRA in addition to any other reporting such as Police or Home Office. This is to enable the MHRA assess risk to public and maintain awareness. For high-risk mislaid stock, it may be better to report this following initial investigation and then later report as found, rather than delay the reporting.

Reports should include:

- the date when the event was first noted;
- products;
- quantities;
- batch numbers (if known);
- details of location;
- contact details;
- police incident number or Home Office reference, where relevant.

Enquiries about potential illegal dealings with medicines should be made to the MHRA Case Referral Centre:

- Telephone (weekdays 9am to 5pm): 020 3080 6330
- Telephone (out-of-hours emergency) for Case Referral Centre/Fakemeds Hotline: 07795 825 727
- E-mail: casereferrals@mhra.gov.uk

or via the Yellow Card Scheme:

- Telephone: 020 3080 6330/020 3080 6701
- E mail: fakemeds@mhra.gov.uk

Sourcing and Exporting Medicinal Products – non-EEA Countries

The GDP guidelines describe the concept that medicinal products may be introduced into the Union that are not intended to be released for free circulation. These are known as introduced medicinal products or products sourced from a country outside of Great Britain for the specific reason of supplying them back to a third country, without entering into the UK supply chain.

"*The provisions applicable to the export of medicinal products from Great Britain and those applicable to the introduction of medicinal products into Great Britain with the sole purpose of exporting them need to be clarified. The provisions applicable to wholesale distributors as well as good distribution practices should apply to all those activities whenever they are performed within Great Britain, including in areas such as free trade zones or free warehouses.*"

UK legislation dictates the need for a wholesale dealer's licence for medicine exported from Great Britain to third countries, and to the sourcing and supply of introduced medicines from and to third countries by way of wholesale.

In the case of wholesale distribution of medicinal products to third countries, GDP provisions pertaining to introduced medicines should apply. Wholesale distributors shall ensure that the medicinal products are obtained only from persons who are authorised or entitled to supply medicinal products in accordance with the applicable legal and administrative provisions of the third country concerned. Where wholesale distributors supply medicinal products to persons in third countries, they shall ensure that such supplies are only made to persons who are authorised or entitled to receive medicinal products for wholesale distribution or supply to the public in accordance with the applicable legal and administrative provisions of the third country concerned.

Introduced medicinal products

For a medicinal product to be an introduced medicinal product it has to be sourced from a third country by a licensed wholesale dealer and supplied to a third country by the same licensed wholesale dealer. An introduced medicinal product will not have a marketing authorisation for the UK. Such products can be held on a licensed site in a free zone or in a bonded warehouse under an appropriate Customs processing procedure.

A medicinal product that is sourced from third country by a licensed wholesale dealer, for the purpose of supply to another legal entity in the UK, is not an introduced medicinal product as it will have been freely circulated to that other legal entity within the community when supplied. In such circumstances the activity will be subject to the need for a manufacturer's licence authorising import as required under The Human Medicines Regulations 2012.

When dealing with introduced medicinal products a licensed wholesale dealer has to ensure that they only source the medicine from a person in the third country who is authorised or entitled to supply medicinal products for wholesale distribution in accordance with the applicable legal and administrative provisions of the third country concerned. A licensed wholesale dealer should also verify that the medicinal products received are not falsified.

A licensed wholesale dealer also has to ensure that they only supply the introduced medicinal product back to a person in the third country who is authorised or entitled to receive medicinal products for wholesale distribution or supply to the public in accordance with the applicable legal and administrative provisions of the third country concerned.

A separate Home Office licence is required for introduced medicines that are also "controlled drugs".

The introduction of a medicinal product can be subdivided into the following categories.

PHYSICAL INTRODUCTION

Introduced medicines are sourced from a third country for the sole purpose of export to a third country. These products by definition will not have a marketing authorisation within GB or the UK. Under the provisions of a wholesale dealer's licence the medicinal product may not be "imported", that is, the customs procedure code quoted on the C88 document cannot include sole or simultaneous entry into free circulation within GB or the UK. A suitable customs procedure code should be declared.

Generally the site of *holding* these products prior to export will be a registered customs warehouse that is the subject of a wholesale dealer's licence.

Further information in respect of the Union Customs Code (UCC) introduced across GB and the UK on 1 May 2016 may be obtained from HMRC.

FINANCIAL INTRODUCTION

Any trade between two third countries being facilitated and invoiced from GB or the UK will be subject to the Good Distribution Practice Guidelines in accordance with Regulation C17 of the Human Medicines Regulations 2012 (GDP) in their entirety.

It is necessary for the supplying licensed wholesale dealer to demonstrate full compliance with GDP Guidelines in accordance with Reg. C17 GB or the UK.

Companies operating this business model will be required to have a wholesale distribution authorisation authorising the activities of *Procurement* and *Supply* as they are buying and selling the product.

This activity should not be confused with brokering. A broker does not at any time take ownership of the product; a broker will bring a buyer and seller together and typically will receive a commission or fee from one or both parties. Brokers are subject to a registration requirement. They must have a permanent address and contact details in the Member State in which they are registered. Brokers are discussed in more detail elsewhere in this guide. See Chapter 5.

Export to a country not on the approved list

A medicinal product that is exported to a third country will be supplied to the specification of the importing country concerned. This might be a medicinal product that is:

- licensed in the UK and has a national marketing authorisation issued by MHRA;
- licensed in Northern Ireland and has a national marketing authorisation issued by the competent authority for medicines of the EEA member state concerned;
- an unlicensed medicine manufactured specifically for export by the holder of a manufacturer's licence;
- an introduced product that the same authorised wholesale dealer has sourced from a third country;
- a medicine that is also a "controlled drug" – requiring a separate Home Office licence. (See section titled "Controls on certain medicinal products" earlier in this chapter.)

An unlicensed medicine known as a "special", manufactured by the holder of a manufacturer's specials licence, cannot be distributed to a third country. This is because to accord with The Human Medicines Regulations 2012 an unlicensed medicine manufactured for export has to be manufactured by the holder of an Manufacturer/Importers Authorisation (MIA) and certified prior to release by the Qualified Person named on that manufacturing authorisation.

A licensed wholesale dealer that exports a medicine that is the subject of a GB or UK marketing authorisation to a third country must obtain their supplies of medicinal products only from persons who are themselves in possession of a GB or Northern Ireland wholesale distribution authorisation or a GB or UK manufacturer's authorisation.

They must also verify that the authorised medicinal product they receive is not falsified by checking the safety feature on the outer packaging in accordance with the requirements laid down in the Human Medicines Regulations 2012.

A licensed wholesale dealer also has to ensure that they supply the authorised medicine only to persons in the third country who are authorised or entitled to receive medicinal products for wholesale distribution or supply to the public in accordance with the applicable legal and administrative provisions of the third country concerned.

The definition of wholesale distribution does not depend on whether the distributor is established or operating in specific customs areas, such as in free zones or in free warehouses. A wholesale distribution authorisation is required and all obligations related to wholesale distribution activities also apply to these distributors.

A number of companies and their sites that were not previously regulated now require a wholesale distribution authorisation. Parties that may be affected include freight consolidators, freight forwarders and logistics services providers in the air, sea or road transport sector when they are "holding" medicinal products.

Customs-approved warehouse facilities "holding" medicinal products are also required to have a wholesale distribution authorisation.

To clear a medicinal product for export, HMRC will need to know exactly what is being shipped. Medicinal products presented for export should therefore be accompanied by the **commercial invoice** fully detailing the commodity to be exported. Use of "proforma invoices" for export purposes are to be avoided.

Customs documentation must be completed fully and legibly. A false or misleading declaration may lead to a fine or to seizure of the item.

The products may be subject to restrictions in the country of destination or there may be trade embargoes or other restrictions preventing certain medicinal products from being exported to certain destinations.

It is the responsibility of the exporter to enquire into import and export regulations (prohibitions, restrictions such as quarantine, pharmaceutical restrictions, etc.) and to find out what documents, if any (commercial invoice, certificate of origin, health certificate, export licence, authorisation for goods subject to quarantine (plant, animal, food products, etc.)) are required in the destination country. See GDP, Chapter 5, Section 5.9:

"Where wholesale distributors supply medicinal products to persons in third countries, they shall ensure that such supplies are only made to persons who are authorised or entitled to receive medicinal products for wholesale distribution or supply to the public in accordance with the applicable legal and administrative provisions of the country concerned."

Export is defined as to *allow GB goods to leave the customs territory*. It is the responsibility of the exporter (consignor) to ensure that:

- medicinal products remain in the legal supply chain;
- export paperwork is completed correctly;
- proof of export is obtained and retained;

- the Consignee is entitled to receive the medicinal products;
- the product has been stored, handled and shipped in accordance with GDP.

HMRC recommends that exporters should routinely provide their freight agents with the following:

- their UK Economic Operator Registration and Identification (EORI) number;
- details of whom the goods are to be consigned to, their name and address in full;
- a commercial reference that can be incorporated into the Declaration Unique Consignment Reference (DUCR) to assist with the export audit trail;
- details of where the goods are to be exported, i.e. country of final destination;
- shipping or flight details (where known);
- correct value of goods in correct currency code;
- the Commodity Code and a clear and unambiguous description of the goods, their quantity marks and numbers;
- any reference numbers already issued by HMRC, e.g. Inward Processing Relief, Outward Processing relief authorisations or previous declarations should also be provided.

Qualification check in third countries

The MHRA recognises that conducting a qualification check in some third countries can be quite difficult. In the first instance suppliers and customers in the third countries concerned should be asked to justify their local entitlement and requirements. However, an authorised wholesale dealer should not just accept information from the supplier or customer that they can supply or import medicines, but should take reasonable steps to verify that the information that they have been provided with is valid and accurate. This may involve making additional checks with the regulatory authority for medicines in the country concerned where possible and documenting the outcome as evidence. Any licences obtained should have been translated into English and authenticated by a notary with appropriate due diligence carried out. The MHRA's expectation is that an authorised wholesale dealer should have oversight of the export of the introduced medicinal product and have all the appropriate documentation to evidence it. See also section on "Qualification of customers and suppliers".

Wholesale obligations for exported and introduced medicinal products

For further obligations of licensed wholesale dealers, see Chapter 2 on Legislation on Wholesale Distribution. You cannot export medicines on the restricted medicines list that have been put on the market for UK patients to other countries in or outside the EEA.

As of 1 January 2021 you may no longer be able to export branded medicines that have been placed on the UK market to countries in the EEA.

Medicines that cannot be exported from the UK

The DHSC has implemented restrictions on some medicines leaving the UK.

WDA(H) holders must implement effective processes to ensure that medicines periodically defined by DHSC are not hoarded exported from GB or UK markets and remain available to facilitate UK patient need.

You can continue to export medicines on the restricted medicines list if you, or a company in your group of companies, holds a marketing authorisation for those medicines and have specifically forecast medicines in GB or UK livery to be exported to meet patient need. The restrictions do not apply.

You can continue to export medicines on the restricted medicines list that are manufactured and intended for markets abroad. The restrictions do not apply.

You can continue to export medicines on the restricted medicines list to:

- ships;
- planes;
- the British, UN and NATO armed forces;
- British citizens abroad;
- British overseas territories and crown dependencies;
- to international humanitarian organisations;
- for clinical trials and other research purposes.

Where companies are actively engaged in export and have orders in place prior to a ban being implemented on a medicine, a final agreed purchase order from an importer must be received before the date of restriction. Open, rolling or frame orders placed by importers before the date of restriction can only be fulfilled if the products have been picked and packed, and transport booked. All orders must be final, evidenced as signed and comply with the above terms.

The restriction for each medicine applies from 00:00am at the start of the date of restriction.

If you export, start hoarding or continue hoarding a medicine on the restricted list it will be considered a breach of regulation 43(2) of the Human Medicines Regulations 2012.

It may lead to regulatory action by the Medicines and Healthcare products Regulatory Agency (MHRA) against the wholesale dealer's licence.

This could include:

- an immediate suspension of the licence or suspension of the supply of certain products under the licence;
- a 28-day notice proposing to vary the licence to restrict or prevent export activity.

Continued breaches could be considered a criminal offence under regulation 34(1), read together with regulation 18(1) of the Human Medicines Regulations 2012.

Please see the website for a list of medicines that cannot be exported from the UK.   https://www.gov.uk/government/publications/medicines-that-cannot-be-parallel-exported-from-the-uk

Incoterms®

Incoterms® 2010 rules are internationally accepted standard definitions of trade terms. Incoterms® were developed by the International Chamber of Commerce, Paris, France in 1936 and have been regularly revised to reflect the changes in transportation and documentation. The current version is Incoterms® 2010.

Full information may be obtained from www.iccwbo.org.

There are 11 Incoterms® that can be broadly split into subgroups according to which party pays for and arranges the main transport. Each group is discussed briefly below.

The first three groups are applicable to products moved by air, road, rail or sea, or by a combination of transport modes.

BUYER ARRANGES MAIN CARRIAGE – EXW

- EXW – EX Works (… named place).

This Incoterm® puts the onus on the customer to complete and pay for the export formalities and for the pre-carriage of the products from the seller's premises to the point of export.

In many cross-border and international transactions this presents practical difficulties. Specifically, the exporter needs to be involved in export reporting formalities and cannot realistically leave these to the buyer.

BUYER ARRANGES MAIN CARRIAGE – FCA

- FCA – Free Carrier (… named place of delivery).

With this Incoterm® the seller has control regarding the transport and customs formalities prior to the goods leaving the Union; the buyer pays for the main transport.

This option crucially gives the seller control over the pre-transport to the point of export and control over the export formalities.

It is the legal responsibility of the declarant to ensure that the goods are accurately declared and presented to HMRC prior to goods leaving the UK. If the exporter is employing a freight agent to declare the goods on his behalf he must ensure he supplies them with the appropriate information to submit a legal declaration.

SELLER ARRANGES MAIN CARRIAGE: CPT; CIP; DAT; DAP; DDP

- CPT – Carriage Paid To (… named place of destination);
- CIP – Carriage and Insurance Paid To (… named place of destination);
- DAT – Delivered At Terminal (… named terminal at destination port);
- DAP – Delivered At Place (… named place of destination);
- DDP – Delivered Duty Paid (… named place of destination).

Here the seller has control over the pre-carriage, customs formalities and the main transport mode.

The following two groups are only applicable when transport is via sea freight or by inland waterways.

BUYER ARRANGES MAIN CARRIAGE: FAS; FOB

- FAS – Free Alongside Ship (… named port of shipment);
- FOB – Free On Board (… named port of shipment).

Pre-carriage and export formalities by seller; the customer pays for the sea freight from the named port of shipment.

SELLER ARRANGES MAIN CARRIAGE: CFR; CIF

- CFR – Cost and Freight (… named port of destination);
- CIF – Cost Insurance and Freight (… named port of destination).

Pre-carriage and export formalities by seller; seller also pays sea freight to the named destination.

When entering into trade negotiations with potential clients, the selection of the appropriate Incoterm® can significantly influence the ability to demonstrate GDP compliance.

Selection of an Incoterm® such as ExW or FCA where the buyer pays for the freight does not absolve the seller of his GDP responsibilities with respect to selection of transport conditions.

As the Consignor, the exporter is legally responsible for the information shown on the customs documentation. The definition of export is *to allow Community goods to leave the customs territory of the Union.*

Import of medicinal products

Import is not a function authorised under a wholesale distribution authorisation from countries not named on a list for the purpose of parallel import. For medicinal products that are imported from a non-listed country, an Article 40 authorisation (Manufacturer's/Importer's Authorisation (MIA)) is required.

Import is briefly discussed in this section for the sake of completeness and to make a clear distinction between the act of Introduction, a GDP activity executed under a wholesale dealer's licence and Importation, a GMP activity requiring an MIA.

Importation of product manufactured in a third country not on the list for parallel import for use in the UK is a GMP activity. This requires a Manufacturing Licence (typically a Manufacturer's/Importer's Authorisation but, in particular circumstances, a Manufacturer's Specials licence may be required). Import activity associated with an MIA requires Q.P. release of product. Full details of these activities may be found in the publication *Rules and Guidance for Pharmaceutical Manufacturers and Distributors* ("The Orange Guide").

Transactions where title is passed from EEA company to non-EEA company

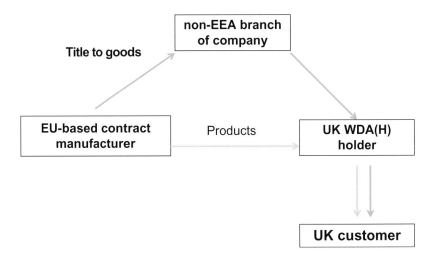

Transactions where title is passed from GB or UK company to non-GB or UK company

In this scenario, licensed medicinal product is manufactured and released within GB or the UK under a Manufacturing Authorisation. The title of the goods is transferred to the *sole UK pre-distribution partner* via a third country while the product physically remains within GB or the UK at suitably licensed premises at all times.

Product transfers directly from the contract manufacturer to the *sole UK pre-distribution partner*. The pre-distributor partner then distributes the products according to their own authorisation.

To accord with regulation 44(1) of the Human Medicines Regulations 2012 the holder of a wholesale dealer's licence may not obtain supplies of medicinal products from anyone except:

(a) the holder of a manufacturer's licence or wholesale dealer's licence in relation to products of that description; or
(b) a person who holds an authorisation granted by another country named on a list authorising the manufacture of products of that description or their distribution by way of wholesale dealing.

Therefore these requirements will prohibit the purchasing of medicines from a company in a third country. This transaction is classed as a *fiscal import* from a third country and therefore is not WDA(H) activity. This business model requires an MIA.

Ensuring you have the correct authorisations for the intended activity

GDP defines wholesale distribution of medicinal products to mean:

"All activities consisting of procuring, holding, supplying or exporting medicinal products, other than supplying these products to the public."[18]

An authorised wholesale dealer may be authorised to undertake one or more of these activities according to the scope of the granted authorisation. Definitions of these activities are provided in the Annex to EU Guidelines on Good Distribution Practice of Medicinal Products for Human Use (GDP)[19] as below:

HOLDING – storing medicinal products. (*The MHRA applies the interpretation that a site is deemed to be holding when either an ambient product is on site for more than 36 hours or there is active refrigeration taking place regardless of dwell time.*)
EXPORT – to allow GB or UK goods to leave customs territory.
A Home Office licence is required to import or export "controlled drugs". Controlled drugs are named in the Misuse of Drugs legislation, and grouped in schedules. Anyone intending to supply a controlled drug must apply for the relevant schedule licence[20].

Exports and customs procedures

YOUR PRODUCT, YOUR DECLARATION

When exporting a medicinal product, a declaration must be made to Her Majesty's Revenue & Customs (HMRC) to indicate exactly what is being

---

[18] Article 1(17).
[19] 2013/C 343/01.
[20] https://www.gov.uk/guidance/controlled-drugs-licences-fees-and-returns

shipped, who is making the shipment and where the product is ultimately going.

The product should be accompanied by a commercial invoice – proforma invoices are to be avoided as this can, and has led to, misleading customs declarations being completed. A false declaration may result in seizure of the product and may also lead to a fine.

It is the responsibility of the exporter to enquire into the import and export regulations (any prohibitions, restrictions, trade embargoes, etc.) that may be in force in relation to the destination country. The exporter must ensure that certificates of origin, export licences and the like that may be required in relation to the trade in the particular commodity within the destination country are applied for and that the correct documentation accompanies the shipment. Copies of this documentation should routinely be retained.

The exporter (consignor) is also responsible for ensuring that:

- medicinal products remain in the legal supply chain;
- export paperwork is correctly completed;
- proof of export is obtained and retained;
- the consignee is entitled to receive the product; and
- the product has been stored, handled and shipped in accordance with GDP.

YOUR FREIGHT FORWARDER OR SHIPPING AGENT IS A KEY PARTNER

It is best practice to routinely provide the freight forwarder, shipping department or freight agent with the following:

- your Economic Operator Registration and Identification (EORI) number;
- details of whom the goods are to be consigned to (name and address in full);
- commercial reference to be incorporated into the Declaration Unique Consignment Reference (DUCR) to assist with export audit trails;
- details of the country of final destination;
- shipping or flight details;
- correct value of goods in the correct currency code;
- the Commodity Code and a clear and unambiguous description of the goods, their quantity, marks and numbers;
- any reference numbers already issued by HMRC – such as any previous declarations made in respect of the product. For example, the declaration made when the product was "introduced".

While on inspection, upon asking for documentation relating to an export to a third country the MHRA is frequently presented with invoices that show the Incoterm® 'Ex Works'. This generally causes traceability issues at inspection as the consignor may have handed the product over for export to a representative of a company appointed by the consignee. Where this is the case, the consignor generally will be unable to demonstrate GDP compliance or indeed produce any paperwork showing the product has been exported as claimed. Companies should obtain copies of the documentation (that is interchangeably referred to as the SAD, C88 or export declaration) from their shipping agent and check this for accuracy.

The Incoterm® EXW (Ex Works) puts the onus on the consignee to arrange the pre-carriage from the seller's premises to the point of export, and to complete and pay for the export formalities. In most export scenarios this presents practical difficulties. Realistically, for all export transactions the exporter needs to be involved in export reporting formalities and cannot leave this to the consignee.

A lesser used but more practical Incoterm® when an exporter does not wish to pay for the carriage of the product, is FCA – Free Carrier (named place of delivery). Generally the named place of delivery will be the port through which the product is leaving. With this Incoterm®, the seller has control regarding the transport and customs formalities prior to the goods leaving the territory, and the buyer pays for the main transport.

As it is the legal responsibility of the declarant to ensure that the goods are accurately declared when presented to HMRC, using this Incoterm® gives the seller the control required. Crucially, the seller also takes responsibility for arranging the transport to the point of shipment (or consolidation) and can therefore control where the goods are held and by whom prior to shipment, hence ensuring that the product remains within the legal supply chain and under GDP control up to the point of main transport, which will have risk assessed according to Chapter 9 of GDP.

Both the GDP and GMP inspectorate will be routinely requesting full export documentation at inspection - and this extends to the CHIEF (Customs Handling of Import and Export Freight) entry – bills of lading or airway bills, export licences where applicable, and any certificates of origin that may be required for that particular commodity to be sent to the destination country. For exports we still expect that you can show the same due diligence. As the exporter, the responsibility in ensuring the information you provide to HMRC rests with you.

Controls on Certain Medicinal Products

Good Distribution Practice (GDP) in accordance with Reg. C17 requires the licence holder and/or the RP to consider extra requirements throughout the wholesale process. The RP must ensure that any additional requirements imposed on certain products by national law are adhered to. This will include ensuring that the correct licences are held for the activities undertaken, ensuring any broker used or any organisation performing outsourced activities are correctly licensed, and that customers are entitled to receive the products supplied. Where products are exported there may be additional national requirements to consider. Supplies made to customers should be monitored to enable any irregularity in the sales patterns of narcotics, psychotropic substances and other dangerous substances to be investigated. Unusual sales patterns may constitute diversion and must be reported to MHRA.

Some products may present additional risks during storage and transport. These could include cytotoxics, radiopharmaceuticals and flammable products. Special destruction requirements may be imposed by national regulation.

Staff may require additional training for the receipt and handling of hazardous products, radioactive materials, products presenting special risks of abuse, as well as temperature-sensitive products. Handling of temperature-sensitive products is addressed elsewhere in this publication.

Transaction arrangements, storage, transport and security measures should all be documented, risk assessed and audited to demonstrate continued suitability and compliance.

GDP frequently refers to 'additional requirements imposed on certain products by national law'. These medicinal products and substances are subject to additional controls not frequently encountered by the licensed wholesale dealer. Further requirements are in place under GDP for:

- medicinal products derived from blood;
- immunological medicinal products;
- narcotic or psychotropic substances;
- radiopharmaceuticals.

These additional controls are managed by the MHRA or other organisations. Some examples are given below.

Controlled drugs and precursor chemicals

The Home Office Drug & Firearms Licensing Unit is the UK Competent Authority for controlled drug and drug precursor chemical licensing. Licences are needed irrespective of the format of the material – whether finished product (licensed medicine or unlicensed 'special'), active substances, starting materials or intermediates – where controlled under the relevant legislation.

'Domestic' Licences are issued to specific 'persons' (i.e. companies) at specific premises, covering a single site. They are not transferrable to different corporate entities or premises. If your company operates at a number of sites you need a licence for each one individually. It is your responsibility to ensure you keep pace with any legislative changes and obtain new licences if needed. You must hold all relevant licences before handling controlled substances.

Prospective licensees must register to use the Drug and Precursor Chemical web application portal and all applications must be submitted electronically. Registration is not automatic and those requesting a user login must be able to show that their business proposals would be lawful and, in principle, have a prospect of success. Prospective licensees looking to handle cannabinoid products should pay particular attention to the Home Office guidance at https://www.gov.uk/government/publications/cannabis-cbd-and-other-cannabinoids-drug-licensing-factsheet. Registrations or applications made without a lawful route to market will be rejected.

If a user registration is accepted it will enable a licensing application to be made, but it is no guarantee that one will succeed. The fees payable are listed here: https://www.gov.uk/government/collections/drugs-licensing

Import–export licences are issued for individual consignments and can only be sought after the company has obtained the relevant domestic licence using the process set out above.

Further information is available at:

Drugs licensing – https://www.gov.uk/government/collections/drugs-licensing

Precursor chemical licensing – https://www.gov.uk/guidance/precursor-chemical-licensing

Use of the mandatory requisition form for Schedule 2 and 3 controlled drugs

On 30 November 2015 legislative provisions came into effect that made it mandatory for specified health and veterinary care professionals, and organisations listed at Regulation 14(4) of the Misuse of Drugs Regulations 2001, to use an approved form for the requisitioning of Schedule 2 and 3 controlled drugs. This change, which the Home Office consulted on in 2011, implemented a final recommendation of the Shipman Inquiry on requisitions.[21]

Following the introduction of the form, the Home Office has been made aware that activities within the hospital sector, which would normally be governed by provisions under Regulation 14(6), and which were not expected to come within the scope of the new requirement, is now captured as a result of changes in the NHS structures in recent years. This is

---

[21] https://www.gov.uk/government/publications/circular-0272015-approved-mandatory-requisition-form-and-home-office-approved-wording/circular-0272015-approved-mandatory-requisition-form-and-home-office-approved-wording

an unintended consequence of the changes to NHS structures and health-care delivery since 2011 rather than a result of a regulatory change.

The Home Office circular that introduced the change made it clear that the requirement to use the mandatory form was to be limited to activities undertaken by health and veterinary care practitioners in the community to enable their requisition activities to be monitored. The requirement to use a mandatory form was not expected to extend to the hospital environment, where traditionally supplies of controlled drugs were undertaken by an on-site pharmacy owned by the hospital and under the Regulation 14(6) provisions.

This additional guidance is therefore being issued to further explain how the provisions governing the use of the new mandatory form may be interpreted. This guidance does not impact on the need for a Home Office licence. The guidance should also not be interpreted as a change in Home Office licensing requirements, which these regulatory and procedural requirements relate to but are not necessarily interdependent on.

(1) The use of the form is mandatory when individual health and veterinary care professionals requisition the relevant controlled drugs in the community, including when such drugs are ordered from pharmaceutical wholesalers and community pharmacies.

(2) It is not the intention of the policy on requisitions forms to capture requisition activities for hospital wards, etc. However, as a number of hospitals wards now obtain the relevant controlled drugs from other trusts or organisations, and therefore across legal entities, these activities do fall within the scope of Regulation 14(2) and therefore the use of the form is mandatory, unless an exemption applies (e.g. registered pharmacies are completely excluded from the requirement to use a requisition when obtaining the relevant controlled drugs). In order to ensure that the regulatory provisions are complied with, it is the view of the Home Office that the person in charge or acting person in charge of a hospital or care home (excluding hospices) can issue a "bulk" or "global" requisition based on previous years' orders to a separate legal entity that supplies its wards. Hospital or Trust wards can then draw on this "bulk" requisition throughout the year using the duplicate order forms as happens presently. Hospital or Trust wards therefore do not need to use the mandatory form when obtaining the relevant controlled drugs from another trust or legal entity. Similarly, the person in charge or acting person in charge of an Ambulance Trust, as defined under the 2001 Regulations, can issue a "bulk" requisition when obtaining the relevant controlled drugs to be supplied directly to employees of the Trust by a separate legal entity. However, those employees, when individually drawing on the "bulk" requisition, must use the mandatory form.

(3) Additionally, pharmaceutical wholesale suppliers (excluding community pharmacies) are exempt under current regulatory provisions from submitting requisitions received for Schedule 2 and 3 controlled drugs to the NHS Business Services Authority (NHSBSA). The only requisition forms that must be submitted to the NHSBSA following the introduction of the mandatory form are those provided by individual healthcare professionals when obtaining the relevant controlled drugs in the community.

The table below provides some examples of how the regulations apply in specific circumstances with reference to Regulations 14(2) and (4). This is only a Home Office view and does not constitute legal advice. Organisations are advised to seek their own independent legal advice where appropriate. This guidance has been developed with the Department of Health and Social Care and the Care Quality Commission.

Supplier	Recipient	Do I need to use the new FP10CDF?	Do I need to submit the FP10 CDF to the NHSBSA?
Wholesaler	Practitioners Paramedics and the other professionals and organisations listed in Regulation 14(4)	Yes, all practitioners and the list of healthcare professionals must use the form when they requisition for stocks	No, the Regulation exempts the submission of requisitions received by wholesalers from being sent to the NHSBSA
Wholesaler	Registered pharmacy (including a hospital registered pharmacy)	NO	N/A
Wholesaler	Hospital, care home or ambulance trust without a registered pharmacy **Excludes hospices	Yes, in line with Regulation 14	No, the regulation exempts the submission of requisitions received by wholesalers from being sent to the NHSBSA
Legal entity A	Legal entity B's hospital wards	Yes, person in charge of legal entity B must issue a yearly global requisition to legal entity A. Wards in legal entity B can then draw on this requisition through the year using duplicate order books	NO
Legal entity A	Legal entity B's registered pharmacy	NO	N/A
Legal entity A	Legal entity B	Yes if organisation is listed at Regulation 14(4)	NO

Controls on strategic goods and drugs useable in execution by lethal injection

The Export Control Organisation (ECO), part of the Department for Business, Innovation and Skills, issues licences for controlling the export of strategic goods. The range of goods and services covered by embargoes and sanctions is extensive, changes from time to time and includes:

- military equipment;
- dual-use goods that can be used for both civil and military purposes;
- products used for torture;
- radioactive sources.

These may apply to medical devices, finished medical products or Active Substances.

ECO also administers controls on trade in certain goods that could be used for capital punishment, torture or other cruel, inhuman or degrading treatment or punishment. This includes the control on the export of certain drugs usable in execution by lethal injection.

As a result of these controls, exporters need to seek appropriate permission from national export control authorities to export to any destination outside the UK, short and intermediate acting barbiturate anaesthetic agents, including, but not limited to, the following:

- amobarbital (CAS RN 57-43-2);
- amobarbital sodium salt (CAS RN 64-43-7);
- pentobarbital (CAS RN 76-74-4);
- pentobarbital sodium salt (CAS 57-33-0);
- secobarbital (CAS RN 76-73-3);
- secobarbital sodium salt (CAS RN 309-43-3);
- thiopental (CAS RN 76-75-5);
- thiopental sodium salt (CAS RN 71-73-8), also known as thiopentone sodium.

The control also applies to products containing one or more of the above. These controls are intended to apply to finished products – in other words, those that are packaged for human or veterinary use. It is not intended that they should apply to raw materials or to intermediate products (i.e. products that require further processing to make them suitable for human or veterinary use).

It is the responsibility of a wholesale dealer to ensure that they export responsibly and within the law. ECO provide training for exporters of strategic goods. Further information on training and licensing can be found on the GOV.UK website[22].

---

[22] https://www.gov.uk/controls-on-torture-goods
https://www.gov.uk/government/organisations/export-control-organisation

Control of lisdexamfetamine, tramadol, zaleplon, zopiclone and reclassification of ketamine

On 10 June 2014, the Parliamentary Order controlling and, in the case of ketamine, reclassifying the following drugs, came into force:

- lisdexamfetamine;
- tramadol;
- zaleplon;
- zopiclone;
- medicines containing these substances.

The Order, available on legislation.gov.uk, controls:

- lisdexamfetamine as a Class B drug;
- tramadol as a Class C drug;
- zopiclone and zaleplon as Class C drugs.

The Order also reclassifies ketamine as a Class B drug under the Misuse of Drugs Act 1971.

Companies that possess, supply or produce lisdexamfetamine, tramadol, zaleplon, zopiclone (or medicines containing these substances) need to get the correct licences from the Home Office.

More information on how to apply for a licence, and how much they cost are available on GOV.UK at https://www.gov.uk/controlled-drugs-licences-fees-and-returns or by calling the Duty Compliance Officer on 020 7035 8972.

Companies without the correct licences are at risk of prosecution.

The listed drugs will be scheduled, alongside their control, as follows to ensure that they remain available for use in healthcare:

- Lisdexamfetamine (a drug that converts to dexamfetamine when administered orally and used as second-line treatment for ADHD) will be listed in Schedule 2 alongside dexamfetamine.
- Tramadol will be listed in Schedule 3 but exempted from the safe custody requirements. Full prescription writing requirements under Regulation 15 will apply to its use in healthcare.
- Zopiclone and zaleplon will be listed in Part 1 of Schedule 4 alongside zolpidem.

Ketamine is not being rescheduled immediately. In line with the Advisory Council on the Misuse of Drugs' (ACMD) advice, the Home Office will carry out a public consultation later this year to assess the impact of rescheduling ketamine to Schedule 2.

A final decision on the appropriate schedule for ketamine will be made after the consultation. Until then, ketamine will remain a Schedule 4 Part 1 drug.

Home Office Circular 008/2014: A change to the Misuse of Drugs Act 1971 – Control of NBOMes, Benzofurans, Lisdexamphetamine, Tramadol, Zopiclone, Zaleplon and Reclassification of Ketamine[23].

Controls and authorisations applying to those handling medicinal products derived from blood

The MHRA is responsible for the controls and authorisations that apply to blood establishments (BEs) and controls that apply to hospital blood banks (HBBs) and sites that collect, test and supply human blood or blood components intended for transfusion. Further information can be obtained from the GOV.UK website[24].

Procurement, storage, distribution and disposal of vaccines

GDP applies to all vaccine wholesale activities. The supply chain in the UK and guidance on who may receive these, how the end user should store them and how they should be disposed of are further described in *Immunisation Against Infectious Disease*, commonly known as the green book. This can be found on the GOV.UK website[25].

In the event of a pandemic there are steps that the government can take to authorise certain activities such as allowing wholesalers to amend expiry dates on frozen products when they are removed from frozen to refrigerated status.

Wholesale of radiopharmaceuticals

Many activities will fall under Good Manufacturing Practice Annex 3, as well as GDP. Further guidance from the marketing authorisation must be followed.

Wholesale of veterinary medicinal products

The Veterinary Medicines Regulations 2013 [SI 2013/2033] came into force on 1 October 2013. A wholesaler of veterinary products will usually be required to hold a WDA(V). The regulations require that the holder must:

---

[23] https://www.gov.uk/government/publications/circular-0082014-changes-to-the-misuse-of-drugs-act-1971

[24] https://www.gov.uk/guidance/blood-authorisations-and-safety-reporting

[25] https://www.gov.uk/government/collections/immunisation-against-infectious-disease-the-green-book#the-green-book

(a) store veterinary medicinal products in accordance with the terms of the marketing authorisation for each product;

(b) comply with the Guidelines on Good Distribution Practice of Medicinal Products for Human Use as if the veterinary medicinal products were authorised human medicinal products;

(c) carry out a detailed stock audit at least once a year; and

(d) supply information and samples to the Secretary of State on demand.

Further information in relation to import and export, the cascade, record keeping, controlled drugs and other veterinary wholesale activities can be found on the GOV.UK website[26].

Sales Representative Samples

Under the legislation on advertising medicines, companies may only provide free samples to persons qualified to prescribe the medicine. Samples may only be supplied in response to a signed and dated request from the prescriber and must be appropriately labelled and accompanied by a copy of the Summary of Product Characteristics (SPC). The company must have adequate procedures for control and accountability for all samples. See section 6.12 of MHRA's Blue Guide for details of the legal requirements.

The MHRA is aware that in some cases sales representatives receive samples to fill prescriber requests and that the medicinal products are delivered to them by colleagues or by couriers. Either way, the storage and delivery arrangements for these medicinal products must be validated to ensure the medicinal product will be transported expeditiously under controlled Good Distribution Practice (GDP) conditions and in accordance with labelled storage requirements at all times. It is highly unlikely that samples requiring refrigeration will meet these requirements. With regard to storage it is not acceptable for samples to be stored in the representative's home (on unlicensed premises, which are not GDP compliant), lacking appropriate storage facilities, security and controls to maintain the quality of the medicines and provide an audit trail.

Likewise, distribution of samples involving delivery in a representative's vehicle that has no provision for maintaining correct storage conditions is also unacceptable. Temperatures in a car boot in high summer could reach 50 degrees Celsius or go below 0 degrees Celsius in winter. The practice of providing sales representatives with samples of medicinal products that they retain for onward distribution is therefore unlikely to be acceptable

---

[26] https://www.gov.uk/government/organisations/veterinary-medicines-directorate

due to the storage and transport difficulties outlined above. The only reason for which sales representatives may hold samples on a long-term basis is for the purpose of product identification. In this regard procedures must be in place to ensure accountability for any such stock and to ensure no packs are provided to healthcare professionals.

Diverted Medicines

Diversion is the term used for the fraudulent activity where medicines destined for non-GB or UK markets re-enter the supply chain and are placed back on to the market at a higher price.

The diversion of medicines involves medicinal products being offered at preferential prices and exported to specific markets (normally third countries) outside GB or the UK. Diversion occurs when unscrupulous traders, on receipt of the medicines, re-export the products back to GB or the UK – with the consequence that patients for whom these preferentially priced medicines were intended, are denied access to them. Such products appearing on the market are then known as "diverted" from their intended market. This represents not only a corrupt diversion for profit, but such activity also poses the risk of inappropriate or unlicensed use, and the risk that the product may also be compromised due to poor storage and transportation.

As with counterfeit and falsified products, wholesale dealers in particular should maintain a high level of vigilance against the procurement or supply of potentially diverted product. Diverted products may be offered for sale below the established market value, therefore appropriate checks should be made on the bona fides of the supplier and the origin of the product should be ascertained.

Chapter 6 Complaints, Returns, Suspected Falsified Medicinal Products and Medicinal Product Recalls

6.1 Principle

All complaints, returns, suspected falsified medicinal products and recalls must be recorded and handled carefully according to written procedures. Records should be made available to the competent authorities. An assessment of returned medicinal products should be performed before any approval for resale. A consistent approach by all partners in the supply chain is required in order to be successful in the fight against falsified medicinal products.

6.2   Complaints

Complaints should be recorded with all the original details. A distinction should be made between complaints related to the quality of a medicinal product and those related to distribution. In the event of a complaint about the quality of a medicinal product and a potential product defect, the manufacturer and/or marketing authorisation holder should be informed without delay. Any product distribution complaint should be thoroughly investigated to identify the origin of or reason for the complaint.

A person should be appointed to handle complaints and allocated sufficient support personnel.

If necessary, appropriate follow-up actions (including CAPA) should be taken after investigation and evaluation of the complaint, including, where required, notification to the national competent authorities.

6.3   Returned medicinal products

Returned products must be handled according to a written, risk-based process taking into account the product concerned, any specific storage requirements and the time elapsed since the medicinal product was originally dispatched. Returns should be conducted in accordance with national law and contractual arrangements between the parties.

Medicinal products which have left the premises of the distributor should only be returned to saleable stock if all of the following are confirmed:

(i)   the medicinal products are in their unopened and undamaged secondary packaging and are in good condition; have not expired and have not been recalled;

(ii)   medicinal products returned from a customer not holding a wholesale distribution authorisation or from pharmacies authorised to supply medicinal products to the public should only be returned to saleable stock if they are returned within an acceptable time limit, for example 10 days;

(iii) it has been demonstrated by the customer that the medicinal products have been transported, stored and handled in compliance with their specific storage requirements;

(iv)   they have been examined and assessed by a sufficiently trained and competent person authorised to do so;

(v)   the distributor has reasonable evidence that the product was supplied to that customer (via copies of the original delivery note or by referencing invoice numbers, etc.) and the batch number for products bearing the safety features is known, and that there is no reason to believe that the product has been falsified.

Moreover, for medicinal products requiring specific temperature storage conditions such as low temperature, returns to saleable stock can

EU GUIDELINES ON GDP AND UK GUIDANCE ON WHOLESALE DISTRIBUTION only be made if there is documented evidence that the product has been stored under the authorised storage conditions throughout the entire time. If any deviation has occurred a risk assessment has to be performed, on which basis the integrity of the product can be demonstrated. The evidence should cover:

(i)   delivery to customer;
(ii)   examination of the product;
(iii) opening of the transport packaging;
(iv)   return of the product to the packaging;
(v)   collection and return to the distributor;
(vi)   return to the distribution site refrigerator.

Products returned to saleable stock should be placed such that the 'first expired first out' (FEFO) system operates effectively.

Stolen products that have been recovered cannot be returned to saleable stock and sold to customers.

6.4   Falsified medicinal products

Wholesale distributors must immediately inform the competent authority and the marketing authorisation holder of any medicinal products they identify as falsified or suspect to be falsified[27]. A procedure should be in place to this effect. It should be recorded with all the original details and investigated.

Any falsified medicinal products found in the supply chain should immediately be physically segregated and stored in a dedicated area away from all other medicinal products. All relevant activities in relation to such products should be documented and records retained[27].

6.5   Medicinal product recalls

The effectiveness of the arrangements for product recall should be evaluated regularly (at least annually).

Recall operations should be capable of being initiated promptly and at any time.

The distributor must follow the instructions of a recall message, which should be approved, if required, by the competent authorities.

Any recall operation should be recorded at the time it is carried out. Records should be made readily available to the competent authorities.

The distribution records should be readily accessible to the person(s) responsible for the recall, and should contain sufficient information on

[27] Article 80(i) of Directive 2001/83/EC.

distributors and directly supplied customers (with addresses, telephone and/or fax numbers inside and outside working hours, batch numbers at least for medicinal products bearing safety features as required by legislation and quantities delivered), including those for exported products and medicinal product samples.

The progress of the recall process should be recorded for a final report.

UK Guidance on Chapter 6 Complaints, Returns, Suspected Falsified Medicinal Products and Medicinal Product Recalls

Handling Returns

Returns of refrigerated medicinal products

Because of the inherent dangers of returning refrigerated products, many licensed wholesale dealers will not consider refrigerated returns for subsequent resale in any event. All such returns are immediately stored in a dedicated and marked area awaiting collection by a licensed disposal company.

In the event of a licensed wholesale dealer accepting a return of a refrigerated product, possibly because of its high monetary value, the product should be returned in accordance with MHRA guidance (below), in an appropriate method of transport, with supporting documentation, such as a returns form. The returns form would normally include the reason for the return, contain details of the product and how it has been stored and should be signed by an authorised and identifiable signatory.

A trained person at the wholesalers should examine the returned product to check for tampering and to confirm that the return has been made in accordance with MHRA guidance. If this examination cannot be undertaken immediately, the product should be stored in a dedicated and marked area in a refrigerator until the checks can be made.

Provided the checks are satisfactory and are documented, the product may then be returned to saleable stock. MHRA guidance on managing returned non-defective (ambient) and refrigerated medicinal products is provided below.

Returns of non-defective medicinal products

Any person acting as a wholesale distributor must hold a wholesale dealer's licence.

Regulation 43(1) of the Human Medicines Regulations 2012[28], as amended, provides that distributors of human medicines must comply with the guidelines for Good Distribution Practice (GDP).

---

[28] SI 2012 No. 1916.

Chapter 6.3 of the GDP Guidelines refers to returned medicinal products, the key elements being that:

"Medicinal products that have left the premises of the distributor should only be returned to saleable stock if …:

(i)   the medicinal products are in their unopened and undamaged secondary packaging and are in good condition; have not expired and have not been recalled;

(ii)   medicinal products returned from a customer not holding a wholesale distribution authorisation or from pharmacies authorised to supply medicinal products to the public should only be returned to saleable stock if they are returned within an acceptable time limit, for example 10 days;

(iii)   it has been demonstrated by the customer that the medicinal products have been transported, stored and handled in compliance with their specific storage requirements;

(iv)   they have been examined and assessed by a sufficiently trained and competent person authorised to do so;

(v)   the distributor has reasonable evidence that the product was supplied to that customer (via copies of the original delivery note or by referencing invoice numbers, etc.) and the batch number for products bearing the safety features is known, and that there is no reason to believe that the product has been falsified."

Definition of licensed and unlicensed sites

The MHRA re-affirms that a licensed site can only be interpreted as being under full GDP control at a licensed wholesale dealer. This applies to all categories of medicines. Medicinal products held in unlicensed storage and distribution sites are not considered to be within the licensed wholesale distribution network.

AMBIENT RETURNS FROM A LICENSED WHOLESALE DEALER'S SITE

The MHRA will adopt a pragmatic approach to the return of non-defective medicinal products for those products returned from a customer operating from a licensed wholesale dealer authorisation (WDA) site.

In such circumstances, the return should be completed as expeditiously as possible and the most expedient and appropriate method of transportation must be used.

The Responsible Person or the authorised person receiving the return, must be able to demonstrate evidence of "full knowledge" of the storage of the returned products throughout the period it has been with the customer, including transportation.

AMBIENT RETURNS FROM AN UNLICENSED SITE

For those non-defective ambient medicinal products returned from an unlicensed site, the return should be completed within 5 days, including transport.

The Responsible Person or the authorised person must be able to demonstrate evidence of "full knowledge" of the storage while at the unlicensed site, including transportation.

REFRIGERATED RETURNS FROM A LICENSED WHOLESALE DEALER'S SITE

The MHRA will adopt a pragmatic approach to the return of non-defective medicinal products for those products returned from a customer operating from a licensed WDA site.

In such circumstances, the return should be completed expeditiously and the most expedient and appropriate method of transportation must be used.

The Responsible Person or the authorised person receiving the return, must be able to demonstrate evidence of "full knowledge" of the storage of the returned products throughout the period it has been with the customer, including transportation.

REFRIGERATED RETURNS FROM AN UNLICENSED SITE

For those non-defective refrigerated medicinal products returned from an unlicensed site, the return should be completed within 24 hours, including transport.

The Responsible Person or the authorised person must be able to demonstrate evidence of "full knowledge" of the storage while at the unlicensed site, including transportation.

Falsified Medicines

A "falsified medicinal product" means any medicinal product with a false representation of:

(a) its identity, including its packaging and labelling, its name or its composition (other than any unintentional quality defect) as regards any of its ingredients, including excipients and the strength of those ingredients;
(b) its source, including its manufacturer, its country of manufacturing, its country of origin or its marketing authorisation holder; or
(c) its history, including the records and documents relating to the distribution channels used.

The supply of falsified medicines is a global phenomenon and one that the MHRA takes very seriously. Falsified medicines represent a threat to the legitimate UK supply chain and to patient safety. They are fraudulent and may be deliberately misrepresented with respect to identity, composition and/or source. Falsification can apply to both innovator and generic products, prescription and self-medication, as well as to traditional herbal remedies. Falsified medicines may include products with the correct ingredients but fake packaging, with the wrong ingredients, without active ingredients or with insufficient active ingredients, and may even contain harmful or poisonous substances.

The supply and distribution of medicines are tightly controlled.

All licensed wholesalers must comply with good distribution practice (GDP) and there exist strict licensing and regulatory requirements in UK domestic legislation to safeguard patients against potential hazards arising from poor distribution practices, e.g. purchasing suspect or falsified products, failing to establish the "bona fides" of suppliers and purchasers, inadequate record keeping, and so on.

Section 6.4 of GDP is of principal importance to wholesale dealers. This states:

"Wholesale distributors must immediately inform the competent authority and the marketing authorisation holder of any medicinal products they identify as falsified or suspect to be falsified[29]. A procedure should be in place to this effect. It should be recorded with all the original details and investigated.

Any falsified medicinal products found in the supply chain should immediately be physically segregated and stored in a dedicated area away from all other medicinal products. All relevant activities in relation to such products should be documented and records retained."

Wholesale dealers in particular should maintain a high level of vigilance against the procurement or supply of potentially falsified product. Such product may be offered for sale below the established market price so rigorous checks should be made on the bona fides of the supplier and the origin of the product. Staff should always be alert to any unusual activities and have a formal mechanism by which they can raise their concerns.

It is known that some wholesalers are themselves developing good practice strategies – such as conducting rigorous physical inspections of packs when grey market purchases are made – and this is encouraged.

Safeguarding examples include the following (this list is not exhaustive):

- what boxes are the stock arriving in – are these unusual in anyway or indicate that maybe they have been stored elsewhere before coming to you?
- deliveries in taxis/personal cars – ask yourself: under what situation would this be acceptable?
- if you reject the delivery and it is returned to the supplier, where is it being returned to – a different address to where you expect?
- significant errors in contents of delivery compared to delivery notes.

---

[29] 83/83/EC.

- large orders becoming unexpectedly available – even if at "normal price". Why would they become available? Where have these come from? Investigate further. Ensure procurement staff are trained to understand indicators of potentially falsified stock.

Any suspicious activity should be reported to:
- **E-mail:** casereferrals@mhra.gov.uk
- **Telephone:** +44 (0)20 3080 6330

To report suspected counterfeit medicines or medical devices:
- **E-mail:** fakemeds@mhra.gov.uk
- **Website:** www.mhra.gov.uk
- **Telephone:** +44 (0)20 3080 6701

Reporting Adverse Reactions

An adverse reaction means a response to a medicinal product that is noxious and unintended. A serious adverse reaction is one that results in a person's death, threatens a person's life, results in hospitalisation, persistent or significant disability/incapacity, or results in a congenital abnormality or birth defect.

Wholesalers supplying special medicinal products (unlicensed products) are under an obligation to keep records of any adverse reaction of which they become aware and report any serious adverse reaction to the MHRA; this should be done by submission of a "Yellow Card"[30] report.

Where the product is an exempt advanced therapy medicinal product, the wholesaler is obliged to inform MHRA of any adverse reaction of which they become aware. All records should be retained for the minimum periods required by UK legislation.

Marketing authorisation, homoeopathic registration and traditional herbal medicinal product licence holders have separate obligations in relation to tracking and reporting adverse reactions.

Product Recall/Withdrawal

Manufacturers, importers and distributors are obliged to inform the MHRA of any suspected quality defect in a medicinal product that could or would result in a recall, or restriction on supply.

A defective medicinal product is one whose quality does not conform to the requirements of its marketing authorisation, specification or for some

---

[30] https://yellowcard.mhra.gov.uk/

other reason of quality is potentially hazardous. A defective product may be suspected because of a visible defect or contamination or as a result of tests performed on it, or because it has caused untoward reactions in a patient or for other reasons involving poor manufacturing or distribution practice. Falsified medicines are considered as defective products.

The Human Medicines Regulations 2012 impose certain obligations on licence holders with regard to withdrawal and recall from sale. The aim of the Defective Medicines Report Centre (DMRC) within the MHRA is to minimise the hazard to patients arising from the distribution of defective (human) medicinal products by providing an emergency assessment and communications system between the suppliers (manufacturers and distributors), the regulatory authorities and the end user. The DMRC achieves this by receiving reports of suspected defective (human) medicinal products, monitoring and, as far as is necessary, directing and advising actions by the relevant licence holder(s) and communicating the details of this action with the appropriate urgency and distribution to users of the products. The communication normally used is a "Medicines Recall/Notification".

Immediately a hazard is identified from any source, it will be necessary to evaluate the level of danger, and the category of recall, if required. Where the reported defect is a confirmed defect, the DMRC will then take one of the following courses of action and obtain a report from the manufacturer on the nature of the defect, their handling of the defect and action to be taken to prevent its recurrence.

Issue a "recall"

Under normal circumstances a recall is always required where a defect is confirmed unless the defect is shown to be of a trivial nature and/or there are unlikely to be significant amounts of the affected product remaining in the market.

It is the licence holder's responsibility to recall products from customers, in a manner agreed with the DMRC. The company should provide copies of draft recall letters for agreement with the DMRC. If the company (licence holder) does not agree to a recall voluntarily, the MHRA, as licensing authority, may be obliged to take compulsory action.

Issue a "Medicines Recall/Notification"

Recall and withdrawal of product from the market are normally the responsibility of the licence holder. However, where a product has been distributed widely and/or there is a serious risk to health from the defect, the MHRA can opt to issue a Medicines Recall/Notification letter. The Medicines Recall/Notification cascade mechanism ensures rapid communication of safety information; it is not a substitute for, but complementary to, any action taken by the licence holder. The text of the Medicines Recall/Notification should be agreed between the MHRA and the company concerned.

In some cases, where a product has been supplied to a small number of known customers, the MHRA may decide that notification will be adequate and a Medicines Recall/Notification is not needed.

The DMRC may also request companies to insert notification in the professional press in certain cases.

Management of the recall

The company should directly contact wholesalers, hospitals, retail pharmacies and overseas distributors supplied. The DMRC is likely to take the lead in notifying Regional Contacts for NHS Trusts and Provider Units and Health Authorities, special and government hospitals and overseas regulatory authorities.

The DMRC will liaise with the company and discuss arrangements for the recall, requesting the dates that supply started and ceased and a copy of any letters sent out by that company concerning the recall. Again, it is desirable that the text of the notices sent via the company and by the DMRC should be mutually agreed.

Management of recall activity by wholesalers

The MHRA expects key personnel, such as the Responsible Person, to keep themselves up to date with medicines safety issues. This can be done, for example, by checking the relevant sections of the MHRA's website daily or alternatively by signing up for relevant MHRA e-mail alerts.

Wholesalers and brokers should retain records of all Medicines Recall/Notifications received and/or reviewed, including those notices for which no action is required.

Recall processes should be designed with quality management in mind, e.g. change control and risk management should be applied for significant changes such as a change of Responsible Person or nominated deputy, changes to product handling/storage or changes to transport arrangements. At such times there should be an assessment of whether a test recall should be performed to provide assurance of the ongoing effectiveness of the company's processes and identify any weaknesses or areas for improvement.

Chapter 6, section 5 of the GDP Guidelines describes the minimum standards for wholesalers in relation to recall activities.

When the wholesaler receives a Medicines Recall/Notification they should take steps to:

- follow the detail of the recall message;
- identify any affected stock on site or in transit (including that returned from customers);
- identify any customers to whom the affected products have been supplied, including where products may have been supplied as samples;
- directly contact those customers, making them aware of the details of the recall and where necessary providing a mechanism for returning affected stock;
- physically segregate and quarantine any affected product in an area away from other medicinal products, ensuring that such stock does not re-enter the supply chain;
- reconcile the quantities of stock purchased, onsite, sent out and returned;
- keep recall notices open for an appropriate period, so as to capture any affected stock still moving through the supply chain.

All recall activities should be documented at the time they occur and at the conclusion of all recall activities the Responsible Person (or their nominated deputy) should produce a report, making an objective assessment of whether the recall process achieved its objectives and identifying any areas requiring improvement.

Testing the recall process

Section 6.5 of the EU GDP Guidelines requires that "the effectiveness of the arrangements for product recall should be evaluated regularly (at least annually)".

The aim of such an evaluation should be to challenge the internal processes of the licence holder as far as practicable. This is particularly important in organisations where recall activities occur infrequently, e.g. where the product range handled is limited in quantity or scope. Where stock is held on behalf of a licence holder at a third-party site then the recall test should extend to covering activities at the third party site; this will require a degree of liaison between both sites' Responsible Persons.

The test process should be described in the company's quality system in sufficient detail to allow staff to perform the test and to be able to assess the progress of the recall process at each step.

It is expected that as a minimum the test process should mimic a real recall but should stop short of contacting the licence holder's customers. The product and batch selected should be typical of those handled by the company in the previous 12 months and where possible provide a worst case scenario (e.g. when key staff are absent or for essential medicines when alternative supplies may need to be made available). Correspondence (e.g. e-mails to staff at a branch level) should, as far as practicable, not indicate that it is being used for test purposes.

The test process should be documented so as to be able to demonstrate that:

- staff can receive information effectively and act on it quickly;
- stock in question can be identified, reconciled and segregated effectively;
- customers supplied with the stock can be identified quickly from records, and their most up-to-date contact details confirmed (including address and telephone details both inside and outside working hours);
- adherence to the company's recall process has taken place;
- the effectiveness of training can be assessed.

For the purposes of a test recall the MHRA does not normally expect licence holders to contact their customers as this could lead to unintended consequences should the customer believe the test recall to be real. Instead, the licence holder should obtain evidence that the contact details (physical address, telephone/fax numbers, e-mail address) they hold for the relevant customers are up to date. Where the licence holder would send a letter/fax/e-mail to their customer with the details of the recall, this should be drafted but not sent.

Where customers are contacted, there should be adequate oversight of the entire test process to ensure that misunderstandings do not occur.

As with all routine recall activities, at the conclusion of test recall activities the Responsible Person should produce a report, making an objective assessment of whether the recall process achieved its objectives and identifying any areas requiring improvement.

It may be possible for a company to use recall activities for non-medicinal products to demonstrate an effective recall process, provided that the process described in the company's quality system covers the handling of both medicinal and non-medicinal products in the same manner and leads to the same outcome.

Follow-up action

The DMRC will monitor the conduct and success of the recall by the manufacturer or distributor. As follow-up action, it may be necessary to consider any or all of the following:

- arrange a visit to the licence holder/manufacturer/distributor;
- arrange a visit to the point of discovery of the defect;
- refer to the Inspectorate to arrange an inspection;
- seek special surveillance of adverse reaction reports;
- refer the matter for adverse licensing and/or enforcement action.

Reporting a suspected defect

Suspected defects can be reported by telephone, e-mail or letter or using our online form:

- **Address:** DMRC, 10 South Colannade, London, E14 4PU, UK
- **Telephone:** +44 (0)20 3080 6574 (08:45–16:45 Monday to Friday)
- **Telephone:** +44 (0)7795 641532 (urgent calls outside working hours, at weekends or on public holidays)
- **E-mail:** dmrc@mhra.gov.uk
- **Online form:** https://yellowcard.mhra.gov.uk/

Wholesale distributors and pharmacovigilance

MHRA Good Distribution Practice (GDP) inspectors have received queries from wholesaler distributors asking in what instances agreements are required between the marketing authorisation holder (MAH) and wholesale distributors for the purposes of fulfilling pharmacovigilance requirements.

If a wholesale distributor could potentially receive safety-related information on behalf of the MAH, or if they are providing a service relating to pharmacovigilance, then they are effectively part of the MAH's pharmacovigilance system. In this situation, contracts or agreements between the MAH and wholesale distributor need to exist, in order for the MAH to ensure that activities performed and services provided by these third parties are in accordance with applicable legislation and guidelines, and in order to ensure that all parties understand and formally agree to the tasks that have been contracted. The terms contract and agreement are used synonymously.

PROVISIONS IN PUBLISHED GUIDELINES TO CONSIDER

The Good Pharmacovigilance Practices (GVP) are a set of measures drawn up to facilitate the performance of pharmacovigilance. UK-specific requirements are described in the "Exceptions and modifications to the EU guidance on good pharmacovigilance practices that apply to UK marketing authorisation holders and the licensing authority."

GVP Module VI.2.2 states that "Each marketing authorisation holder shall have in place a system for the collection and recording of all reports of suspected adverse reactions which are brought to its attention". As indicated earlier, wholesale distributors may be a potential source of safety information. Hence, the MAH will need to have a mechanism to collect reports of adverse reactions received by wholesaler distributors.

GVP Module VI.B.7 outlines the reason why agreements between the MAH and wholesale distributors may be required "Where the marketing authorisation holder has set up contractual arrangements with a person or an organisation, explicit procedures and detailed agreements should exist between the marketing authorisation holder and the person/organisation to ensure that the marketing authorisation holder can comply with the reporting obligations. These procedures should in particular specify the processes for exchange of safety information, including timelines and regulatory reporting responsibilities and should avoid duplicate reporting to the competent authorities".

As reports of suspected adverse reactions may be brought to the attention of wholesale distributors, agreements between the MAH and the wholesale distributor support the fulfilment of the collection and recording of these reports by the MAH.

Indeed, section 6.3 of the Good Distribution Practice of medicinal products for human use states "In the event of a complaint about the quality of a medicinal product and a potential product defect, the manufacturer and/or marketing authorisation holder should be informed without delay". Complaints received by wholesale distributors may include reports of suspected adverse drug reactions and should be forwarded to the MAH; the implementation of an agreement between the parties may help facilitate this activity.

FACTORS INFLUENCING WHETHER AN AGREEMENT IS REQUIRED

The MAH needs to assess if the wholesale distributor they have engaged with is a potential source of safety information (such as reports of adverse reactions, medical enquiries or product quality complaints), and/or are providing pharmacovigilance services on behalf of the MAH, and whether an agreement is required to fulfil pharmacovigilance requirements. Some factors that are likely to result in an agreement being required include:

- if the name and/or contact details of the wholesale distributor appears on product packaging, the patient information leaflet (PIL) or the MAH's website;
- if the MAH does not have a contactable presence in the market where the product is being distributed, which may increase the likelihood of the wholesale distributor becoming a point of contact by a member of the public or healthcare professionals (HCPs);
- if the wholesale distributor is providing services that may increase their interaction with HCPs and the likelihood of receiving safety information, such as actively promoting products via a sales team;
- if the wholesale distributor is performing pharmacovigilance services on behalf of the MAH, e.g. undertaking follow-up of adverse events in their territory on behalf of the MAH, undertaking local literature searching activities or distributing risk minimisation materials.

The above list is not intended to be exhaustive and the MAH should consider all factors that may result in the wholesale distributor becoming part of the MAH's pharmacovigilance system.

There may be situations when an agreement is not required, e.g. if the wholesale distributor is not in a contractual relationship with the MAH and would not be regarded as a potential source of safety information and thus would not form part of the MAH's pharmacovigilance system.

CONTENT OF AGREEMENTS

If an agreement between the MAH and the wholesale distributor is required, it should contain sufficient detail to ensure that pharmacovigilance requirements are met. It is the responsibility of the MAH to decide what provisions need to be included in these agreements, particularly considering the content required in agreements may vary depending on the parties involved. Some provisions that the MAH may wish to consider in agreements are outlined below; however, this list is not intended to be exhaustive and the MAH should use their judgement when deciding what information should be included in agreements:

- the roles and responsibilities of each party;
- the types of safety information that should be collected and forwarded to the MAH by the wholesale distributor (e.g. suspected adverse reactions, lack of efficacy reports, product quality complaints, etc.);
- timeframes for the exchange of safety information between parties and case confirmation and/or reconciliation provisions;
- contact details of where the wholesale distributor should send safety information received to;
- how the transfer of outstanding safety information to the MAH will be handled should commercial arrangements be terminated;
- provision for the oversight of the wholesale distributor by the MAH (e.g. in process compliance measures and the right of the MAH to audit the wholesale distributor).

The MAH should consider how to ensure all parties are complying with the terms of the agreements, such as including wholesale distribution partners on the MAH's risk-based audit programme, or implementing routine checks of pharmacovigilance relevant wholesale distributor activity, such as periodic reconciliation of reports of adverse events between the distributor and the MAH that may identify discrepancies in information exchanged.

CONCLUSION

In conclusion, when deciding if an agreement between the MAH and the wholesale distributor is required, the MAH needs to consider if the wholesale distributor is a potential source of safety information and/or performing pharmacovigilance tasks on behalf of the MAH, and implement agreements as appropriate. Provided the aforementioned factors have been considered, it is anticipated that there may be instances where an agreement between the MAH and the wholesale distributor is not required. The MAH should ensure that where an agreement is required, these agreements contain sufficient detail and provisions relative to the relationship between the MAH and the partner.

Chapter 7 Outsourced Activities

7.1 Principle

Any activity covered by the GDP guide that is outsourced should be correctly defined, agreed and controlled in order to avoid misunderstandings which could affect the integrity of the product. There must be a written contract between the contract giver and the contract acceptor which clearly establishes the duties of each party.

7.2 Contract giver

The contract giver is responsible for the activities contracted out.

The contract giver is responsible for assessing the competence of the contract acceptor to successfully carry out the work required and for ensuring by means of the contract and through audits that the principles and guidelines of GDP are followed. An audit of the contract acceptor should be performed before commencement of, and whenever there has been a change to, the outsourced activities. The frequency of audit should be defined based on risk depending on the nature of the outsourced activities. Audits should be permitted at any time.

The contract giver should provide the contract acceptor with all the information necessary to carry out the contracted operations in accordance with the specific product requirements and any other relevant requirements.

7.3 Contract acceptor

The contract acceptor should have adequate premises and equipment, procedures, knowledge and experience, and competent personnel to carry out the work ordered by the contract giver.

The contract acceptor should not pass to a third party any of the work entrusted to him under the contract without the contract giver's prior evaluation and approval of the arrangements and an audit of the third party by the contract giver or the contract acceptor. Arrangements made between the contract acceptor and any third party should ensure that the wholesale distribution information is made available in the same way as between the original contract giver and contract acceptor.

The contract acceptor should refrain from any activity which may adversely affect the quality of the product(s) handled for the contract giver.

The contract acceptor must forward any information that can influence the quality of the product(s) to the contract giver in accordance with the requirement of the contract.

UK Guidance on Chapter 7 Outsourced Activities

Naming of third-party sites on UK Wholesale Dealer's Licence

Regulation 18(3) of the Human Medicines Regulations 2012, as amended, provides that:

> "Distribution of a medicinal product by way of wholesale dealing, or possession for the purpose of such distribution, is not to be taken to be in accordance with a wholesale dealer's licence unless the distribution is carried on, or as the case may be the product held, at premises located in the UK and specified in the licence."

The need for a third-party site to hold a Wholesale Dealer's Licence of their own and be named on another party's licence will rest on the activities being carried out, in particular whether licensable activities (procurement, holding, supply or export) are being undertaken on behalf of the holder of a Wholesale Dealer's Licence. There are instances where such arrangements can be clear cut (e.g. long-term holding) but there are also instances where the need to hold a Wholesale Dealer's Licence and name sites may be less clear (e.g. certain customer or supplier qualification activities or invoicing).

Other exemptions in law or policies operated by the MHRA's Inspectorate may impact on the need for a site to be licensed. One example is the exemption provided for in Regulation 19(4)(b) of the Human Medicines Regulations 2012, in relation to import agents; another example is the policy operated by the MHRA Inspectorate in relation to the short-term holding of ambient storage products (sometimes commonly referred to as the "36-hour rule") This exemption does not apply to cold chain products.

Historically, it has been possible for the holder of a Wholesale Dealer's Licence or Manufacturer's licence to use third-party storage and distribution sites located within the European Economic Area (EEA); these sites have never been named on the face of a UK Wholesale Dealer's Licence but will hold Wholesale Distribution Authorisations (WDA(H)) in their own right in the relevant territory. This MHRA policy continues to be implemented following the UK's exit from the European Union.

Clearly, the detail of arrangements between the parties involved is key in determining the need for licensing and naming, and responsibilities should be clearly laid out in written agreement(s) signed and dated by key personnel representing both parties. The Responsible Person has a key role in the oversight of outsourced activities, particularly in relation to ensuring compliance with Good Distribution Practice. Even where a licence may not be required or the third-party site needs to be named on the contract giver's licence, the activities are still subject to the requirements of Chapter 7 and Chapter 1 ("Management of Outsourced Activities") of Good Distribution Practice.

Chapter 8 Self-inspections

8.1　Principle

Self-inspections should be conducted in order to monitor implementation and compliance with GDP principles and to propose necessary corrective measures.

8.2　Self-inspections

A self-inspection programme should be implemented covering all aspects of GDP and compliance with the regulations, guidelines and procedures within a defined time frame. Self-inspections may be divided into several individual self-inspections of limited scope.

Self-inspections should be conducted in an impartial and detailed way by designated competent company personnel. Audits by independent external experts may also be useful but may not be used as a substitute for self-inspection.

All self-inspections should be recorded. Reports should contain all the observations made during the inspection. A copy of the report should be provided to the management and other relevant persons. In the event that irregularities and/or deficiencies are observed, their cause should be determined and the corrective and preventive actions (CAPA) should be documented and followed up.

UK Guidance on Chapter 8 Self-inspections

Self-inspections must be implemented as a key component to maintain compliance with principles of GDP. The main objective of self-inspections is to perform an impartial assessment of compliance with GDP and recognise the possible need for corrective actions and provide a means of identifying potential improvements. The self-inspection programme should be reflective of the business model, site-specific operations and the size of the organisation. The self-inspection programme should be conducted in an independent and objective manner.

An annual self-inspection schedule must be implemented as part of the QMS. The audit can be conducted as a single exercise or it can be spread throughout the year. The ultimate decision should be made with regard to minimising disruption to operations.

The self-inspection process must be robust enough to identify any symptomatic and sporadic non-compliance with GDP. The self-inspection programme must take into consideration all applicable areas of GDP, the full scope of the QMS, a review of all relevant records, personnel, premises, equipment, computerised systems and compliance with the current legislation. Particular attention should be paid to:

- the documented procedures and their suitability for the specific business model;
- whether QMS outputs are raised contemporaneously and closed within the periods as set out in the organisation's relevant procedures;
- accuracy and availability of records;
- effectiveness of the QMS;
- an audit of transaction records;
- any changes in legislation and impact on the licensable activities.

The scope of the self-inspection programme must extend to assessing any outsourced activities. The review of audit findings of relevant contract acceptors should form part of the self-inspection process.

The observations and outcomes of the self-inspection must be documented. A report containing sufficient level of detail must be made available for review by management and other relevant personnel.

If any areas of non-compliance are identified, investigations must be conducted with the intention of establishing the root cause and implementing appropriate CAPAs. Investigators must consider beyond the initial probable root cause of an incident and confirm or rule out other plausible potential root causes. It is important to review previous incidents to identify potentially recurring issues. Risk assessments may also be necessary depending on the type of non-compliance identified.

Decisions to implement corrective actions should be based on the observations made during the self-inspection process and the outcomes of any related investigations.

A well-managed self-inspection system

The system supporting investigation activities should be monitored with trending to obtain meaningful information that can be used to drive routine improvements and to ensure that approved timescales are met. This includes scrutiny during the management review of the outcomes of the self-inspection and escalation where needed to ensure the system remains in control and an effective means of protecting patients and the integrity of the medicines when things have gone wrong.

Chapter 9 Transportation

9.1 Principle

It is the responsibility of the supplying wholesale distributor to protect medicinal products against breakage, adulteration and theft, and to ensure that temperature conditions are maintained within acceptable limits during transport.

Regardless of the mode of transport, it should be possible to demonstrate that the medicines have not been exposed to conditions that may compromise their quality and integrity. A risk-based approach should be utilised when planning transportation.

9.2 Transportation

The required storage conditions for medicinal products should be maintained during transportation within the defined limits as described by the manufacturers or on the outer packaging.

If a deviation such as temperature excursion or product damage has occurred during transportation, this should be reported to the distributor and recipient of the affected medicinal products. A procedure should also be in place for investigating and handling temperature excursions.

It is the responsibility of the wholesale distributor to ensure that vehicles and equipment used to distribute, store or handle medicinal products are suitable for their use and appropriately equipped to prevent exposure of the products to conditions that could affect their quality and packaging integrity.

There should be written procedures in place for the operation and maintenance of all vehicles and equipment involved in the distribution process, including cleaning and safety precautions.

Risk assessment of delivery routes should be used to determine where temperature controls are required. Equipment used for temperature monitoring during transport within vehicles and/or containers, should be maintained and calibrated at regular intervals at least once a year.

Dedicated vehicles and equipment should be used, where possible, when handling medicinal products. Where non-dedicated vehicles and equipment are used procedures should be in place to ensure that the quality of the medicinal product will not be compromised.

Deliveries should be made to the address stated on the delivery note and into the care or the premises of the consignee. Medicinal products should not be left on alternative premises.

For emergency deliveries outside normal business hours, persons should be designated and written procedures should be available.

Where transportation is performed by a third party, the contract in place should encompass the requirements of Chapter 7. Transportation providers should be made aware by the wholesale distributor of the relevant transport conditions applicable to the consignment. Where the transportation route includes unloading and reloading or transit storage at a transportation hub, particular attention should be paid to temperature monitoring, cleanliness and the security of any intermediate storage facilities.

Provision should be made to minimise the duration of temporary storage while awaiting the next stage of the transportation route.

9.3   Containers, packaging and labelling

Medicinal products should be transported in containers that have no adverse effect on the quality of the products, and that offer adequate protection from external influences, including contamination.

Selection of a container and packaging should be based on the storage and transportation requirements of the medicinal products; the space required for the amount of medicines; the anticipated external temperature extremes; the estimated maximum time for transportation including transit storage at customs; the qualification status of the packaging; and the validation status of the shipping containers.

Containers should bear labels providing sufficient information on handling and storage requirements and precautions to ensure that the products are properly handled and secured at all times. The containers should enable identification of the contents of the containers and the source.

9.4   Products requiring special conditions

In relation to deliveries containing medicinal products requiring special conditions such as narcotics or psychotropic substances, the wholesale distributor should maintain a safe and secure supply chain for these products in accordance with requirements laid down by the Member States concerned. There should be additional control systems in place for delivery of these products. There should be a protocol to address the occurrence of any theft.

Medicinal products comprising highly active and radioactive materials should be transported in safe, dedicated and secure containers and vehicles. The relevant safety measures should be in accordance with international agreements and national legislation.

For temperature-sensitive products, qualified equipment (e.g. thermal packaging, temperature-controlled containers or temperature-controlled vehicles) should be used to ensure correct transport conditions are maintained between the manufacturer, wholesale distributor and customer.

If temperature-controlled vehicles are used, the temperature monitoring equipment used during transport should be maintained and calibrated at regular intervals. Temperature mapping under representative conditions should be carried out and should take into account seasonal variations.

If requested, customers should be provided with information to demonstrate that products have complied with the temperature storage conditions.

If cool packs are used in insulated boxes, they need to be located such that the product does not come in direct contact with the cool pack. Staff must be trained on the procedures for assembly of the insulated boxes (seasonal configurations) and on the re-use of cool packs.

There should be a system in place to control the re-use of cool packs to ensure that incompletely cooled packs are not used in error. There should be adequate physical segregation between frozen and chilled ice packs.

The process for delivery of sensitive products and control of seasonal temperature variations should be described in a written procedure.

UK Guidance on Chapter 9 Transportation

MHRA expectations in regard to control and monitoring of temperature during transportation

Following dispatch from a manufacturing facility, the distribution chain for medicinal products can be complex, potentially involving a number of storage locations, wholesalers and modes of transport, before the product finally reaches the patient.

The transportation arrangements from one location to another are regarded as an extension of the storage activities and distributors are expected to treat each journey as unique with the length and complexity, as well as any seasonal variations, being considered when choosing the packing method and mode of distribution.

Temperature should be monitored and controlled throughout the transportation chain. When planning transport routes, allowances should be made for potential impact on the shipment due to delays or the possibility that the customer may refuse the load and the product needs to be transported back to site. For impact on specific products, the supplier or customer may assess the impact of the temperature excursion on individual medicines in the load or profile them as products with equivalent temperature requirements, physical attributes, formulation and packaging. The acceptable temperature range relates to the labelled conditions for the specific product. MHRA expectations for this are defined below.

With respect to the transport of medicines, the Guidelines on Good Distribution Practice for Medicinal Products clearly require that: "The required storage conditions for medicinal products should be maintained during transportation within the defined limits as described by the manufacturers on the outer packaging. It is the responsibility of the supplying wholesale distributor to ensure that vehicles and equipment used to distribute, store or handle medicinal products are suitable for their use and appropriately equipped to prevent exposure of the products to conditions that could affect their quality and packaging integrity."

This guidance is also applicable to the Manufacturer or Marketing Authorisation Holder and should be adhered to when supplying medicinal products.

Packing of consignments and temperature management during transportation

Before being transported, medicinal products should be appropriately packed in such a way as to ensure that the required temperatures are maintained throughout the journey to ensure the medicines are transported in accordance with their labelling requirements in accordance with Chapter 9.3 of the GDP Guidelines.

Phase change materials, stabilised to the correct temperature range according to the packaging instructions, may be added to the packaging to maintain appropriate temperatures throughout the transport. The positioning of these packs within the consignment is extremely important and phase change materials must not be allowed into direct contact with the medicinal products being shipped.

Bespoke packaging with compartments for the phase change materials (also referred to as passive transport systems) are available. It is important to note that these systems will require validating by the wholesaler for the purposes of the transport. While these systems are often sold with studies indicating the thermal capabilities of these systems, they are not "pre validated" and there is an expectation that the wholesaler will have verified the systems through their own documented validation programme.

Larger volumes of refrigerated products will generally be shipped via temperature controlled or "active" transport.

Whichever method of transport is used, it is expected that the supplying wholesaler can show that the required temperatures ranges have been maintained.

The implementation of temperature monitoring as a matter of routine for all refrigerated deliveries is considered best practice. Temperatures should be strictly controlled and monitored with calibrated equipment of a suitable sensitivity, to provide temperature data for the entire journey. Some countries require that all imported consignments of medicinal products include a temperature monitor.

Data pertaining to temperature during transport should be retained by the supplying wholesaler for the required 5 years.

Where transhipment or cross docking is necessary, daily minimum and maximum temperature monitoring and recording should also be carried out at these locations. The recording devices should be calibrated and the data be available to the supplying wholesaler as part of the route planning exercise.

Wholesale dealers should review and maintain all temperature records and there should be procedures in place for implementing corrective action in the case of adverse events. Wholesalers should also ensure that consignments are clearly labelled with the required storage and transport conditions to be maintained as stated above.

Mean kinetic temperature (MKT) has been incorrectly applied by wholesalers in attempts to justify temperature excursions caused by lack of control. In the very rare occasions where use of MKT was appropriate, continuous and consistent temperature monitoring was carried out from the point of manufacturer batch release and supported by appropriate designation of acceptable MKT limits and methodology.

Controlled-temperature shipments

Controlled transport is generally referred to in terms of "active" or "passive" systems. In general terms, an active system is a temperature-controlled environment such as a mechanical refrigeration system often seen in specialised pharmaceutical delivery vans, refrigerated shipping containers or aircraft holds. A "passive" solution would rely on the use of phase change materials within an insulated box.

Controlled-temperature transport is equally applicable to cold-chain (generally store between 2 and 8 degrees celsius) "ambient" products (which generally have the storage instruction do not store above 25 or sometimes 30 degrees celsius). "Do not refrigerate" products (it is generally accepted that these should not be stored or transported below 8 degrees celsius) or frozen products (for which the temperature range is usually product specific).

Regardless of whether active or passive solutions are utilised, general principles and expectations apply. In general, it should be ensured that the cooling capacity is capable of handling the peak stock level of the time and temperature-sensitive pharmaceutical products. When packing the load, or loading the vehicle, it is expected that the time for the necessary "conditioning" is known. This conditioning time will vary with the external conditions and should be evaluated as part of the qualification.

For example, during the winter months, the vehicle compartments may need to be warmed to attain the correct loading temperature, whereas in the summer months, the cooler unit will be activated in order to attain and maintain the same target temperature.

When phase change materials are used, it is important that there is a protocol in place for any re-conditioning of the material if indeed it is reusable and many of these systems are specified as single-use systems.

The general requirements for these systems is that they are:

- capable of maintaining temperatures within a defined temperature range;
- equipped with calibrated temperature-monitoring equipment (either continuous or at a selected (and justifiable) sampling rate such as once every 10 minutes);
- equipped with an alarm system to alert to temperature deviations;
- that the sensors are of a calibrated accuracy of ±0.5 degrees celsius and can resolve to 0.1 degrees celsius;
- that the sensors are placed according to a mapping study.

The World Health Organization (WHO) estimates that approaching 30% of all pharmaceuticals that are disposed of are directly due to temperature excursions during transport and that up to 35% of vaccines have reduced efficacy that can be directly attributed to incorrect handling during shipping and transportation.

Qualification/validation/verification studies

It is expected that transport systems will be subject to validation studies to show that the chosen system or systems to be fit for purpose. The expectation is that sufficient data will be obtained in order that a robust risk assessment for ongoing monitoring may be put in place. Typically, these initial studies will be conducted over the course of one full calendar cycle in real delivery scenarios. The object of the exercise is to ascertain (a) that medicinal products are being transported according to their labelled storage conditions and (b) under what circumstances additional control measures may be required. These circumstances may be predicted heat-waves or other extreme weather events, the potential for disruption to planned transport lanes due to industrial action or issues at the border in relation to additional freight checks following changes in border control.

Uncontrolled ambient transport

This is a phrase used to describe a transport system where there is neither active nor passive control measures in place and the environmental conditions are not controlled. Such a transport system can rarely be shown to be GDP compliant where products have specific storage temperature requirements.

Transport providers

When wholesale dealers employ the services of a third-party transport service, they must satisfy themselves that the activities are compliant with Good Distribution Practice (e.g. driver training) and are competent to provide the service for which they are engaged.

The selection of third party service providers is very important and roles and responsibilities must be defined by a written contract. Chapter 7 of the EU GDP Guidelines (Outsourced Activities) provides advice in this area and Chapter 1.3 covers the management of outsourced activities.

During transport, a dedicated temperature-controlled fleet should be utilised or the services of a specialist third-party logistics provider may be contracted. As with uncontrolled ambient transport, it is unlikely that a "general courier service" will be able to provide a GDP-compliant service.

GDP guidelines state that, where possible, dedicated vehicles should be used to transport medicinal products; this cannot be achieved by utilising a general courier service (see also security during transport).

Reverse logistics consideration

Some companies operate on a "supplier collects model". This model is only appropriate where the products stay within GB (due to the formalities at the borders which are the obligation of the wholesaler to fulfil). Where a supplier collection model is in place, provision should be made to facilitate the "reverse logistics" in order that control may be demonstrated in respect to any returned products. Many wholesalers operating on this model find the simplest way to control this aspect is by not accepting returns from their customer. This generally forms part of the transport agreement between the two parties.

Hygiene and contamination

Shipping practices should ensure that the medicinal product does not become contaminated. The majority of measures will be taken during packaging operations, such as control of use of recycled pallets or recycled packing filler and wrapping of product. Some considerations associated with transportation include:

- use of transport hub refrigerators also used to hold raw meat products;
- co-transport of volatile products, e.g. coffee beans, industrial chemicals;

- co-transport with poisons, e.g. pesticides;
- co-transport with active substances, e.g. industrial chemicals, active pharmaceutical ingredients;
- decontamination of shipping containers.

Care should be taken when the load is to be consolidated to inform the shipping company or transport provider of that nature of the product and to avoid the load being consolidated with product that could compromise or cross-contaminate the medicines.

Where possible, dedicated vehicles should be utilised for the transport of medicinal products.

Transport lanes

In order to ensure that appropriate transport conditions are applied in the most efficient manner during transportation, some wholesalers apply a transport lane validation approach. This enables knowledge of routes and quality risk management to be applied to proportionate development of controls. In the most basic form, the validation plan approach may consist of palletised shipments between sites within a single company or to a small group of customers being grouped in one transport lane, with the remaining transport chains supplying tote quantities to many customers being grouped in a second lane. More commonly, transport lane validation plans are much more extensive with lanes developed according to destination territories, transport modes, transportation chains with specific complexities or where a range of medicinal products are especially vulnerable to particular types of risk. The risk profiling and control measures allocated to each lane will maximise efficiency of management of transportation and monitoring. Transport lane validation is most useful where similar transport chains are used by a wholesaler on a routine basis.

General steps in development of a lane validation approach are provided below, which, in practice, is likely to vary depending on the organisation and their chosen approach.

STEP 1. DEVELOPMENT OF A VALIDATION PLAN

The aim and development process for the transport lane validation plan should be documented and describe its aim and how it is to be applied. Any individual protocols or route assessments should refer back to this document.

STEP 2. RISK IDENTIFICATION

A variety of approaches to describe risk categories during supply of medicines may be used, such as those associated with medicine type, customer type, geographical regions and transport modes. This can be broad in scope and be further developed at a later stage for higher risk areas; e.g., if delays are an important consideration for a specific customer, the risk can be broken down to delays at the consolidator, border control, en route for multi-drop shipments, intermodal transfer or be weather-related. For this customer, they can be placed into a transport lane where these risks have been previously characterised.

The risks generated as a direct consequence of transportation should be identified, for example, temperature excursions, delay, mis-delivery, loss including theft, damage due to high humidity, damage due to vibration, compromised associated document trail and compromised chain of custody.

STEP 3. ROUTE PROFILING

The various transport chains are next grouped into transport lanes to reflect similar common characteristics, e.g.:

Lane 1   National intra-company distribution of palletised ambient and cold chain medicines using two approved logistics providers.

Lane 2   National inter-company distribution of palletised and non-palletised ambient and cold chain using six logistics providers and one customer-collect transport.

Lane 3   Export to EMEA region within a temperature controlled container of medicines by sea freight using freight forwarder "X".

Lane 4   Export to EMEA by air freight of medicinal product using freight forwarder "Y".

Alternatively, they may be defined according to common risk profiles. Having assigned transport routes to transport lanes, a review of the routes and risks should be carried out to confirm they are compatible.

STEP 4. RISK MITIGATION AND MONITORING

Having collated information of different transport chains within a lane, a single mitigation can be developed for each of the risks, e.g. a single packaging qualification representative of all transport chains within a lane to protect against temperature excursions for shipments to a specified geographical region.

The validation plan should be routinely reviewed to confirm validity of the lane criteria and to assess any deviations that may apply to the integrity of the validation.

Advantages of a transport lane validation approach

Transport and packaging qualification and risk assessments can be directed at groups of transport chains rather than for each individual chain, thereby enabling knowledge transfer between lanes and reducing duplication of effort.

The extent of qualification and risk assessment can be reduced for any new transport chain introduced into an established transport lane.

Risks and risk mitigation can be trended easily.

Transport validation plans tend to drive collation of performance data and knowledge of transport chains resulting in more efficient supply chains.

Maintaining security during transportation

The largest risk of medicine theft in the UK occurs during road transportation. This is due to a number of factors dependant on transportation chain and vehicle type. Routine deliveries can enable thieves to plan thefts, both by the pallet load for vehicles parked overnight in motorway lorry parks or prior to a booked delivery slot, or on a smaller scale for deliveries to pharmacies where multiple deliveries are made and parking may be some way from the delivery point. Selection of vehicle build can mitigate some of these risks, such as use of solid-sided trailers with intrusion sensors or smaller vans that have good quality locks and alarms. Training drivers in practices to minimise security risk not only protects the consignment, but importantly helps protect the driver.

Safe custody of Controlled Drugs as defined in the Misuse of Drugs Act 1971 should also be considered. For specific guidance on transportation of controlled drugs, please refer to the Home Office.

Other transport modes have vulnerabilities specific to them, and different risk profiles apply across geographical areas. The supplying wholesaler should be aware of the risks that apply to them and apply appropriate control measures when planning transport. An example of application of quality risk management to transportation is provided in MHRA Guidance to Chapter 1.

Examples of some risks applied to transportation

The following are examples of how risks vary across transport modes. It is the responsibility of the supplying wholesaler to develop a good understanding of pertinent risks that apply to their supply chain.

ROAD TRANSPORT

- Relative ease for thieves to track and access vehicles and remove stock.
- Only one driver is normally present.
- There is risk of opportune theft such as the slash and grab model in addition to targetted theft.
- Variable operational standards are applied by transport providers, and not all are aligned with GDP expectations – it is however the responsi-

bility of the wholesaler to select a transport partner who can provide a service that is suitable for the product type.

- Restriction of driver hours leads to forced rest stops, especially with deliveries from mainland Europe, with the consequence that some locations have become theft hotspots for parked vehicles.
- Curtain-sided trailers afford poor temperature control and are more vulnerable to theft.
- Cross-docking poses additional high risks which should be assessed and mitigated.

AIR FREIGHT

Generally, air freight is very secure; however, internal flight transfers within some third countries are vulnerable to theft.

Time on tarmac can provide significant risk of temperature excursions.

Failure to specify hold conditions can lead to damage from low temperature or low air pressure.

See also the IATA Time and Temperature Guidance.

SEA FREIGHT

The relatively long journey time increases risk of an event relevant to the medicine occurring in transit, e.g. temperature excursion duration or medicine recall.

Supply chain delays can extend to days or weeks, e.g. adverse weather, civil unrest and piracy.

Failure to use temperature-controlled shipping containers commonly known as reefers leads to vulnerability to exposure of container to heat or cold.

RAIL FREIGHT

Rail is not yet commonly used in the UK; however, there has been significant investment in the rail infrastructure for both national and international movements. Some parts of South America are known for the risk of hijacking of rail freight. In other countries it provides a relatively secure service but can be vulnerable to environmental temperature extremes unless temperature-controlled systems are used.

FINAL MILE

Suppliers should be aware of vulnerabilities associated with all stages of their transport chain, including trans-modal operations. The final leg of the journey can prove particularly challenging in remote areas or those regions which experience extreme environments. There has been a slow but steady increase in the use of drones to fly medicines to the final destination. These may be convenient, but pose risks of physical damage, theft or weakness in the documented chain of custody.

Other Guidance – United Kingdom Exit from the European Union, and Northern Ireland

The UK's new relationship with the EU

The United Kingdom (UK) left the European Union (EU) on 31 January 2020 and moved into a transition period that ended on 31 December 2020, with the UK and EU agreeing to a Trade and Cooperation Agreement on 24 December 2020.

During the transition period the UK continued to follow EU legislation and regulations, but this changed on 1 January 2021. From 1 January 2021 Northern Ireland (NI) has continued to be aligned to EU legislation and regulations in respect of medicines and medical devices as a requisite of the Ireland/ Northern Ireland Protocol and Great Britain (GB) has not.

The Ireland/Northern Ireland Protocol, which came into effect from 1 January 2021, has resulted in changes to regulations regarding medicines in relation to importation requirements and compliance with Falsified Medicines Directive. The UK and EU agreed to a phased in approach of these regulatory requirements until 31 December 2021 to allow time for industry to prepare.

Separate to regulatory differences, under the Protocol, new customs rules and procedures for the movement of all goods from GB to NI apply from 1 January 2021.

As a consequence of the UK leaving the Single Market and Customs Union, the way businesses in Great Britain trade goods with the EU has changed. To export goods to the EU businesses now need to comply with new customs procedures, including UK export declarations and import requirements on entry to EU Member States. For importing medicines into GB from EU Member States new requirements are in place.

The Human Medicines Regulations 2012 refers to lists of approved countries for:

- importation of medicines under a wholesale dealer's licence ("approved country for import list");
- batch testing of medicines ("approved country for batch testing list");
- manufacturing of active substances with regulatory standards equivalent to the UK ("approved country for active substances list").

The UK will accept certification by a Qualified Person and Active Substance manufacture from countries specified in these lists. These lists will initially include EEA countries and other countries with whom regulatory equivalence has been confirmed. The lists will be reviewed at least every 3 years.

The UK's acceptance of batch testing done in EEA countries will be reviewed before 31 December 2022. A 2-year notice period will be given in the case of changes.

Approved Country for Import List

Regulation 18A of the Human Medicines Regulations 2012 will allow importation of human medicines into Great Britain under a UK wholesale dealer's licence from the following countries, provided that the UK wholesale dealer confirms that each batch has been certified by a Qualified Person (QP) in a listed country.

EU countries

- Austria
- Belgium
- Bulgaria
- Croatia
- Republic of Cyprus
- Czech Republic
- Denmark
- Estonia
- Finland
- France
- Germany
- Greece
- Hungary
- Ireland
- Italy
- Latvia
- Lithuania
- Luxembourg
- Malta
- Netherlands
- Poland
- Portugal
- Romania
- Slovakia
- Slovenia
- Spain
- Sweden

The European Economic Area (EEA)

EU countries, plus Iceland, Liechtenstein and Norway.

Sourcing medicines for the UK Market

Importing Medicines from an EEA State that is on An Approved Country for Import List

Qualified Person (QP) certified medicines from the European Economic Area (EEA) are accepted in Great Britain (England, Wales and Scotland) if certain checks are made. These checks are explained in guidance on acting as a Responsible Person for Import.

These medicines will not require re-testing or re-certification by a UK Qualified Person (QP) if imported and checked by a wholesale dealer in Great Britain.

A manufacturer or wholesaler from a country that is on an approved country for import list may only supply a licensed medicine to a wholesaler in Great Britain. The sale and supply to an authorised person (hospital, doctor or retailer) must be from a UK-licensed wholesaler.

Importing UK or Great Britain Authorised Human Medicines from a Country on the List for Use In Great Britain

If you import a UK or Great Britain authorised medicine from a country on the list, you will need to hold a wholesale dealer's licence that authorises import.

This licence will need to cover the following activities of handling medicinal products:

- 1.1 With "an authorisation" (a UK, Great Britain or Northern Ireland Marketing Authorisation, certificate of registration or traditional herbal registration).

Your licence must authorise wholesale distribution operations, including:

- products imported from countries on a list;
- products certified under Article 51 of Directive 2001/83/EC.

You will need a Responsible Person (import).

Importing Human Medicines from a Country On the List for Use as a Special Medicinal Product

If you import a medicine from a country on the list, for use as a special medicinal product, you will need to hold a wholesale dealer's licence that authorises import.

IMPORTING MEDICINES LICENSED IN THE LISTED COUNTRY

If the medicine is licensed in the listed country, you will need an RPi.

Your wholesale dealer's licence will need to cover the following activities of handling medicinal products:

- 1.2 Without "an authorisation" (a UK, Great Britain or Northern Ireland Marketing Authorisation, certificate of registration or traditional herbal registration) in Great Britain or EEA and intended for the UK market.

This licence will also need to authorise wholesale distribution operations covering:

- products imported from countries on a list;
- products certified under Article 51 of Directive 2001/83/EC.

The current notification of intent to import an unlicensed medicine remains the same (https://www.gov.uk/guidance/import-a-human-medicine).

IMPORTING MEDICINES NOT LICENSED IN THE LISTED COUNTRY

If the medicine is not licensed in the UK or a listed country, you will need an ordinary Responsible Person and not an RPi.

Your wholesale dealer's licence will need to cover the following activities of handling medicinal products.

- 1.2 Without "an authorisation" (a UK, Great Britain or Northern Ireland Marketing Authorisation, certificate of registration or traditional herbal registration) in Great Britain or EEA and intended for the UK market.

Your licence will also need to authorise wholesale distribution operations covering:

- products imported from countries on a list;
- products not certified under Article 51 of Directive 2001/83/EC.

The current notification of intent to import an unlicensed medicine remains the same (https://www.gov.uk/guidance/import-a-human-medicine).

Importing Human Medicines from a Country on the List for Export

If you import a medicine from a country on the list, that you will export, you will need to hold a wholesale dealer's licence that authorises import and export.

Introduced medicine is a term used previously for the category 1.3. To be clear, a wholesaler could not "import" from a third country as that is a manufacturing activity. A wholesaler could, with the correct customs procedures, "introduce" the product for direct supply to a customer in a third country.

IMPORTING MEDICINES LICENSED IN THE LISTED COUNTRY

If the medicine is licensed in the UK or a listed country, you will need a RPi.

For medicines licensed in the UK: your wholesale dealer's licence will need to cover the following activities of handling medicinal products:

- 1.1 With "an authorisation" (a UK, Great Britain or Northern Ireland Marketing Authorisation, certificate of registration or traditional herbal registration).

Your licence will also need to authorise wholesale distribution operations covering:

- products imported from countries on a list;
- products certified under Article 51 of Directive 2001/83/EC;
- export.

For medicines licensed in a listed country: your wholesale dealer's licence will need to cover the following activities of handling medicinal products:

- 1.3 Without "an authorisation" (a UK, Great Britain or Northern Ireland Marketing Authorisation, certificate of registration or traditional herbal registration) in the UK and not intended for the UK market.

Your licence will also need to authorise wholesale distribution operations covering:

- products imported from countries on a list;
- products certified under Article 51 of Directive 2001/83/EC;
- export.

IMPORTING MEDICINES NOT LICENSED IN THE LISTED COUNTRY OR THE UK

If the medicine is not the subject of a marketing authorisation in the UK or a listed country then you will need an ordinary Responsible Person and not an RPi to import it into Great Britain for export outside the UK.

Your wholesale dealer's licence will need to cover the following activities of handling medicinal products.

- 1.3 Without "an authorisation" (a UK, Great Britain or Northern Ireland Marketing Authorisation, certificate of registration or traditional herbal registration) in the UK and not intended for the UK market.

Your licence will also need to authorise wholesale distribution operations covering:

- products imported from countries on a list;
- products not certified under Article 51 of Directive 2001/83/EC;
- export.

Importing Medicines from a Country on the List for Supply to the United Kingdom Parallel Import Market

If you import a medicine from a country on the list, for relabelling / repackaging as a parallel import, for supply to the UK Parallel Import market you will need to hold a wholesale dealer's licence that authorises import.

The imported medicine must have the appropriate marketing authorisation in a country on the list for the designated Product Licence Parallel Import (PLPI).

Your licence will need to cover the following activities of handling medicinal products:

- 1.4 With a Marketing Authorisation in EEA member state(s) and intended for the GB parallel import market.

Your licence will also need to authorise wholesale distribution operations covering:

- products imported from countries on a list;
- products certified under Article 51 of Directive 2001/83/EC.

You will need an RPi if located in Great Britain.

EU GUIDELINES ON
GDP AND UK GUIDANCE ON
WHOLESALE DISTRIBUTION

Sourcing a medicine from Northern Ireland to Great Britain

SOURCING FOR WHOLESALE

Medicinal products sourced from Northern Ireland for wholesale purposes are permitted under the supervision of an ordinary Responsible Person (RP) and not an RPi.

If you hold a WDA with sites in Northern Ireland and Great Britain, an RPi will be required for activities conducted in Great Britain.

PRODUCTS GRANTED AN AUTHORISATION UNDER THE UNFETTERED ACCESS SCHEME

To facilitate unfettered access for Northern Ireland products to the Great Britain market, medicines authorised within Northern Ireland will be granted an authorisation in Great Britain. The product licence numbers will be marked with a "(UA)" suffix on the packaging and summary of product characteristics.

If you source a medicine with a "(UA)" suffix it may only be purchased from:

- a Northern Ireland manufacturer or wholesaler (a "qualifying business");
- a wholesale dealer in Great Britain.

SOURCING FOR PARALLEL TRADE IN GREAT BRITAIN

If you source a medicine with a marketing authorisation from Northern Ireland for supply to the Great Britain Parallel Import market or for export to a third country, you will need a wholesale dealer's licence. You will need an ordinary Responsible Person and not an RPi.

SOURCING BIOLOGICAL MEDICINES

A Northern Ireland manufacturer or wholesaler who supplies a biological medicines to Great Britain will need to confirm that a national batch release certificate has been issued by NIBSC for each batch.

Products Supplied from the European Union to Great Britain

Wholesale dealers in Great Britain that import biological medicines from the EEA will be required to check that each batch has an appropriate NIBSC or Mutual Recognition Agreement certificate before placing on the market in Great Britain. This information can be obtained from the product's Marketing Authorisation Holder.

PRODUCTS SUPPLIED FROM NORTHERN IRELAND TO GREAT BRITAIN

Products supplied from Northern Ireland to Great Britain will require the supplying manufacturer or wholesale dealer in Northern Ireland to confirm that a NIBSC or Mutual Recognition Agreement certificate is available before supplying a Great Britain wholesaler or other authorised person in Great Britain, such as a hospital.

BIOLOGICAL MEDICINES IMPORTED INTO GREAT BRITAIN UNDER A PARALLEL IMPORT LICENCE

Products placed on the market in Great Britain under a Parallel Import Licence will require a NIBSC certificate. Please follow the guidance above for batches for Great Britain, including the requirement to provide a UK Marketing Information Form and NIBSC certificate in advance of the product being placed on the market.

The Falsified Medicines Directive

The EU Falsified Medicines Directive (2011/62/EU) (FMD) was adopted in 2011 and introduced new harmonised measures to ensure that medicines in the European Union (EU) are safe and that trade in medicines is properly controlled.

The final part of the Directive, the 'safety features' Delegated Regulation (EU) 2016/161 came into force on 9 February 2019, and applies to certain categories of prescription only medicines (POM) and certain named non-prescription medicines.

Following the UK's departure from the EU, the 'safety features' Delegated Regulation (EU) 2016/161 no longer applies in Great Britain (England, Scotland and Wales) but still applies in Northern Ireland.

These safety features are:

- a unique identifier (a 2D data matrix code and human readable information) which will be placed on medical products that can be scanned at fixed points along the supply chain
- tamper evident features (anti-tampering devices) on the pack

The unique identifier comprises:

- a product code which allows the identification of at least:
  - the name of the medicine,
  - the common name
  - the pharmaceutical form
  - the strength, the pack size
  - the pack type
- a serial number which is a numeric or alphanumeric sequence of a maximum of 20 characters randomly generated
- a batch number
- an expiry date

If the member state to which the medicine is being supplied requires it, the unique identifier will also need to include the national reimbursement number. This is not applicable in the UK.

The unique identifier must be printed on the pack in a 2D data-matrix code and be printed in a way in which the information can be read by the human eye.

The choice of tamper-evident feature to be used is for the marketing authorisation holder (MAH) to decide. A European Standard is available with guidance on the types of tamper-evident features which could be considered by MAHs. This is titled 'Tamper verification features for medicinal product packaging EN 16679:2014'.

MAHs are required to place the safety features on the packaging of medicines which fall within the remit of the delegated regulation and upload the data into European Medicines Verification System (EMVS) prior to placing the product on the market.

The 2D barcode is scanned at various points in the supply chain to verify that it is an 'authentic' medicine.

Upon supply to the patient in the EU or Northern Ireland, the unique identifier must be 'decommissioned' via a scan from the FMD system, to prevent any duplication of a legitimate identifier for use on a falsified medicine. This will be checked against data in the national repository, which for Northern Ireland is the UKNI Medicines Verification System (UKNI-MVS) run by SecurMed UK.

Guidance and useful resources

Supply of medicines to GB and NI

Medicines with a marketing authorisation valid only in Great Britain (PLGB) do not require a Unique Identifier. However, we encourage companies to retain the tamper evident device.

Medicines with a marketing authorisation (MA) valid in Northern Ireland (PL and PLNI) require a unique identifier and a tamper evident device on each pack.

Marketing authorisation holders with valid marketing authorisations for Northern Ireland can continue uploading serialisation data into the European Medicines Verification System (EMVS).

A derogation from the delegated regulation is in effect meaning that the unique identifiers on packs with a marketing authorisation valid in NI, supplied by a manufacturer or wholesaler in the EEA do not require decommissioning when exported to the UK. This supports the flow of products through Great Britain to Northern Ireland. Unique identifiers on these packs should be decommissioned in Northern Ireland as required by EU Delegated Regulation 2016/161.

The above derogation on decommissioning upon export from the EEA is in place until 31st December 2024.

Export of medicines to non-EEA countries

Holders of wholesale dealer authorisations in Great Britain no longer have access to the UKNI MVS and are therefore no longer obliged to decommission packs upon export.

Holders of wholesale dealer authorisations in Northern Ireland continue to have access to the UKNI MVS and should continue to decommission packs upon export to non-EEA countries, including Great Britain, in line with the delegated regulation.

Implementation and enforcement

In accordance with the Northern Ireland Protocol the Northern Ireland market should follow the EU acquis. This is as set out in the draft EU Unilateral Declaration in the Withdrawal Agreement Joint Committee. The UK is committed to meeting the requirements of EU FMD safety features Delegated Regulation in Northern Ireland, and we expect all stakeholders in the supply chain comply with these requirements.

Despite the significant work undertaken to date in the UK and given the complexities associated with setting up the medicines verification system across the EU, it is anticipated issues will arise. It is important that these issues do not compromise confidence in the medicines supply chain. The Government's priority is the continued supply of safe medicines to patients.

For example, several Member States have formally advised those who may receive 'unknown' error messages to dispense anyway. Therefore, the MHRA and DHNI will also be taking a pragmatic, flexible approach to how we enforce the legal requirements, as long as the normal checks are carried out and there is no reason to think that the medicine is falsified. This position will be kept under review.

Error messaging and false alerts

Medicinal products manufactured and released before 9 February 2019 may have had the safety features applied but may not have been uploaded to the repositories system. There are also packs of medicines already on the UK market which contain 2D barcodes that do not relate to the FMD safety features due to other international initiatives.

Attempts to verify or verify and decommission these products will trigger system alerts. This situation may continue for a period of time due to the shelf life of medicinal products, in some cases up to five years.

Any instances of suspected falsification (including physical signs of tampering) are to be reported in the usual way via the Yellow Card reporting system.

Where the MAH is notified by the alerting system that a data error has occurred, they are to notify the MHRA if upon further investigation, falsification is suspected.

Further information and explanation of explaining the alert management process may be found on the EMVO website.

Reporting suspected falsified medicines

Any falsified medicines identified should be reported through the Yellow Card reporting system [Report a FAKE or Counterfeit]. For FMD applicable Prescription only Medicines (POM) products containing the Unique Identifier (UI) 2D bar code the following information is needed: A report of an alert for one of these packs should include:

- the alert number in the following format: "GB-xxxxxxxx-xxxx-xxxx-xxxx-xxxxxxxxxxxx" and the following details from the pack itself:
  – GTIN
  – serial number
  – batch id
  – expiry date

Ideally this would be with images of the pack showing all 4 elements in human readable format AND the 2D barcode. The alert could be generated for any of the following codes upon verification or decommissioning;

- NMVS_FE_LOT_03
- NMVS_FE_LOT_12
- NMVS_FE_LOT_13
- NMVS_NC_PC_01
- NMVS_NC_PC_02
- NMVS_NC_PCK_19
- NMVS_NC_PCK_22

For FMD applicable products without a Unique Identifier (UI) 2D bar code from Italy or Greece the following is needed:

- supplier details
- product particulars
- photographs (to include the side where the adhesive stickers / labels should have been present
- date received

Wholesale dealers licences for sites in Northern Ireland

The MHRA issues WDA(H) for the UK and these reflect the wording as relevant for Great Britain according to the Human Medicines Regulations. For WDA(H) that name sites in Northern Ireland the licences issued to companies do not reflect the European format and wording. For example, in Great Britain the category 1.1. states "With 'an authorisation' (a UK, Great Britain or Northern Ireland Marketing Authorisation, an Article 126a authorisation, a certificate of registration or traditional herbal registration)", and the EEA format states: "1.1 with a Marketing Authorisation in EEA country(s)".

For WDA(H) based in Northern Ireland they continue to be listed on EUDRAGMDP and as such the functions are mapped on that database to the European format.

Export of medicines to approved countries for import

According to Article 40(3) of Directive 2001/83/EC and Article 44(3) of Directive 2001/82/EC, the competent authorities of the Union are to ensure that the import of medicinal products into their territory is subject to an authorisation. The authorisation is granted when a number of conditions, as defined in Articles 41 and 42 of Directive 2001/83/EC and Articles 45 and 46 of Directive 2001/82/EC, are fulfilled (e.g. availability of a qualified person within the EU, GMP inspection). As of the end of the transition period, medicinal products shipped from Great Britain to the EU will be imported medicinal products, and the requirements for importers apply.

SUPPLIES OF CATEGORY 4 DRUG PRECURSOR CHEMICALS (THESE ARE NOT CONTROLLED DRUGS UNDER THE MISUSE OF DRUGS ACT OR REGULATIONS) FROM GREAT BRITAIN

Import and export licences are required for companies for the movement of any drug precursor chemicals that are imported or exported to and from Great Britain and, in some cases, Northern Ireland (NI).

For the purposes of drug precursor chemical control, NI will continue to apply European Union regulations, while Great Britain will not. This means NI companies trading with European Union Member States will not require import or export licences as this is considered "intra-community trade".

However, trade between Great Britain and NI will be subject to licensing in accordance with the requirements in Precursor chemical export and import authorisation. This includes "category 4" drug precursor chemicals, namely **medicinal preparations of ephedrine and pseudoephedrine**.

The Drug and Firearms Licensing Unit continues to act as the UK Competent Authority for drug precursor chemical control. Both Great Britain and NI companies should apply to the Drugs and Firearms Licensing Unit of the Home Office for their licences.

International collaboration

PHARMACEUTICAL INSPECTORATE CO-OPERATION SCHEME (PIC/S)

The MHRA is a member of the Pharmaceutical Inspectorate Co-operation Scheme (PIC/S), and has contributed to harmonising inspection standards since 1999.

PIC/S and its members continue close international cooperation between pharmaceutical authorities across GMP and GDP areas.

The MHRA maintains membership of the PIC/S Expert Circle on Good Distribution Practice (GDP), which was established in 2013. During this time, the Expert Circle has undertaken training of Inspectors by providing advanced training courses imparting GDP Inspectors with the knowledge and competence to inspect the global supply chain in a harmonised way. The Expert Circle has also developed a number of PIC/S GDP guidance documents, including the PIC/S GDP Guide of which the MHRA contributes.

The MHRA continues to promote the harmonisation of GDP practices and actively works with colleagues to ensure continuing development of regulations.

The goals of the Expert Circle on Good Distribution Practice (GDP) are to:

- design, develop and implement an advanced training course for GDP Inspectors;
- develop a question and answer document;
- identify, design and develop GDP PIC/S guidance documents.

The MHRA actively contributes to the development of guidance and the identification of emerging regulatory trends.

The Application and Inspection Process: "What to Expect"

Application

To sell or supply medicines to anyone other than the patient using the medicine, you need a wholesale dealer's licence – also known as a wholesale distribution authorisation or WDA(H).

Applicants for a new wholesale dealer's licence or existing licence holders wishing to vary their licence should follow MHRA guidance and instructions and make their application using the MHRA Process Licensing Portal accessible via the GOV.UK website.

The MHRA, acting as the licensing authority, will only issue a wholesale dealer's licence when it is satisfied, following an inspection of the site(s), that the information contained in the application is accurate and in compliance with the requirements of the legislation.

When appropriate, the MHRA may refuse to grant a wholesale dealer's licence or may grant a wholesale dealer's licence otherwise than as applied for. In such cases the licensing authority will notify the applicant of its proposals. The notification will set out the reasons for its proposals and give the applicant a period of not less than 28 days to respond (https://pclportal.mhra.gov.uk/).

APPLY FOR A LICENCE FOR HUMAN OR VETERINARY MEDICINES

The licence applicant must provide the following:

- A separate application for a human medicines wholesale dealer's licence and a veterinary medicines wholesale dealer's licence.
- An application fee (which includes the fee relating to the first inspection).

- Company and site details.
- Nomination of one or more people to be named as Responsible Person (RP) or Responsible Person for import (RPi) for a human medicines wholesale dealer's licence or a wholesale dealer's Qualified Person on a veterinary medicines wholesale dealer's licence. This should be supported with CV, references and identification details for each named person.
- Details of the activities to be carried out and the medicinal products to be wholesaled. For all activities and products included in the application there must be sufficient provisions on site to support the application.

The licence applicant should also consider if any of the following are required (separate applications are required for each):

- Broker registration;
- Active Substance registration.

APPLY TO VARY A LICENCE

The licence holder is required to keep their licence up to date. Any changes to named personnel, sites, activities or categories of products wholesaled require a licence variation. This variation may trigger an inspection, which must take place before the variation can be approved. Wholesale from a new site, new activities or new products may not commence until the replacement licence is received.

https://www.gov.uk/guidance/apply-for-manufacturer-or-wholesaler-of-medicines-licences

Inspection

PLANNING

Fee-bearing inspections of licensed wholesale dealers are carried out to assess the degree of compliance to standards of Good Distribution Practice (GDP) and compliance with the provisions of the licence.

Inspections of licensed wholesale dealers are undertaken as part of the risk-based inspection programme, further details of which can be found later in this guide.

NOTIFICATION

Advance notice of inspection is normally given to a company, unless circumstances require that an unannounced inspection should take place. The timing of the inspection would normally be notified in writing by the inspector.

In accordance with the GDP risk-based inspection process, sites will be required to complete a Compliance Report in advance of inspection. Further information and guidance can be found in the risk-based inspections section.

CONDUCT

The major stages of the inspection process are:
- the introductory or opening meeting;
- the detailed site inspection;
- the summary or closing meeting.

INTRODUCTORY OR OPENING MEETING

The purpose of the meeting is for the inspector to meet with the appropriate key personnel from the company to discuss the arrangements for the inspection. The inspector would typically confirm the nature of the business, premises and security arrangements, areas to be visited and any documentation that may be required.

SITE INSPECTION

The purpose of the site inspection is to determine the degree of conformity of the operations to the requirements of GDP and to assess compliance with the terms and conditions of licences issued under the appropriate legislation or with details submitted in support of an application for a licence. The inspection will typically involve visits to goods receipt, storage and dispatch areas (including ambient and refrigerated), returns/quarantine area, interviews with key personnel and a review of stock movement and quality system documentation, including product recalls. Any observations, recommendations and deficiencies noted during the inspection would normally be discussed with the company representatives at the time.

During inspections of manufacturing and wholesale operations, samples of starting materials, work in progress and finished products may be taken for testing if an inspector considers that this might assist in the detection of quality deficiencies. Occasionally, samples may be taken when these cannot be obtained from other sources, for routine surveillance purposes.

The inspection will also assess if the named RP meets the knowledge, experience and responsibility requirements. This will be more noticeable when a person has been newly nominated or if their role has changed substantially.

The licence applicant/licence holder must be prepared to demonstrate that all proposed sites, activities, products and personnel are suitable, within the scope of the licence and accurately reflected on the licence. A table is provided in Appendix 4 to assist the licence holder/applicant in ensuring they have the correct licence when planning to import or export.

SUMMARY OR CLOSING MEETING

The purpose of the meeting is for the inspector to provide the company with a verbal summary of the inspection findings and to allow the company to correct at this stage any misconceptions. The inspector would typically summarise the definition and classification of deficiencies they propose to report and the company are encouraged to give an undertaking to resolve the deficiencies and to agree a provisional timetable for corrective action. The inspector would also describe the arrangements for the formal notification of the deficiencies to the company (the post-inspection letter) and what is expected as a response.

Deficiencies are classified as follows:

- Critical deficiency:

  Any departure from Guidelines on GDP resulting in a medicinal product causing a significant risk to the patient and public health. This includes an activity increasing the risk of falsified medicines reaching the patients. A combination of a number of major deficiencies that indicates a serious systems failure. An example of a critical deficiency could be: purchase from or supply of medicinal products to a non-authorised person; storage of products requiring refrigeration at ambient temperatures; rejected or recalled products found in sellable stock.

- Major deficiency:

  A non-critical deficiency:
  – that indicates a major deviation from GDP; **or**
  – that has caused or may cause a medicinal product not to comply with its marketing authorisation, in particular its storage and transport conditions; **or**
  – that indicates a major deviation from the terms and provisions of the wholesale distribution authorisation; **or** a combination of several other deficiencies, none of which on their own may be major, but which may together represent a major deficiency.

- *Other deficiency*:

  A deficiency that cannot be classified as either critical or major but that indicates a departure from guidelines on GDP.

The choice of company representatives at the meeting is primarily for the company to decide but should normally include the senior staff who were present during the inspection and the RP.

Depending upon the inspection findings and the response from the company during and following the inspection, the inspector may take one of a number of actions ranging from:

- issuing a GDP certificate confirming essential compliance with GDP; to
- referral to the compliance escalation process or the Inspection Action Group (IAG) for consideration for adverse licensing action where serious non-compliance is found.

Further information on the Compliance escalation process and IAG can be found in this publication.

The inspected site is expected to provide a written response (by letter or e-mail) to the post-inspection letter within the required timeframe. The response should consider the context of the deficiency within the overall quality system rather than just the specific issue identified. The response should include proposals for dealing with the deficiencies, together with a timetable for their implementation. The response should be structured as follows:

- restate the deficiency number and the deficiency as written below;
- state the proposed corrective action;
- state the proposed target date for the completion of the corrective action(s);
- include any comment the company considers appropriate;
- provide evidence supporting any corrective action where it is considered appropriate.

Once the inspector is satisfied that any necessary remedial action has been taken or is in hand and that the site is essentially in compliance with GDP, an inspection report and GDP certificate are finalised.

Risk-based Inspection Programme

Introduction

The MHRA has been incorporating elements of risk management into its inspection programme for a number of years. A formal risk-based inspection (RBI) programme was implemented on 1 April 2009 and covers all aspects of good practices associated with the inspection of clinical, pre-clinical and quality control laboratories, clinical trials, manufacturers, wholesalers and pharmacovigilance systems. The primary aim of the RBI programme is to enable inspectorate resources to focus on areas that maximise protection of public health while reducing the overall administrative and economic burden to stakeholders.

GDP risk-based inspection (RBI) programme

The GDP risk-based inspection process commenced for all wholesale dealer's licence holders on 1 April 2009. Inspections may be conducted on site, remotely or as a hybrid combination of the two.

Compliance Report

Sites will be required to complete a Compliance Report in advance of inspection: this will be prompted by the inspector. Guidance to completing the report can be found within the document. The Compliance Report should be returned to your inspector prior to the inspection.

Risk rating process

Inspectors use the inspection outputs along with a number of other factors to identify a risk rating for the site, which equates to a future inspection frequency. As this process is not concluded until the inspection is closed the risk ratings *will not* be discussed at the closing meetings. However, a copy of the full inspection report, which includes the full risk rating rationale, is provided to sites once the inspection has been closed.

The issue of a certificate of GDP compliance and/or support of the site on the relevant licence is indication of meeting the minimum level of GDP compliance. Risk ratings identify the degree of surveillance required within the licensing and inspection programme. There is no intention that sites be rated against each other as a result of risk ratings assigned by MHRA. Risk ratings can change following inspection resulting in either increased or decreased risk. Inspection risk ratings will not be published by MHRA.

There will be no formal process of appeal against risk ratings and future inspection frequency. However, any rating that results in an increased inspection frequency from the previous standard will be peer reviewed before conclusion by a GDP operations manager. The MHRA does have a formal complaints process if sites wish to log an issue; however, any concerns regarding the inspection process should be raised with the inspector.

Conditions of Holding a Wholesale Dealer's Licence

The holder of a wholesale dealer's licence must comply with certain conditions in relation to the wholesale distribution of medicinal products. These conditions are set out in regulations 43–45 (in the case of a wholesale dealer's licence held in Northern Ireland) or regulations 43 to 45AA (in the case of a wholesale dealer's licence held in Great Britain) of the Human Medicines Regulations 2012 [SI 2012/1916] ("the Regulations"). They require that the licence holder shall:

- comply with the guidelines on Good Distribution Practice; in the case of a licence holder in Great Britain, published under, or that apply by virtue of, regulation C17 of the Regulations and in the case of a licence holder in Northern Ireland, published by the European Commission in accordance with Article 84 of the 2001 Directive.

- ensure, within the limits of their responsibility as a distributor of medicinal products, the appropriate and continued supply of such medicinal products to pharmacies and persons who may lawfully sell such products by retail or who may lawfully supply them in circumstances corresponding to retail sale, so that the needs of patients in the UK are met;
- provide and maintain such staff, premises, equipment and facilities for the handling, storage and distribution of the medicinal products under the licence as are necessary to maintain the quality of, and ensure proper distribution of, the medicinal products;
- inform the licensing authority of any proposed structural alteration to, or discontinued use of, premises to which the licence relates or premises that have been approved by the licensing authority;
- inform the licensing authority of any change to the Responsible Person;
- not sell or offer for sale or supply in the case of a product for sale or supply in Great Britain, there is a UKMA(GB), UKMA(UK), a COR(GB), a COR(UK), a THR(GB) or a THR(UK), or in Northern Ireland there is a UKMA(NI), UKMA(UK), a COR(NI), a COR(UK), a THR(NI), a THR(UK) and EU marketing authorisation or an Article 126a authorisation, in force in relation to the product and the sale or supply, or offer for sale or supply, is in accordance with that authorisation. This restriction on the holder of a wholesale dealer's licence shall not apply to:
  - the sale or supply, or offer for sale or supply, of a special medicinal product in the United Kingdom;
  - the export from Northern Ireland to an EEA State, or supply for the purposes of such export, of a medicinal product which may be placed on the market in that State without a marketing authorisation, Article 126a authorisation, certificate of registration or traditional herbal registration by virtue of legislation adopted by that State under Article 5(1) of the 2001 Directive;
  - the export from Great Britain to an approved country for import, or supply for the purposes of such export, of a medicinal product which may be placed on the market in that country without:
    (i) a marketing authorisation, certificate of registration or traditional herbal registration within the meaning of the 2001 Directive, by virtue of legislation adopted by that country under Article 5(1) of that Directive, where the approved country for import is an EEA State, or
    (ii) such equivalent authorisation, certificate or registration in the approved country for import, under legislation in that country that makes provision that is equivalent to Article 5(1) of the 2001 Directive, where the approved country for import is not an EEA State;
  - the sale or supply, or offer for sale or supply, of an unauthorised medicinal product where the Secretary of State has temporarily authorised the distribution of the product under regulation 174; or

– the wholesale distribution of medicinal products:
  (i) from Northern Ireland to a person in a country other than Great Britain or a country other than an EEA State; or
  (ii) from Great Britain to a person in a country other than Northern Ireland or a country other than an approved country for import.

The holder of a wholesale dealer's licence shall:
- keep such documents relating to the sale of medicinal products to which their licence relates as will facilitate the withdrawal or recall from sale of medicinal products in accordance with an emergency plan referred to below;
- have in place an emergency plan that will ensure effective implementation of the recall from the market of any relevant medicinal products where such recall is:
- ordered by the licensing authority
  – in the case of a licence holder in Great Britain, by an appropriate authority for the licensing of medicinal products in an approved country for import;
  – in the case of a licence holder in Northern Ireland, by the competent authority of any EEA State
- carried out in co-operation with the manufacturer of, or the holder of:
  – in the case of a product for sale or supply in Great Britain, the UKMA(GB) or UKMA(UK), certificate of registration or traditional herbal registration, or
- in the case of a product for sale or supply in Northern Ireland, the UKMA(NI) or UKMA(UK), EU marketing authorisation, Article 126a authorisation, certificate of registration or traditional herbal registration for the product;
- keep records in relation to the receipt, dispatch or brokering of medicinal products, of the date of receipt, the date of despatch, the date of brokering, the name of the medicinal product, the quantity of the product received, dispatched or brokered, the name and address of the person from whom the products were received or to whom they are dispatched, and where the receipt, dispatch or brokering of medicinal products takes places in Northern Ireland, the batch number of medicinal products bearing safety features referred to in point (o) of Article 54 of the 2001 Directive.

Where the holder of a wholesale dealer's licence in Northern Ireland imports from another EEA State for which they are not the holder of the marketing authorisation, Article 126a authorisation, certificate of registration or a traditional herbal registration of the product, then they shall notify the holder of that authorisation of their intention to import that product. In the case where the product is the subject of a marketing authorisation granted under Regulation (EC) No 726/2004, the holder of the wholesale dealer's licence shall notify the EMA or for any other authorisation they shall notify the licensing authority. In both cases they will be required to pay a fee to the EMA in accordance with Article 76(4) of the 2001 Directive or the licensing authority as the case may be, in accordance with the Fees Regulations. These requirements will not apply in relation to the wholesale distribution of medicinal products to a person in a non-EEA country.

Where the licence holder imports into Great Britain a medicinal product, other than for the sole purpose of wholesale distribution of that product to a person in a country other than the United Kingdom but is not the holder of a UK marketing authorisation, certificate of registration or traditional herbal registration in respect of that product they must notify he holder of any authorisation, certificate or registration, granted by an authority in the country from which the product is exported, to sell or supply that product in that country, and the licensing authority, of the intention to import that product and pay a fee to the licensing authority in accordance with the Fees Regulations.

The licence holder, for the purposes of enabling the licensing authority to determine whether there are grounds for suspending, revoking or varying the licence, must permit a person authorised in writing by the licensing authority, on production of identification, to carry out any inspection, or to take any samples or copies, that an inspector could carry out or take under Part 16 (enforcement) of the Regulations.

The holder of a wholesale dealer's licence permitting wholesale dealings in Northern Ireland must verify that any medicinal products they receive that are required by Article 54a of the Directive to bear safety features are not falsified. This does not apply in relation to the distribution of medicinal products received from a third country by a person for supply to a person in a third country. Any verification is carried out by checking the safety features on the outer packaging, in accordance with the requirements laid down in the delegated acts adopted under Article 54a(2) of the 2001 Directive medicinal products that are required to bear safety features pursuant to Article 54a of the 2001 Directive. Before supplying a medicinal product to person in Northern Ireland who falls within one of the classes specified below the licence holder must verify the safety features and decommission the unique identifier of that medicinal product in accordance with the requirements laid down in Commission Regulation 2016/161. The classes of person mentioned here are:

- persons authorised or entitled to supply medicinal products to the public who do not operate within a healthcare institution or within a pharmacy;
- persons who receive the product for the purpose of selling, supplying or administering it as a veterinary medicinal product;
- dentists;
- registered optometrists or registered dispensing opticians;

- registered paramedics;
- persons who are members of Her Majesty's armed forces;
- the Police Service of Northern Ireland;
- government institutions maintaining stocks of medicinal products for the purposes of civil protection or disaster control;
- universities or other institutions concerned with higher education or research, other than healthcare institutions;
- a prison service;
- persons carrying on the business of a school;
- nursing homes;
- hospices.

The licence holder must maintain a quality system setting out responsibilities, processes and risk-management measures in relation to their activities.

The licence holder must also immediately inform the licensing authority and, where applicable, the marketing authorisation holder or EU marketing authorisation holder, of medicinal products which the licence holder receives or is offered which the licence holder knows or suspects, or has reasonable grounds for knowing or suspecting, to be falsified.

Where the medicinal product is obtained through brokering, a licence holder in Great Britain must verify that the broker involved fulfils the requirements set out in regulation 45A(1)(b) and a licence holder in Northern Ireland must verify that the broker involved is validly registered with the licensing authority or the competent authority of an EEA State.

The licence holder must not obtain supplies of medicinal products from anyone except:

(a) the holder of a manufacturer's licence or wholesale dealer's licence in relation to products of that description;

(b) the person who holds an authorisation granted by (an approved country for import (in the case of a licence holder in Great Britain) or by an EEA State (in the case of a licence holder in Northern Ireland) authorising the manufacture of products of the description of their distribution by way of wholesaling dealing; or

(c) where the medicinal product is directly received:

    (i) in the case of a licence holder in Great Britain, from a country that is not an approved country for import ("A") for export to a country that is not an approved country for import ("B"), and

    (ii) in the case of a licence holder in Northern Ireland, from a state other than an EEA State ("A") for export to another state other than an EEA State ("B"),

the supplier of the medicinal product in country A is a person who is authorised or entitled to supply such medicinal products in accordance with the legal and administrative provisions in country A. This does not apply to in the case of a licence holder in Great Britain, products received from Northern Ireland and, in the case of a licence holder in Northern Ireland, products received from Great Britain.

From 28 October 2013, where the medicinal product is directly received from a non-EEA country for export to a non-EEA country, the licensed wholesale dealer must check that the supplier of the medicinal product in the exporting non-EEA country is authorised or entitled to supply such medicinal products in accordance with the legal and administrative provisions in that country.

The holder of a wholesale dealer's licence must verify that the wholesale dealer who supplies the product complies with the principles and guidelines of good distribution practices, or the manufacturer or importer who supplies the product holds a manufacturing authorisation.

The holder of a wholesale dealer's licence may distribute medicinal products by way of wholesale dealing only to:

- the holder of a wholesale dealer's licence relating to those products;
- the holder of an authorisation granted by in the case of a licence holder in Great Britain, the appropriate authority of an approved country for import in the case of a licence holder in Northern Ireland, the competent authority of an-other EEA State, that is responsible for authorising the supply of those products by way of wholesale dealing;
- the holder of a wholesale dealer's licence relating to those products, the holder of an authorisation granted by the competent authority of another EEA State authorising the supply of those products by way of wholesale dealing, a person who may lawfully sell those products by retail or may lawfully supply them in circumstances corresponding to retail sale, or a person who may lawfully administer those products. This does not apply in relation to medicinal products that are distributed by way of wholesale dealing to a person in a non-EEA country.
- In relation to supply in the case of a licence holder in Great Britain to persons in countries other than approved countries for import, a person who is authorised or entitled to receive medicinal products for wholesale distribution or supply to the public in accordance with the applicable legal and administrative provisions of the country to which the product is supplied and, in the case of a licence holder in Northern Ireland, to persons in a state other than an EEA State, a person who is authorised or entitled to receive medicinal products for wholesale distribution or supply to the public in accordance with the applicable legal and administrative provisions of the state other than an EEA State concerned. This does not apply to in the case of a licence holder in Great Britain, products supplied to Northern Ireland, and in the case of a licence holder in Northern Ireland, products supplied to Great Britain.

From 28 October 2013, where the medicinal product is supplied directly to persons in a non-EEA country the licensed wholesale dealer must check that the person who receives it is authorised or entitled to receive medicinal products for wholesale distribution or supply to the public in accordance with the applicable legal and administrative provisions of the non-EEA country concerned.

Where any medicinal product is supplied to any person who may lawfully sell those products by retail or who may lawfully supply them in circumstances corresponding to retail sale, the licence holder shall enclose with the product a document which makes it possible to ascertain:

- the date on which the supply took place;
- the name and pharmaceutical form of the product supplied;
- the quantity of product supplied;
- the names and addresses of the person or persons from whom the products were supplied to the licence holder; and
- the batch number of the medicinal products bearing the safety features referred to in point (o) of Article 54 of the 2001 Directive in the case of a licence holder in Northern Ireland.

The holder of a wholesale dealer's licence shall keep a record of the information supplied where any medicinal product is supplied to any person who may lawfully sell those products by retail or who may lawfully supply them in circumstances corresponding to retail sale for a minimum period of 5 years after the date on which it is supplied and ensure, during that period, that the record is available to the licensing authority for inspection.

A licence holder in Great Britain may only obtain a medicinal product in respect of which a UKMA(GB) was granted under the unfettered access route if the product satisfies the definition of qualifying Northern Ireland goods.

The wholesale dealer's licence holder shall at all times have at their disposal the services of a Responsible Person who, in the opinion of the licensing authority, has knowledge of the activities to be carried out and of the procedures to be performed under the licence which is adequate for performing the functions of Responsible Person; and has experience in those procedures and activities which is adequate for those purposes.

The functions of the Responsible Person shall be to ensure, in relation to medicinal products, that the conditions under which the licence has been granted have been, and are being, complied with and ensuring that the quality of medicinal products handled by the licence holder is being maintained in accordance with the requirements of in the case of a licence holder in Great Britain, the UK marketing authorisations, certificates of registration or traditional herbal registrations, and in the case of a licence holder in

Northern Ireland, the marketing authorisations, Article 126a authorisations, certificates of registration or traditional herbal registrations, applicable to those products.

The licence holder must notify the licensing authority of any change to the Responsible Person; and the name, address, qualifications and experience of the Responsible Person. They must not permit any person to act as a Responsible Person other than the person named in the licence or another person notified to the licensing authority.

A Responsible Person (import) is required where a licence holder in Great Britain imports a medicinal product from an approved country for import under a wholesale dealer's licence. This requirement does not apply where an unlicensed medicinal product imported from an approved country for import for the sole purpose of distribution by way of wholesale dealing as a special medicinal product; or for the sole purpose of wholesale distribution of that product to a person in a country other than an approved country for import. The licence holder must ensure that there is available at all times at least one Responsible Person (import) whose name is included in the register established by the licensing authority.

A Responsible Person (import) must carry out the functions of a Responsible Person unless a Responsible Person is performing those functions in respect of the licence; and they must ensure that there is appropriate evidence to confirm that each production batch of a medicine imported from an approved country for import under the licence has been certified as provided for in Article 51 of the 2001 Directive, or such equivalent certification procedure as applies in the approved country for import and ensure that each production batch of a medicinal product that is subject to the batch testing condition and that is imported into Great Britain from an approved country for import has been certified as being in conformity with the approved specifications in the UK marketing authorisation by the appropriate authority, or where the batch testing exemption applies, a laboratory in a country that has an agreement with the United Kingdom to the effect that the appropriate authority will recognise that certificate in place of the appropriate authority's own examination.

The licence holder must apply to vary the licence if a change is proposed to the Responsible Person (import) and they must not permit any person to act as a Responsible Person (import) other than the person named in the licence.

The standard provisions for wholesale dealer's licences, that is, those provisions which may be included in all licences unless the licence specifically provides otherwise, insofar as those licences relate to relevant medicinal products, shall be those provisions set out in Part 4 of Schedule 4 of the Regulations.

The licence holder shall not use any premises for the purpose of the handling, storage or distribution of relevant medicinal products other than those specified in their licence or notified to the licensing authority by them and approved by the licensing authority.

The licence holder shall provide such information as may be requested by the licensing authority concerning the type and quantity of any relevant medicinal products that they handle, store or distribute.

Where and insofar as the licence relates to special medicinal products to which regulation 167 of the Regulations apply, which do not have a marketing authorisation and are commonly known as "specials" (refer to MHRA Guidance Note 14), the licence holder shall only import such products from another in the case of an import into Great Britain, an approved country for import and in the case of an import into Northern Ireland, an EEA State in response to an order that satisfies the requirements of regulation 167 of the Regulations; and where the following conditions are complied with:

- No later than 28 days prior to each importation of a special medicinal product, the licence holder shall give written notice to the licensing authority stating their intention to import that special medicinal product and stating the following particulars:
  - the name of the medicinal product, being the brand name or the common name, or the scientific name, and any name, if different, under which the medicinal product is to be sold or supplied in the United Kingdom;
  - any trademark or name of the manufacturer of the medicinal product;
  - in respect of each active constituent of the medicinal product, any international non-proprietary name or the British approved name or the monograph name or, where that constituent does not have an international non-proprietary name, a British-approved name or a monograph name, the accepted scientific name or any other name descriptive of the true nature of that constituent in English;
  - the quantity of medicinal product that is to be imported that shall not exceed more, on any one occasion, than such amount as is sufficient for 25 single administrations, or for 25 courses of treatment where the amount imported is sufficient for a maximum of 3 months' treatment; and
  - the name and address of the manufacturer or assembler of that medicinal product in the form in which it is to be imported and, if the person who will supply that medicinal product for importation is not the manufacturer or assembler, the name and address of such supplier.
  - Subject to the next bullet point below, the licence holder shall not import the special medicinal product if, before the end of 28 days from the date on which the licensing authority sends or gives the licence holder an acknowledgement in writing by the licensing authority that they have received the notice referred to in the bullet point above, the licensing authority have notified them in writing that the product should not be imported.

- The licence holder may import the special medicinal product referred to in the notice where they have been notified in writing by the licensing authority, before the end of the 28-day period referred to in the bullet point above, that the special medicinal product may be imported.
- Where the licence holder sells or supplies special medicinal products, they shall, in addition to any other records that they are required to make by the provisions of their licence, make and maintain written records relating to the batch number of the batch of the product from which the sale or supply was made and details of any adverse reaction to the product so sold or supplied of which they become aware.
- The licence holder shall import no more on any one occasion than such amount as is sufficient for 25 single administrations, or for 25 courses of treatment where the amount imported is sufficient for a maximum of 3 months' treatment, and on any such occasion shall not import more than the quantity notified to the licensing authority in the notification of intention to import.
- The licence holder shall inform the licensing authority forthwith of any matter coming to their attention that might reasonably cause the licensing authority to believe that the medicinal product can no longer be regarded either as a product that can safely be administered to human beings or as a product that is of satisfactory quality for such administration.
- The licence holder shall not issue any advertisement, catalogue or circular relating to the special medicinal product or make any representations in respect of that product.
- The licence holder shall cease importing or supplying a special medicinal product if they have received a notice in writing from the licensing authority directing that, as from a date specified in that notice, a particular product or class of products shall no longer be imported or supplied.

A licence holder in Great Britain may only supply a special medicinal product to a person in Northern Ireland, and in Northern Ireland may only supply a special medicinal product to a person in Great Britain in response to an order which satisfies the requirements of regulation 167.

The licence holder shall take all reasonable precautions and exercise all due diligence to ensure that any information they provide to the licensing authority that is relevant to an evaluation of the safety, quality or efficacy of any medicinal product for human use which they handle, store or distribute is not false or misleading in a material particular.

Where a wholesale dealer's licence relates to exempt advanced therapy medicinal products the licence holder shall keep the data for the system for the traceability of the advanced therapy medicinal products for such period, being a period of longer than 30 years, as may be specified by the licensing authority.

The Standard Provisions also require the holder of a wholesale dealer's licence that relates to exempt advanced therapy medicinal products to obtain supplies of exempt advanced therapy medicinal products only from the holder of a manufacturer's licence in respect of those products or the holder of a wholesale dealer's licence in respect of those products.

The licence holder must:

- distribute an exempt advanced therapy medicinal product by way of wholesale dealing only to the holder of a wholesale dealer's licence in respect of those products; or a person who may lawfully administer those products, and solicited the product for an individual patient;
- establish and maintain a system ensuring that the exempt advanced therapy medicinal product and its starting and raw materials, including all substances coming into contact with the cells or tissues it may contain, can be traced through the sourcing, manufacturing, packaging, storage, transport and delivery to the establishment where the product is used;
- inform the licensing authority of any adverse reaction to any exempt advanced therapy medicinal product supplied by the holder of the wholesale dealer's licence of which the holder is aware;
- keep the data for ensuring traceability for a minimum of 30 years after the expiry date of the exempt advanced therapy medicinal product or longer as specified by the licensing authority;
- ensure that the data for ensuring traceability will, in the event that the licence is suspended, revoked or withdrawn or the licence holder becomes bankrupt or insolvent, be held available to the licensing authority by the holder of a wholesale dealer's licence for the same period that the data has to be kept; and
- not import or export any exempt advanced therapy medicinal product.

(1) Guidelines on Good Distribution Practice of Medicinal Products for Human Use (2013/C 343/01) http://eur-lex.europa.eu/LexUriServ/LexUriServ.do?uri=OJ:C:2013:343:0001:0014:EN:PDF.

(2) Point (o) of Article 54 was inserted by Directive 2011/62/EU of the European Parliament and of the Council (OJ No L 174, 1.7.2011, p.74).

(3) Article 76(4) was inserted by Directive 2011/62/EU of the European Parliament and of the Council (OJ No L 174, 1.7.2011, p.74).

(4) Article 54a was inserted by Directive 2011/62/EU of the European Parliament and of the Council (OJ No L 174, 1.7.2011, p.74).

Matters Relating to Unlicensed Medicines

Unless exempt, a medicinal product must be the subject of a marketing authorisation before being placed on the market.

Regulation 167 of the Human Medicines Regulations 2012 provides an exemption from the need for a marketing authorisation for a medicinal product that is supplied:

- in response to an unsolicited order;
- manufactured and assembled in accordance with the specification of a person who is a doctor, dentist, nurse independent prescriber, pharmacist independent prescriber or supplementary prescriber;
- for use by a patient for whose treatment that person is directly responsible in order to fulfil the special needs of that patient; and meets the conditions specified in Regulation 167(2)–(8).

In the interest of public health the exemption is narrowly drawn because these products, unlike licensed medicinal products, may not have been assessed by the licensing authority against the criteria of safety, quality and efficacy.

See MHRA Guidance Note 14 on the supply of unlicensed medicinal products "specials" which contains additional guidance for those who want to manufacture, import, distribute or supply unlicensed medicines for human use for the treatment of an individual patient.

Supply of unlicensed medicines when an equivalent licensed product becomes available

Unlicensed medicines may only be supplied against valid special clinical needs of a patient. This requires that there is no authorised equivalent available on the national market. Supply for reasons of cost, institutional need or convenience is not acceptable and is not a special clinical need.

Examples of inappropriate reasons for supply have included preference for a non-parallel imported product, cost, more convenient presentation and longer shelf-life of the unlicensed product. None of these reasons is acceptable.

While requests for procurement of unlicensed medicines are not regulated by MHRA, the supply of unlicensed medicines falls under the Human Medicines Regulations 2012 [SI 2012/1916]. Importers and suppliers must be able to demonstrate compliance with these regulations. This includes supply of unlicensed medicines only to meet valid special clinical needs. Appropriate evidence of supply against such needs should be retained.

https://www.gov.uk/government/publications/supply-unlicensed-medicinal-products-specials

https://www.gov.uk/guidance/import-a-human-medicine

Brokering of Medicines

4

UK Legislation on Brokering Medicines

Contents

The Human Medicines Regulations 2012 [SI 2012/1916]

Editor's note	These extracts from the Human Medicines Regulations 2012 [SI 2012/1916] as amended are presented for the reader's convenience. Reproduction is with the permission of HMSO and the Queen's Printer for Scotland. For any definitive information reference must be made to the original amending Regulations. The numbering and content within this section correspond with the regulations set out in the published Statutory Instrument [SI 2012/1916] as amended.

Citation and commencement

1 (1) These Regulations may be cited as the Human Medicines Regulations 2012.

   (2) These Regulations come into force on 14th August 2012.

General interpretation

8 (1) In these Regulations (unless the context otherwise requires) "brokering" means all activities in relation to the sale or purchase of medicinal products, except for wholesale distribution, that do not

include physical handling and that consist of negotiating independently and on behalf of another legal or natural person;

"falsified medicinal product" means any medicinal product with a false representation of:

(a) its identity, including its packaging and labelling, its name or its composition (other than any unintentional quality defect) as regards any of its ingredients including excipients and the strength of those ingredients;
(b) its source, including its manufacturer, its country of manufacturing, its country of origin or its marketing authorisation holder; or
(c) its history, including the records and documents relating to the distribution channels used.

Brokering in medicinal products

45A (1) A person may not broker a medicinal product in Great Britain unless:
  (a) the product is covered by an authorisation granted:
    (i) by the licensing authority, or
    (ii) by an appropriate authority responsible for the licensing of medicinal products in an approved country for import, and
  (b) that person:
    (i) is validly registered as a broker with the licensing authority,
    (ii) has a permanent address in the United Kingdom, and
    (iii) complies with the guidelines on good distribution practice which apply under, or by virtue of, regulation C17 insofar as those guidelines apply to brokers.
(1A) A person may not broker a medicinal product in Northern Ireland unless:
  (a) the product is covered by an authorisation granted:
    (i) under Regulation (EC) No 726/2004,
    (ii) by the licensing authority, or
    (iii) by a competent authority of a member State, and
  (b) that person:
    (i) is validly registered as a broker with the licensing authority or a competent authority of a member State,
    (ii) except where the person is validly registered with the competent authority of an EEA state, has a permanent address in the United Kingdom, and
    (iii) complies with the guidelines on good distribution practice published by the European Commission in accordance with Article 84 of the 2001 Directive insofar as those guidelines apply to brokers.
(2) A person is not validly registered for the purpose of paragraph (1)(b) or (1A)(b) if:

(a) the person's permanent address is not entered into a register of brokers kept by a competent authority of a member State or the licensing authority (as appropriate);

(b) the registration is suspended; or

(c) the person has notified the competent authority of a member State or the licensing authority (as appropriate) to remove that person from the register.

Application for brokering registration

45B (1) The licensing authority may not register a person as a broker unless paragraphs (2) to (7) are complied with.

(2) An application for registration must be made containing:

(a) the name of the person to be registered;

(b) the name under which that person is trading (if different to the name of that person);

(c) that person's:
   (i) permanent address in the United Kingdom,
   (ii) e-mail address, and
   (iii) telephone number;

(d) a statement of whether the medicinal products to be brokered are:
   (i) prescription only medicines,
   (ii) pharmacy medicines, or
   (iii) medicines subject to general sale;

(e) an indication of the range of medicinal products to be brokered;

(f) evidence that that person can comply with regulations 45A(1)(b)(iii), 45E(3)(a) to (f) and 45F(1); and

(g) any fee payable in connection with the application in accordance with the Fees Regulations.

(3) Where the address at which the emergency plan, documents or record necessary to comply with regulation 45E(3)(b) to (d) are kept is different from the address notified in accordance with sub-paragraph (2)(c)(i), the application must contain:

(a) that address where the plan or records are to be kept;

(b) the name of a person who can provide access to that address for the purpose of regulation 325 (rights of entry); and

(c) that person's:
   (i) address,
   (ii) e-mail address, and
   (iii) telephone number.

(4) Unless paragraph (6) applies, the application for registration must:

(a) be in English; and

(b) be signed by the person seeking a brokering registration.

(5) The pages of the application must be serially numbered.

(6) Where the application is made on behalf of the person seeking a brokering registration by another person ("A"), the application must:

(a) contain the name and address of A; and

(b) be signed by A.

Criteria of broker's registration

45E (1) Registration of a broker is conditional on that broker:

(a) complying with regulation 45A(1); and

(b) satisfying:

(i) the criteria in paragraphs (3), (4) and (7), and

(ii) such other criteria as the licensing authority considers appropriate and notifies the broker of.

(2) The criteria referred to in paragraph (1)(b)(ii) may include (but are not limited to) the criteria specified in paragraphs (5) and (6).

(3) The broker must:

(a) have a permanent address in the United Kingdom;

(b) maintain an emergency plan to ensure effective implementation of the recall from the market of a medicinal product where recall is:

(i) ordered by:

(aa) in the case of a broker in Great Britain, the licensing authority or by an appropriate authority responsible for the licensing of medicinal products in an approved country for import, or

(bb) in the case of a broker in Northern Ireland, the licensing authority or by the competent authority of any EEA State, or

(ii) carried out in co-operation with the manufacturer of, or the holder of the marketing authorisation, for the product;

(c) keep documents relating to the sale or supply of medicinal products under the licence which may facilitate the withdrawal or recall from sale of medicinal products in accordance with sub-paragraph (b);

(d) record in relation to the brokering of each medicinal product:

(i) the name of the medicinal product,

(ii) the quantity of the product brokered,

(iii) the batch number where the sale or supply of the medcinal product is in Northern Ireland of the medicinal product bearing the safety features referred to in point (o) of Article 54 of the 2001 Directive,

(iv) the name and address of the:

(a) (aa) supplier, or

(b) (bb) consignee, and

    (v) the date on which the sale or purchase of the product is bro-
     kered;
   (e) maintain a quality system setting out responsibilities, processes
    and risk management measures in relation to their activities; and
   (f) keep the documents or record required by sub-paragraph (c) or
    (d) available to the licensing authority for a period of 5 years; and
   (g) comply with regulation 45F(1), (2) and (4).

(4) Where the address at which the plan or records necessary to comply
  with paragraph (3)(b) to (d) are kept is different from the address
  notified in accordance with regulation 45B(2)(c)(i), the broker must:
  (a) ensure that the plan or records are kept at an address in the United
   Kingdom; and
  (b) inform the licensing authority of the address at which the plan or
   records are kept.

(5) The broker must provide such information as may be requested by
  the licensing authority concerning the type and quantity of medicinal products brokered within the period specified by the licensing
  authority.

(6) The broker must take all reasonable precautions and exercise all due
  diligence to ensure that any information provided by that broker to
  the licensing authority in accordance with regulation 45F is not false
  or misleading.

(7) For the purposes of enabling the licensing authority to determine
  whether there are grounds for suspending, revoking or varying the
  registration, the broker must permit a person authorised in writing by
  the licensing authority, on production of identification, to carry out
  any inspection, or to take any copies, which an inspector may carry
  out or take under regulations 325 (rights of entry) and 327 (powers of
  inspection, sampling and seizure).

Provision of information

45F (1) A broker registered in the UK must immediately inform:
   (a) the licensing authority; and
   (b) in the case of a broker in:
    (i) Great Britain, either:
     (aa) the UK marketing authorisation holder, or
     (bb) where applicable, the holder of the licence or authori-
      sation granted by an appropriate authority responsible
      for the licensing of medicinal products in an approved
      country for import, or
    (ii) Northern Ireland, either:
     (aa) the UK marketing authorisation holder, or

        (bb) where applicable, the EU marketing authorisation holder, of medicinal products which the broker identifies as, suspects to be, or has reasonable grounds for knowing or suspecting to be, falsified.

(2) On or before the date specified in paragraph (3), a broker who is, or has applied to the licensing authority to become, a registered broker in the United Kingdom must submit a report to the licensing authority, which:

(a) includes a declaration that the broker has in place an appropriate system to ensure compliance with regulations 45A, 45B and this regulation; and

(b) details the system which the broker has in place to ensure such compliance.

(3) The date specified for the purposes of this paragraph is:

(a) in relation to any application made before 31 March 2014, the date of the application; and

(b) in relation to each subsequent reporting year, 30 April following the end of that year.

(4) The broker must without delay notify the licensing authority of any changes to the matters in respect of which evidence has been supplied in relation to paragraph (2) which might affect compliance with the requirements of this Chapter.

(5) Any report or notification to the licensing authority under paragraph (2) or (4) must be accompanied by the appropriate fee in accordance with the Fees Regulations.

(6) The licensing authority may give a notice to a registered broker requiring that broker to provide information of a kind specified in the notice within the period specified in the notice.

(7) A notice under paragraph (6) may not be given to a registered broker unless it appears to the licensing authority that it is necessary for the licensing authority to consider whether the registration should be varied, suspended or revoked.

(8) A notice under paragraph (6) may specify information which the licensing authority thinks necessary for considering whether the registration should be varied, suspended or revoked.

(9) In paragraph (3)(b), "reporting year" means a period of twelve months ending on 31 March.

5

EU Guidelines on GDP and UK Guidance on Brokering Medicines

Contents

Introduction

Persons procuring, holding, storing, supplying or exporting medicinal products are required to hold a wholesale distribution authorisation in accordance with the Human Medicines Regulations 2012.

However, the distribution network for medicinal products may involve operators who are not necessarily authorised wholesale distributors. To ensure the reliability of the supply chain, the Human Medicines Regulations 2012 regulates not only wholesale distributors, whether or not they physically handle the medicinal products, but also brokers who are involved in the sale or purchase of medicinal products without selling or purchasing those products themselves, and without owning and physically handling the medicinal products.

Brokers of medicines must comply with Chapter 10 of the European Commission's Guidelines on Good Distribution Practice of medicinal products for human use. This chapter sets out the guidelines alongside the expectations for UK brokers.

Chapter 10 – Specific Provisions for Brokers[1]

10.1 Principle

A "broker" is a person involved in activities in relation to the sale or purchase of medicinal products, except for wholesale distribution, that do not include physical handling and that consist of negotiating independently and on behalf of another legal or natural person[2].

Brokers are subject to a registration requirement. They must have a permanent address and contact details in the Member State where they are registered[3]. They must notify the competent authority of any changes to those details without unnecessary delay.

By definition, brokers do not procure, supply or hold medicines. Therefore, requirements for premises, installations and equipment as set out in Directive 2001/83/EC do not apply. However, all other rules in Directive 2001/83/EC that apply to wholesale distributors also apply to brokers.

10.2 Quality system

The quality system of a broker should be defined in writing, approved and kept up to date. It should set out responsibilities, processes and risk management in relation to their activities.

The quality system should include an emergency plan which ensures effective recall of medicinal products from the market ordered by the manufacturer or the competent authorities, or carried out in cooperation with the manufacturer or marketing authorisation holder for the medicinal product concerned[4]. The competent authorities must be immediately informed of any suspected falsified medicines offered in the supply chain[5].

10.3 Personnel

Any member of personnel involved in the brokering activities should be trained in the applicable EU and national legislation and in the issues concerning falsified medicinal products.

---

[1] Article 85b(3) of Directive 2001/83/EC.
[2] Article 1(17a) of Directive 2001/83/EC.
[3] Article 85b of Directive 2001/83/EC.
[4] Article 80(d) of Directive 2001/83/EC.
[5] Article 85b(1), third paragraph of Directive 2001/83/EC.

10.4 Documentation

The general provisions on documentation in Chapter 4 apply.

In addition, at least the following procedures and instructions, along with the corresponding records of execution, should be in place:

(i)   Procedure for complaints handling.
(ii)   Procedure for informing competent authorities and marketing authorisation holders of suspected falsified medicinal products.
(iii)   Procedure for supporting recalls.
(iv)   Procedure for ensuring that medicinal products brokered have a marketing authorisation.
(v)   Procedure for verifying that their supplying wholesale distributors hold a distribution authorisation, their supplying manufacturers or importers hold a manufacturing authorisation, and their customers are authorised to supply medicinal products in the Member State concerned.
(vi)   Records should be kept either in the form of purchase/sales invoices or on computer, or in any other form for any transaction in medicinal products brokered and should contain at least the following information: date; name of the medicinal product; quantity brokered; name and address of the supplier and the customer; and batch number at least for products bearing the safety features.

Records should be made available to the competent authorities, for inspection purposes, for the period stated in national legislation but at least 5 years.

UK Guidance on Chapter 10 – Specific Provisions for Brokers

Directive 2011/62/EU, known as the Falsified Medicines Directive (FMD), was transposed into UK law on 20 August 2013. It amended Directive 2001/83/EC by including measures aimed at preventing the entry of falsified medicines into the legal supply chain.

To accord with legislation, brokers of medicinal products are required to register their activities with the National competent authority. In the UK, this is the MHRA.

Brokers can negotiate between:

- the manufacturer and a wholesaler;
- or one wholesaler and another wholesaler;
- or the manufacturer or wholesale dealer with a person who may lawfully sell those products by retail or may lawfully supply them in circumstances corresponding to retail sale or a person who may lawfully administer those products.

Also:

- brokers may only broker medicinal products that are the subject of a marketing authorisation granted by the national competent authority;
- brokers must adhere to certain requirements of the registration including compliance with Chapter 10 of the Guidelines on Good Distribution Practice.

The Human Medicines (Amendments) Regulations 2013, UK Statutory Instruments 2013 No. 1855 Part 2 Regulation 16 "Chapter 3", introduced "Brokering in Medicinal Products" under Regulations 45A to 45L.

Following the changes on 1 January 2021, further amendments to Regulation have been implemented. The Human Medicines (Amendment etc.) (EU Exit) Regulations 2020, SI 2020 No. 1488, amended Regulations 45A, 45E and 45F of the Human Medicines Regulations 2012.

Background

A "broker" is a person involved in all activities in relation to the sale or purchase of medicinal products, except for wholesale distribution, that do not include physical handling and that consist of negotiating independently and on behalf of another legal or natural person.

Brokers are subject to a registration requirement. They must have a permanent address and contact details in the (UK) or approved country where they are registered. They must notify the competent authority of any changes to those details without unnecessary delay.

Brokers do not procure, supply or hold medicines. Therefore, requirements for premises, installations and equipment, as set out in legislation, do not apply. However, many other rules in legislation that apply to wholesale distributors also apply to brokers.

A broker based in the UK needs to be registered with the MHRA. If a UK wholesaler wishes to engage with a client of an EEA broker, they will need to check if that broker is legally entitled to broker in that country, and if their client is legally entitled to receive the medicine.

List of approved countries for authorised human medicines – GOV.UK https://www.gov.uk/government/publications/list-of-approved-countries-for-authorised-human-medicines/list-of-approved-countries.

Based on the above definition, the key factors that distinguish the activity of brokering of medicinal products from wholesale distribution include the following:

- Brokering is a financial activity focused only on purchasing and selling. Wholesaling involves a wider range of activities and participation in the supply chain.
- Brokering does not involve taking title for the medicinal products.

- Brokering is limited to negotiation of the relevant financial transactions. It is an intermediary role where the broker acts on behalf of another operator within that supply chain.
- Brokering does not involve the operator physically handling the medicinal products.

Application assessments are normally carried out as a desktop review by nominated MHRA Inspectors. The assessment consists of a review of the Broker's quality-management system submitted with the application. Once the Inspector is content that the applicant is compliant with GDP and the Human Medicines Regulations 2012, they are entered on to the Register of Brokers.

Some wholesalers may apply for a WDA(H) and broker registration at the same time. If so, both aspects will be looked at on inspection rather than by desktop review.

If an inspection is carried out, a broker will be inspected against Chapter 10 of the GDP Guidelines and Regulation 45A of the Human Medicines Regulations 2012.

The requirements for brokers are set out in the Human Medicines Regulations 2012 Regulations 45A, B, E and F. Brokers must also comply with GDP Chapter 10.

The Register of Brokers is maintained by MHRA Data Processing Team and is posted on the MHRA website at the following location:

https://www.gov.uk/government/publications/register-of-brokers-authorised-to-deal-in-human-medicines.

How to apply

Brokers apply to be registered through the MHRA Submissions portal: https://www.gov.uk/guidance/medicines-register-as-a-broker.

Once the application has been received, the information is downloaded, processed and passed to the GDP Inspectorate for assessment.

Annually from 1 April, brokers must submit a declaration confirming compliance with the Regulations. This annual declaration is passed to the GDP Inspectorate for assessment. The annual declaration is requested by MHRA.

Any changes to the broker registration must be communicated via a variation to the MHRA and significant changes are passed to GDP Inspectorate for assessment.

Changes passed for assessment would be an issue that potentially affects how the company operates, such as a change in personnel or adding additional sites.

Specific provisions for brokers

Brokers are required to:

- maintain a quality system;
- adhere to some good distribution practice requirements; and
- maintain a sufficient level of documentation relating to transactions carried out, to assist with ensuring full traceability for medicinal products across the supply chain.

Legislation sets out specific provisions with which brokers must comply. These include the following requirements:

- Maintain an emergency plan that ensures effective implementation of any recall from the market ordered by the Competency Authority or carried out in cooperation with the manufacturer or marketing authorisation holder for the medicinal product concerned.
- Keep records either in the form of purchase/sales invoices or on computer, or in any other form, giving for any transaction in medicinal products received, dispatched or brokered at least the following information: date; name of the medicinal product; quantity brokered; name and address of the supplier and consignee; batch number of the medicinal products, at least for products bearing the safety features referred to in point (o) of Article 54 of the Directive.
- Keep the records referred to available to the MHRA, for inspection purposes, for a period of 5 years.
- Comply with the principles and guidelines of Good Distribution Practice for medicinal products.
- Maintain a quality system setting out responsibilities, processes and risk-management measures in relation to their activities.
- Immediately inform the MHRA and, where applicable, the Marketing Authorisation Holder, of medicinal products identified as falsified or suspected to be falsified.

Quality management system (QMS)

When completing the application via the MHRA Submissions portal, there is a requirement to submit the following standard operating procedures for review by the GDP Inspectorate:

STANDARD OPERATING PROCEDURES

The SOPs to be attached are those listed in EU GDP in Chapter 10.4 as follows:

(i)   Procedure for complaints handling.
(ii) Procedure for informing competent authorities and marketing authorisation holders of suspected falsified medicinal products.

(iii) Procedure for supporting recalls.

(iv) Procedure for ensuring that medicinal products brokered have a marketing authorisation.

(v) Procedure for verifying that their supplying wholesale distributors hold a distribution authorisation, their supplying manufacturers or importers hold a manufacturing authorisation and their customers are authorised to supply medicinal products in the Member State concerned.

(vi) Records should be kept either in the form of purchase/sales invoices or on computer, or in any other form for any transaction in medicinal products brokered and should contain at least the following information: date; name of the medicinal product; quantity brokered; name and address of the supplier and the customer; and batch number at least for products bearing the safety features.

In addition to the standard operating procedures, a full description of the intending brokering business model should be included in the documentation provided on the Submissions portal. This provides the opportunity for the assessing Inspector to review all submitted documentation and determine if the company is compliant with the proposed business operational model.

The MHRA will inform the company by way of e-mail they have been approved.

The company *does not* receive any form of licence; they are added to the Broker Register on the MHRA website.

If a physical inspection is carried out, the organisation receives a GDP Broker Certificate of Compliance.

Providing inaccurate information leads to delaying the approval process. For example:

NO PROCEDURES

- There is a requirement to provide relevant standard operating procedures as described on the application.

LACK OF INFORMATION

- The information submitted falls extensively short of the requirements for approval.

LACK OF CLARITY ON THE INTENDED BUSINESS MODEL

- To ensure I have a clear understanding of your intended business model, would you please confirm that is it your intention to conduct brokering activities as described below:

A *"broker" is a person involved in activities in relation to the sale or purchase of medicinal products, except for wholesale distribution, that*

EU GUIDELINES ON GDP AND UK GUIDANCE ON BROKERING MEDICINES

*"do not include physical handling" and that consist **only** of "negotiating independently" and on behalf of another legal or natural person. Therefore, by definition, brokers do not **procure, supply or hold medicines**.*

- Reference is made to the Responsible Person in several of your procedures and QMS. A Responsible Person is not a requirement of the Broker registration. The scope of the business model appears to relate to the wholesale distribution of medicinal product.

If an application is incomplete, and a company fails to respond or it becomes clear that the company is not a broker but is a wholesaler, they will be invited to withdraw the application by the Inspector. If the invitation to withdraw is not accepted and the company is unsuitable to be registered, the application will be referred to the MHRA Inspection Action Group (IAG) for consideration of removal.

Additional UK Guidance

Criteria of Broker's Registration

A person may not broker a medicinal product unless that product is covered by the licensing authority, or by an appropriate authority responsible for the licensing of medicinal products in an approved country for import, and that person is validly registered as a broker with the licensing authority, has a permanent address in the United Kingdom and complies with the guidelines on Good Distribution Practice that apply under, or by virtue of, regulation C17 of the Human Medicines Regulations 2012 insofar as those guidelines apply to brokers.

A person may not broker a medicinal product in Northern Ireland unless the product is covered by an authorisation granted under Regulation (EC) No 726/2004, by the licensing authority or by a competent authority of a Member State, and that person is validly registered as a broker with the licensing authority or a competent authority of a Member State, except where the person is validly registered with the competent authority of an EEA state, has a permanent address in the United Kingdom and complies with the guidelines on Good Distribution Practice published by the European Commission in accordance with Article 84 of the 2001 Directive insofar as those guidelines apply to brokers. Brokers must satisfy all the conditions of brokering and:

- have a permanent address in the UK;
- have an emergency plan that ensures effective implementation of any recall from the market ordered by, in the case of a broker in Great

Britain, the licensing authority or by an appropriate authority responsible for the licensing of medicinal products in an approved country for import, or in the case of a broker in Northern Ireland, the licensing authority or by the competent authority of any EEA State;

- keep records either in the form of purchase/sales invoices or on computer, or in any other form, giving for any transaction in medicinal products brokered at least the following information:

  - date on which the sale or purchase of the product is brokered;
  - name of the medicinal product;
  - quantity brokered;
  - name and address of the supplier or consignee, as appropriate;
  - batch number, where the sale or supply of the medicinal product is in Northern Ireland, of the medicinal products at least for products bearing the safety features referred to in point (o) of Article 54 of Directive 2001/83/EC;

- keep the records available to the competent authorities, for inspection purposes, for a period of 5 years;
- comply with the principles and guidelines of Good Distribution Practice for medicinal products as laid down in Article 84 of Directive 2001/83/ EC;
- maintain a quality system setting out responsibilities, processes and risk-management measures in relation to their activities.

Where the address at which the plan or records necessary to comply with the provisions of brokering are kept is different from the address notified in accordance with the application, the broker must ensure that the plan or records are kept at an address in the UK and inform the licensing authority of the address at which the plan or records are kept.

The broker must provide such information as may be requested by MHRA concerning the type and quantity of medicinal products brokered within the period specified by MHRA.

The broker must take all reasonable precautions and exercise all due diligence to ensure that any information provided by that broker to MHRA is not false or misleading.

For the purposes of enabling the MHRA to determine whether there are grounds for suspending, revoking or varying the registration, the broker must permit a person authorised in writing by MHRA, on production of identification, to carry out any inspection, or to take any copies, that an inspector may carry out or take under the provisions of the Human Medicines Regulations 2012 [SI 2012/1916].

Provision of Information

Once registered, a broker will have to notify the MHRA of any changes to the details for registration that might affect compliance with the requirements of the legislation in respect of brokering without unnecessary delay. This notification will be subject to a variation procedure. The responsibility for notifying the MHRA of any changes lies with the person responsible for management of the brokering activities.

The person responsible for management of the brokering activities shall be required to submit a report that shall include:

- a declaration that the broker has in place appropriate systems to ensure compliance with the requirements for brokering;
- the details of the systems that it has in place to ensure such compliance.

An annual compliance report will need to be submitted in relation to any application made before 31 March 2014, the date of the application and in relation to each subsequent reporting year, by 30 April following the end of that year. The annual compliance report will be subject to a variation procedure so that the broker can change the original details provided.

The broker must, without delay, notify the licensing authority of any changes to the matters in respect of which evidence has been supplied in relation to the compliance report that might affect compliance with the requirements of brokering.

The broker must immediately inform the MHRA and, in the case of a broker in Great Britain, either the UK marketing authorisation holder, or, where applicable, the holder of the licence or authorisation granted by an appropriate authority responsible for the licensing of medicinal products in an approved country for import, or Northern Ireland, either the UK marketing authorisation holder, or, where applicable, the EU marketing authorisation holder.

Management of Recall Activity by Brokers

Chapter 10 of the EU GDP Guidelines deals with brokers, and includes the requirement for the broker to have in place "...an emergency plan which ensures effective recall of medicinal products from the market...". The guidelines go on to specify that brokers should have a written procedure for supporting recalls, alongside an obligation to maintain relevant documentation.

As brokers do not hold or handle stock the scope of their recall activities are somewhat more limited than wholesalers.

A broker should:

- follow the detail of the recall message;
- identify those persons or companies involved in relevant brokered deals;
- directly contact those customers, making them aware of the details of the recall;
- keep recall notices open for an appropriate period, so as to capture any affected stock still moving through the supply chain.

As with wholesalers all recall activities should be documented at the time they occur, and at the conclusion of all recall activities the broker should produce a report, making an objective assessment of whether the recall process achieved its objectives and identifying any areas requiring improvement.

Supply and brokering to countries outside of the UK

Where wholesale stock has been supplied or brokered to countries outside the UK, there are the same obligations to contact the relevant customers to make them aware of the recall. It should be noted that certainly within approved countries, dependent on the nature of the recall and its impact on product availability and patient health, different countries may take varying levels of action. The wholesaler or broker should confirm with the relevant competent authority the particular terms of a recall in a particular territory.

Manufacture, Importation and Distribution of Active Substances

6

UK Legislation on the Manufacture, Importation and Distribution of Active Substances

Contents

The Human Medicines Regulations 2012 (SI 2012/1916)

> **Editor's note**   These extracts from the Human Medicines Regulations 2012 [SI 2012/1916] as amended are presented for the reader's convenience. Reproduction is with the permission of HMSO and the Queen's Printer for Scotland. For any definitive information reference must be made to the original Regulations. The numbering and content within this section correspond with the regulations set out in the published Statutory Instrument [SI 2012/1916] as amended.

Citation and commencement

1   (1)   These Regulations may be cited as the Human Medicines Regulations 2012.

(2)   These Regulations come into force on 14th August 2012.

General interpretation

8   In these Regulations (unless the context otherwise requires):

"active substance" means any substance or mixture of substances intended to be used in the manufacture of a medicinal product and that, when used in its production, becomes an active ingredient of that product intended to exert a pharmacological, immunological or metabolic action with a view to restoring, correcting or modifying physiological functions or to make a medical diagnosis;

"assemble", in relation to a medicinal product or an active substance, includes the various processes of dividing up, packaging and presentation of the product or substance, and "assembly" has a corresponding meaning;

"excipient" means any constituent of a medicinal product other than the active substance and the packaging material;

"export" means export, or attempt to export, from the United Kingdom, whether by land, sea or air;

"falsified medicinal product" means any medicinal product with a false representation of:

(a) its identity, including its packaging and labelling, its name or its composition (other than any unintentional quality defect) as regards any of its ingredients including excipients and the strength of those ingredients;

(b) its source, including its manufacturer, its country of manufacturing, its country of origin or its marketing authorisation holder; or

(c) its history, including the records and documents relating to the distribution channels used;

"import" means import, or attempt to import, into the United Kingdom, whether by land, sea or air and "imported" is to be construed accordingly;

"the licensing authority" has the meaning given by regulation 6(2):

Subject to regulation C17(6), references in these Regulations to:

(a) good manufacturing practice for active substances relate to the principles and guidelines for good manufacturing practice adopted by the European Commission under the third paragraph of Article 47[1] of the 2001 Directive;

(b) good distribution practice for active substances relate to the guidelines on good distribution practices for active substances adopted by the European Commission under the fourth paragraph of Article 47 of the 2001 Directive.

---

[1] Paragraphs 3 and 4 of Article 47 were substituted by Directive 2011/62/EU of the European Parliament and of the Council (OJ No L 174, 1.7.2011, p74).

Interpretation

A17   In this Part "manufacture", in relation to an active substance, includes any process carried out in the course of making the substance and the various processes of dividing up, packaging and presentation of the active substance.

Chapter 1A Good Manufacturing Practice and Good Distribution Practice

Guidelines on good manufacturing practice and good distribution practice

C17   (1)   The licensing authority may publish in relation to the manufacture or assembly of a medicinal product in, or import to, Great Britain:

(a)   detailed guidelines of good manufacturing practice in respect of medicinal products, and investigational medicinal products, referred to in Article 46(f) of the 2001 Directive, including guidelines as to the formalised risk assessment for ascertaining the appropriate good manufacturing practice for excipients;

(b)   principles and guidelines of good manufacturing practice for active substances, referred to in the first paragraph of point (f) of Article 46 and in Article 46b of that Directive;

(c)   principles and guidelines of good distribution practice referred to in the first paragraph of point (f) of Article 46, and Article 84, of that Directive.

(2)   Guidelines or principles under paragraph (1) may replace, amend or otherwise modify any guidelines or principles published or adopted by the European Commission under the second, third, fourth or fifth paragraph of Article 47, or Article 84, of the 2001 Directive.

(3)   Unless replaced by principles or guidelines published under paragraph (1), principles and guidelines published or adopted by the European Commission under the second, third, fourth or fifth paragraph of Article 47, or Article 84, of the 2001 Directive, as they applied immediately before IP completion day, continue to apply on and after IP completion day (subject to any amendments or modifications published under paragraph (1)).

(4)   Before exercising the power under paragraph (1), the licensing authority must consult such persons as it considers appropriate.

(5)   The licensing authority may only exercise its power under paragraph (1) if it considers that it is necessary in order to take account of technical or scientific progress.

(6)   If the licensing authority publishes principles and guidelines under paragraph (1), any reference in these Regulations to any principle or guideline adopted under the provisions of the 2001 Directive specified in those paragraphs is instead to be read as a reference to the principle or guideline published under paragraph (1), or that principle or guideline as amended or modified (as the case may be).

Criteria for importation, manufacture or distribution of active substances

45M (1) A person may not:
(a) import,
(b) manufacture or
(c) distribute
(d) an active substance unless that person is registered with the licensing authority in accordance with regulation 45N and the requirements in regulation 45O are met.
(2) Paragraph (1) applies in relation to an active substance that is to be used in an investigational medicinal product only:
(a) if
  (i) in the case of a product for sale or supply in Great Britain, the product has a UK marketing authorisation, certificate of registration or traditional herbal registration, or
  (ii) in the case of a product for sale or supply in Northern Ireland, the product has a marketing authorisation, Article 126a authorisation, certificate of registration or traditional herbal registration, and
(b) to the extent that the manufacture of the active substance is in accordance with the terms and conditions of that authorisation, certificate or registration.
(3) Paragraph (1)(a) does not apply to a person who, in connection with the importation of an active substance:
(a) provides facilities solely for transporting the active substance; or
(b) acting as an import agent, imports the active substance solely to the order of another person who holds a certificate of good manufacturing practice issued by the licensing authority.

Registration in relation to active substances

45N (1) For registration in relation to active substances, the licensing authority must have received a valid registration form from the applicant for import, manufacture or, as the case may be, distribution of the active substance and:
(a) 60 days have elapsed since receipt and the licensing authority have not notified the applicant that an inspection will be carried out; or
(b) the licensing authority:
  (i) notified the applicant within 60 days of receipt of a registration form that an inspection will be carried out; and
  (ii) within 90 days of that inspection the licensing authority have issued that person with a certificate of good manufacturing practice or, as the case may be, of good distribution practice; and

(c) that person has not instructed the licensing authority to end that person's registration.

(2) The person applying for registration under paragraph (1) must notify the licensing authority of any changes that have taken place as regards the information in the registration form:

(a) immediately where such changes may have an impact on quality or safety of the active substances that are manufactured, imported or distributed;

(b) in any other case, on each anniversary of the receipt of the application form by the licensing authority.

(3) For the purpose of paragraph (2), changes that are notified in accordance with that paragraph shall be treated as incorporated in the application form.

(4) Any notification to the licensing authority under paragraph (2) must be accompanied by the appropriate fee in accordance with the Fees Regulations.

(5) A registration form is valid for the purpose of paragraph (1) if:

(a) it is provided to the licensing authority; and

(b) is completed in the way and form specified in Schedule 7A.

(6) Paragraph (1) does not apply until 20 October 2013 in relation to a person who had, before 20 August 2013, commenced the activity for which the person would, apart from this provision, need to send a registration form to the licensing authority.

Requirements for registration as an importer, manufacturer or distributor of an active substance

45O (1) Where principles and guidelines of good manufacturing practice have been published under, or apply by virtue of, regulation C17, that apply to an active substance manufactured in Great Britain, a manufacturer in Great Britain must comply with those principles and guidelines of good manufacturing practice in relation to that active substance.

(1A) Where the Commission has adopted principles and guidelines of good manufacturing practice under the third paragraph of Article 47[2] of the 2001 Directive that applies to an active substance manufactured in Northern Ireland, a manufacturer in Northern Ireland must comply with those principles and guidelines of good manufacturing practice in relation to that active substance.

(2) Where principles and guidelines of good distribution practice have been published under, or apply by virtue of, regulation C17, that apply

---

[2] Article 47 was amended by Directive 2011/62/EU of the European Parliament and of the Council (OJ No L 174, 1.7.2011, p74).

to an active substance distributed in Great Britain, a distributor in Great Britain must comply with those principles and guidelines of good distribution practice in relation to that active substance.

(2A) Where the Commission has adopted principles and guidelines of good distribution practice under the fourth paragraph of Article 47 of the 2001 Directive that applies to an active substance distributed in the Northern Ireland, a distributor in Northern Ireland must comply with those principles and guidelines of good distribution practice in relation to that active substance.

(3) Without prejudice to regulation 37(4) (manufacture and assembly in relation to active substances) and paragraph 9A of Schedule 8 (material to accompany an application for a UK marketing authorisation in relation to an active substance), where principles and guidelines of good manufacturing practice have been published under, or apply by virtue of, regulation C17, that apply to an active substance imported into Northern Ireland and where an active substance is imported into Northern Ireland from a country other than an EEA State so imported:

(a) the importer must comply with good manufacturing practice and good distribution practice in relation to the active substance;

(b) the active substances must have been manufactured in accordance with standards that are at least equivalent to good manufacturing practice; and

(c) the active substances must be accompanied by a written confirmation from the competent authority of the exporting country of the following:

(i) the standards of manufacturing practice applicable to the plant manufacturing the exported active substance are at least equivalent to good manufacturing practice,

(ii) the manufacturing plant concerned is subject to regular, strict and transparent controls, and to the effective enforcement of standards of manufacturing practice at least equivalent to good manufacturing practice, including repeated and unannounced inspections, so as to ensure a protection of public health at least equivalent to that in Northern Ireland, and

(iii) in the event of findings relating to non-compliance, information on such findings is supplied by the exporting country to the licensing authority without any delay.

(3A) Without prejudice to regulation 37(4) (manufacture and assembly in relation to active substances) and paragraph 9A of Schedule 8 (material to accompany an application for a UK marketing authorisation in relation to an active substance), where principles and guidelines of good manufacturing practice have been published under, or apply by virtue of, regulation C17, which apply to an active substance imported into Great Britain other than from Northern Ireland and where an active substance is so imported:

(a) the importer must comply with good manufacturing practice and good distribution practice in relation to the active substance,

(b) the active substances must have been manufactured in accordance with standards that are at least equivalent to good manufacturing practice, and

(c) the active substances must be accompanied by a written confirmation from the competent authority of the exporting country of the following:

   (i) the standards of manufacturing practice applicable to the plant manufacturing the exported active substance are at least equivalent to good manufacturing practice,

   (ii) the manufacturing plant concerned is subject to regular, strict and transparent controls, and to the effective enforcement of standards of manufacturing practice at least equivalent to good manufacturing practice, including repeated and unannounced inspections, so as to ensure a protection of public health at least equivalent to that in Great Britain, and

   (iii) in the event of findings relating to non-compliance, information on such findings is supplied by the exporting country to the licensing authority without any delay.

(4) Paragraph (3)(c) or 3A(c) do not apply:

(a) where the country from where the active substance is exported is included in the list referred to in Article 111b of the 2001 Directive (in the case of an import into Northern Ireland) or paragraph (6) (in the case of an import into Great Britain); or

(b) for a period not exceeding the validity of the certificate of good manufacturing practice, where:

   (i) in relation to a plant where active substances are manufactured where the competent authority of a member State or licensing authority (in the case of an import into Northern Ireland) or licensing authority or an appropriate authority responsible for the licensing of medicinal products in a country included in a list under paragraph (6) (in the case of an import into Great Britain) has found, upon inspection, that a plant complies with the principles and guidelines of good manufacturing practice, and

   (ii) the licensing authority is of the opinion that it is necessary to waive the requirement to ensure availability of the active substance.

(5) The criteria in this regulation apply regardless of whether an active substance is intended for export.

(6) The licensing authority may publish a list of countries that it is satisfied have a regulatory framework applicable to active substances

exported to Great Britain that is equivalent to the regulatory framework in Great Britain, in that the respective control and enforcement activities in those countries ensures an equivalent level of protection of public health.

(7) Before including a country in the list under paragraph (6), the licensing authority must assess the equivalence referred to in that paragraph by:

(a) reviewing relevant documentation; and

(b) unless the country is included in the approved country for batch testing list, carrying out:

(i) an on-site review of the country's regulatory system, and

(ii) if the licensing authority considers it necessary, an inspection of one or more of that country's manufacturing sites for active substances.

(8) In carrying out an assessment under paragraph (7) the licensing authority must, in particular, take account of the:

(a) country's rules for good manufacturing practice;

(b) regularity of inspections to verify compliance with good manufacturing practice;

(c) effectiveness of enforcement of good manufacturing practice; and

(d) regularity and rapidity of information provided by that country relating to non-compliant producers of active substances.

(9) The licensing authority must:

(a) review the list under paragraph (6) to determine if a country included in it still satisfies the requirements for inclusion in the list, and if it is not so satisfied, remove that country; and

(b) undertake such a review at least every 3 years, beginning with the date on which a country is included in the list.

Provision of information

45P (1) In this regulation:

"R" means a person who is, or has applied to the licensing authority to become, a registered importer, manufacturer or distributor of active substances;

"reporting year" means a period of 12 months ending on 31 March.

(2) On or before the date specified in paragraph (3), R must submit a report to the licensing authority that:

(a) includes a declaration that R has in place an appropriate system to ensure compliance with regulations 45N, 45O and this regulation; and

(b) details the system that R has in place to ensure such compliance.

(3) The date specified for the purposes of this paragraph is:

(a) in relation to any application made before 31 March 2014, the date of the application; and

(b) in relation to each subsequent reporting year, 30 April following the end of that year.

(4) R must without delay notify the licensing authority of any changes to the matters in respect of which evidence has been supplied in relation to paragraph (2) that might affect compliance with the requirements of this Chapter.

(5) Any report or notification to the licensing authority under paragraph (2) or (4) must be accompanied by the appropriate fee in accordance with the Fees Regulations.

(6) The licensing authority may give a notice to R, requiring R to provide information of a kind specified in the notice within the period specified in the notice.

(7) A notice under paragraph (6) may not be given to R unless it appears to the licensing authority that it is necessary for the licensing authority to consider whether the registration should be varied, suspended or removed from the active substance register.

(8) A notice under paragraph (6) may specify information which the licensing authority thinks necessary for considering whether the registration should be varied, suspended or removed from the active substance register.

Schedule 7A Information to be provided for registration as an importer, manufacturer or distributor of active substances

(1) The name and address of the applicant.

(2) The name and address of the person (if any) making the application on the applicant's behalf.

(3) The address of each of the premises where any operations to which the registration relates are to be carried out.

(4) The address of any premises not mentioned by virtue of the above requirement, where:

(a) the applicant proposes to keep any living animals, from which substance(s) used in the production of the active substance(s) to which the application relates are to be derived;

(b) materials of animal origin from which an active substance is to be derived, as mentioned in the above sub-paragraph, are to be kept.

(5) The address of each of the premises where active substances are to be stored, or from which active substances are to be distributed.

(6) The address of each of the premises where any testing associated with the manufacture or assembly of active substances to which the registration relates.

(7) The name, address, qualifications and experience of the person whose duty it will be to supervise any manufacturing operations, and the name and job title of the person to whom they report.

(8) The name, address, qualifications and experience of the person who will have responsibility for the quality control of active substances, and the name and job title of the person to whom they report.

(9) The name, address, qualifications and experience of the person whose duty it will be to supervise any importation, storage or distribution operations, and the name and job title of the person to whom they report.

(10) The name, address and qualifications of the person to be responsible for any animals kept as mentioned in paragraph 4(a).

(11) The name, address and qualifications of the person to be responsible for the culture of any living tissue for use in the manufacture of an active substance.

(12) For each active substance to be manufactured, imported, or distributed:
  (a) the CAS registration number[3] assigned to that active substance by the Chemical Abstracts Service, a division of the American Chemical Society;
  (b) where applicable, the Anatomical Therapeutic Category code[4] assigned to that active substance under the Anatomical Therapeutic Chemical Classification System used for the classification of drugs by the World Health Organization's Collaborating Centre for Drug Statistics Methodology;
  (c) either:
    (i) the International Union of Pure and Applied Chemistry nomenclature, or
    (ii) the common name; and
  (d) the intended quantities of each active substance to be manufactured, imported or distributed.

(13) Details of the operations to which the registration relates, including a statement of whether they include:
  (a) the manufacture of active substances;
  (b) the importation of active substances from third countries;
  (c) the storage of active substances; or
  (d) the distribution of active substances.

(14) A statement of the facilities and equipment available at each of the premises where active substances are to be manufactured, stored or distributed.

---

[3] Further information is available from the website of the Chemical Abstracts Service at www.cas.org

[4] Further information is available from the website of the WHO Collaborating Centre for Drug Statistics Methodology at www.whocc.no

(15) A statement as to whether the particular active substances are intended for:

(a) use in a medicinal product with an EU marketing authorisation;

(b) use in a special medicinal product; or

(c) export to a third country.

(16) A separate statement in respect of each of the premises mentioned in the application of:

(a) the manufacturing, storage or distribution operations carried out at those sites, and the specific active substances to which those activities relate; and

(b) the equipment available at those premises for carrying out those activities.

(17) A statement of the authority conferred on the person responsible for quality control to reject unsatisfactory active substances.

(18) A description of the arrangements for the identification and storage of materials before and during the manufacture of active substances.

(19) A description of the arrangements for the identification and storage of active substances.

(20) A description of the arrangements at each of the premises where the applicant proposes to store active substances for ensuring, as far as practicable, the turnover of stocks of active substances.

(21) A description of the arrangements for maintaining:

(a) production records, including records of manufacture and assembly;

(b) records of analytical and other tests used in the course of manufacture or assembly for ensuring compliance of materials used in manufacture, or of active substances, with the specification for such materials or active substances;

(c) records of importation;

(d) records of storage and distribution.

(22) A description of the arrangements for keeping reference samples of:

(a) materials used in the manufacture of active substances; and

(b) active substances.

(23) Where the application relates to active substances intended for use in an advanced therapy medicinal product, an outline of the arrangements for maintaining records to allow traceability containing sufficient detail to enable the linking of an active substance to the advanced therapy medicinal product it was used in the manufacture of and vice versa.

(24) Details of:

(a) any manufacturing, importation, storage or distribution operations, other than those to which the application for registration relates, carried on by the applicant on or near each of the premises, and

(b) the substances or articles to which those operations relate.

Guidelines of 19 March 2015 on Principles of Good Distribution Practice of Active Substances for Medicinal Products for Human Use (2015/C 95/01)

Contents

Introduction

These guidelines are based on the fourth paragraph of Article 47 of Directive 2001/83/EC[1].

They follow the same principles that underlie the guidelines of EudraLex Volume 4, Part II, Chapter 17, with regard to the distribution of active substances and the Guidelines of 5 November 2013 on Good Distribution Practice of medicinal products for human use[2].

These guidelines provide standalone guidance on Good Distribution Practice (GDP) for importers and distributors of active substances for medicinal products for human use. They complement the rules on distribution set out in the guidelines of EudraLex Volume 4, Part II, and apply also to distributors of active substances manufactured by themselves.

[1] Directive 2001/83/EC of the European Parliament and of the Council of 6 November 2001 on the Community code relating to medicinal products for human use (OJ L 311, 28.11.2001, p. 67).

[2] OJ C 343, 23.11.2013, p. 1.

Any manufacturing activities in relation to active substances, including re-packaging, re-labelling or dividing up, are subject to Commission Delegated Regulation (EU) No 1252/2014[3] and EudraLex Volume 4, Part II.

Additional requirements apply to the importation of active substances, as laid down in Article 46b of Directive 2001/83/EC.

Distributors of active substances for medicinal products for human use should follow these guidelines as of 21 September 2015.

CHAPTER 1 SCOPE

1.1   These guidelines apply to distribution of active substances, as defined in Article 1(3a) of Directive 2001/83/EC, for medicinal products for human use. According to that provision, an active substance is any substance or mixture of substances intended to be used in the manufacture of a medicinal product and that, when used in its production, becomes an active ingredient of that product intended to exert a pharmacological, immunological or metabolic action with a view to restoring, correcting or modifying physiological functions or to make a medical diagnosis.

1.2   For the purpose of these guidelines, distribution of active substances shall comprise all activities consisting of procuring, importing, holding, supplying or exporting active substances, apart from brokering.

1.3   These guidelines do not apply to intermediates of active substances.

CHAPTER 2 QUALITY SYSTEM

2.1   Distributors of active substances should develop and maintain a quality system setting out responsibilities, processes and risk-management principles. Examples of the processes and applications of quality risk management can be found in EudraLex Volume 4, Part III: GMP related documents, ICH guideline Q9 on Quality Risk Management (ICH Q9).

2.2   The quality system should be adequately resourced with competent personnel, and suitable and sufficient premises, equipment and facilities. It should ensure that:

---

[3]   Commission Delegated Regulation (EU) No 1252/2014 of 28 May 2014 supplementing Directive 2001/83/EC of the European Parliament and of the Council with regard to principles and guidelines of good manufacturing practice for active substances for medicinal products for human use (OJ L 337, 25.11.2014, p. 1).

(i)   active substances are procured, imported, held, supplied or exported in a way that is compliant with the requirements of GDP for active substances;

(ii)   management responsibilities are clearly specified;

(iii) active substances are delivered to the right recipients within a satisfactory time period;

(iv)   records are made contemporaneously;

(v)   deviations from established procedures are documented and investigated;

(vi)   appropriate corrective and preventive actions, commonly known as "CAPA", are taken to correct deviations and prevent them in line with the principles of quality risk management;

(vii) changes that may affect the storage and distribution of active substances are evaluated.

2.3   The size, structure and complexity of the distributor's activities should be taken into consideration when developing or modifying the quality system.

CHAPTER 3 PERSONNEL

3.1   The distributor should designate a person at each location where distribution activities are performed who should have defined authority and responsibility for ensuring that a quality system is implemented and maintained. The designated person should fulfil his responsibilities personally. The designated person can delegate duties but not responsibilities.

3.2   The responsibilities of all personnel involved in the distribution of active substances should be specified in writing. The personnel should be trained on the requirements of GDP for active substances. They should have the appropriate competence and experience to ensure that active substances are properly handled, stored and distributed.

3.3   Personnel should receive initial and continuing training relevant to their role, based on written procedures and in accordance with a written training programme.

3.4   A record of all training should be kept, and the effectiveness of training should be periodically assessed and documented.

CHAPTER 4 DOCUMENTATION

4.1   Documentation comprises all written procedures, instructions, contracts, records and data, in paper or in electronic form. Documentation should be readily available or retrievable. All documentation related to compliance of the distributor with these guidelines should be made available on request of competent authorities.

4.2   Documentation should be sufficiently comprehensive with respect to the scope of the distributor's activities and in a language understood by personnel. It should be written in clear, unambiguous language and be free from errors.

4.3   Any alteration made in the documentation should be signed and dated; the alteration should permit the reading of the original information. Where appropriate, the reason for the alteration should be recorded.

4.4   Each employee should have ready access to all necessary documentation for the tasks executed.

Procedures

4.5   Written procedures should describe the distribution activities that affect the quality of the active substances. This could include receipt and checking of deliveries, storage, cleaning and maintenance of the premises (including pest control), recording of the storage conditions, security of stocks on site and of consignments in transit, withdrawal from saleable stock, handling of returned products, recall plans, etc.

4.6   Procedures should be approved, signed and dated by the person responsible for the quality system.

4.7   Attention should be paid to the use of valid and approved procedures. Documents should be reviewed regularly and kept up to date. Version control should be applied to procedures. After revision of a document a system should exist to prevent inadvertent use of the superseded version. Superseded or obsolete procedures should be removed from workstations and archived.

Records

4.8   Records should be clear, be made at the time each operation is performed and in such a way that all significant activities or events are traceable. Records should be retained for at least 1 year after the expiry date of the active substance batch to which they relate. For active substances with retest dates, records should be retained for at least 3 years after the batch is completely distributed.

4.9   Records should be kept of each purchase and sale, showing the date of purchase or supply, name of the active substance, batch number and quantity

GUIDELINES ON
PRINCIPLES OF GDP OF
ACTIVE SUBSTANCES

received or supplied, and name and address of the supplier and of the original manufacturer, if not the same, or of the shipping agent and/or the consignee. Records should ensure the traceability of the origin and destination of products, so that all the suppliers of, or those supplied with, an active substance can be identified. Records that should be retained and be available include:

(i)   identity of supplier, original manufacturer, shipping agent and/or consignee;
(ii)   address of supplier, original manufacturer, shipping agent and/or consignee;
(iii)   purchase orders;
(iv)   bills of lading, transportation and distribution records;
(v)   receipt documents;
(vi)   name or designation of active substance;
(vii) manufacturer's batch number;
(viii) certificates of analysis, including those of the original manufacturer;
(ix)   re-test or expiry date.

CHAPTER 5 PREMISES AND EQUIPMENT

5.1   Premises and equipment should be suitable and adequate to ensure proper storage, protection from contamination, e.g. narcotics, highly sensitising materials, materials of high pharmacological activity or toxicity, and distribution of active substances. They should be suitably secure to prevent unauthorised access. Monitoring devices that are necessary to guarantee the quality attributes of the active substance should be calibrated according to an approved schedule against certified traceable standards.

CHAPTER 6 OPERATIONS

Orders

6.1   Where active substances are procured from a manufacturer, importer or distributor established in the EU, that manufacturer, importer or distributor should be registered according to Article 52a of Directive 2001/83/EC.

Receipt

6.2   Areas for receiving active substances should protect deliveries from prevailing weather conditions during unloading. The reception area should be separate from the storage area. Deliveries should be examined at receipt in order to check that:

(i)   containers are not damaged;

(ii)   all security seals are present with no sign of tampering;

(iii)   correct labelling, including correlation between the name used by the supplier and the in-house name, if these are different;

(iv)   necessary information, such as a certificate of analysis, is available; and

(v)   the active substance and the consignment correspond to the order.

6.3   Active substances with broken seals, damaged packaging or suspected of possible contamination should be quarantined either physically or using an equivalent electronic system and the cause of the issue investigated.

6.4   Active substances subject to specific storage measures, e.g. narcotics and products requiring a specific storage temperature or humidity, should be immediately identified and stored in accordance with written instructions and with relevant legislative provisions.

6.5   Where the distributor suspects that an active substance procured or imported by him is falsified, they should segregate it either physically or using an equivalent electronic system and inform the national competent authority of the country in which they are registered.

6.6   Rejected materials should be identified and controlled and quarantined to prevent their unauthorised use in manufacturing and their further distribution. Records of destruction activities should be readily available.

Storage

6.7   Active substances should be stored under the conditions specified by the manufacturer, e.g. controlled temperature and humidity when necessary, and in such a manner to prevent contamination and/or mix up. The storage conditions should be monitored and records maintained. The records should be reviewed regularly by the person responsible for the quality system.

6.8   When specific storage conditions are required, the storage area should be qualified and operated within the specified limits.

6.9   The storage facilities should be clean and free from litter, dust and pests. Adequate precautions should be taken against spillage or breakage, attack by micro-organisms and cross-contamination.

6.10   There should be a system to ensure stock rotation, e.g. "first expiry (retest date), first out", with regular and frequent checks that the system is operating correctly. Electronic warehouse management systems should be validated.

6.11   Active substances beyond their expiry date should be separated, either physically or using an equivalent electronic system, from approved stock and not be supplied.

GUIDELINES ON PRINCIPLES OF GDP OF ACTIVE SUBSTANCES

6.12   Where storage or transportation of active substances is contracted out, the distributor should ensure that the contract acceptor knows and follows the appropriate storage and transport conditions. There must be a written contract between the contract giver and contract acceptor, which clearly establishes the duties of each party. The contract acceptor should not sub-contract any of the work entrusted to him under the contract without the contract giver's written authorisation.

Deliveries to customers

6.13   Supplies within the EU should be made only by distributors of active substances registered according to Article 52a of Directive 2001/83/EC to other distributors, manufacturers or to dispensing pharmacies.

6.14   Active substances should be transported in accordance with the conditions specified by the manufacturer and in a manner that does not adversely affect their quality. Product, batch and container identity should be maintained at all times. All original container labels should remain readable.

6.15   A system should be in place by which the distribution of each batch of active substance can be readily identified to permit its recall.

Transfer of information

6.16   Any information or event that the distributor becomes aware of, which have the potential to cause an interruption to supply, should be notified to relevant customers.

6.17   Distributors should transfer all product quality or regulatory information received from an active substance manufacturer to the customer and from the customer to the active substance manufacturer.

6.18   The distributor who supplies the active substance to the customer should provide the name and address of the original active substance manufacturer and the batch number(s) supplied. A copy of the original certificate of analysis from the manufacturer should be provided to the customer.

6.19   The distributor should also provide the identity of the original active substance manufacturer to competent authorities upon request. The original manufacturer can respond to the competent authority directly or through its authorised agents. (In this context "authorised" refers to authorised by the manufacturer.)

6.20   The specific guidance for certificates of analysis is detailed in Section 11.4 of Part II of Eudralex Volume 4.

CHAPTER 7 RETURNS, COMPLAINTS AND RECALLS

Returns

7.1 Returned active substances should be identified as such and quarantined pending investigation.

7.2 Active substances which have left the care of the distributor, should only be returned to approved stock if all of the following conditions are met:

(i) the active substance is in the original unopened container(s) with all original security seals present and is in good condition;

(ii) it is demonstrated that the active substance has been stored and handled under proper conditions. Written information provided by the customer should be available for this purpose;

(iii) the remaining shelf life period is acceptable;

(iv) the active substance has been examined and assessed by a person trained and authorised to do so;

(v) no loss of information/traceability has occurred.

This assessment should take into account the nature of the active substance, any special storage conditions it requires, and the time elapsed since it was supplied. As necessary, and if there is any doubt about the quality of the returned active substance, advice should be sought from the manufacturer.

7.3 Records of returned active substances should be maintained. For each return, documentation should include:

(i) name and address of the consignee returning the active substances;

(ii) name or designation of active substance, active substance batch number and quantity returned;

(iii) reason for return;

(iv) use or disposal of the returned active substance and records of the assessment performed.

7.4 Only appropriately trained and authorised personnel should release active substances for return to stock. Active substances returned to saleable stock should be placed such that the stock rotation system operates effectively.

Complaints and recalls

7.5 All complaints, whether received orally or in writing, should be recorded and investigated according to a written procedure. In the event of a complaint about the quality of an active substance the distributor should review the complaint with the original active substance manufacturer in order to determine whether any further action, either with other customers who may have received this active substance or with the competent authority, or both, should be initiated. The investigation into the cause for the complaint should be conducted and documented by the appropriate party.

7.6   Complaint records should include:

(i)   name and address of complainant;

(ii)   name, title, where appropriate, and phone number of person submitting the complaint;

(iii)   complaint nature, including name and batch number of the active substance;

(iv)   date the complaint is received;

(v)   action initially taken, including dates and identity of person taking the action;

(vi)   any follow-up action taken;

(vii)   response provided to the originator of complaint, including date response sent;

(viii) final decision on active substance batch.

7.7   Records of complaints should be retained in order to evaluate trends, product-related frequencies and severity with a view to taking additional, and if appropriate, immediate corrective action. These should be made available during inspections by competent authorities.

7.8   Where a complaint is referred to the original active substance manufacturer, the record maintained by the distributor should include any response received from the original active substance manufacturer, including date and information provided.

7.9   In the event of a serious or potentially life-threatening situation, local, national and/or international authorities should be informed and their advice sought.

7.10   There should be a written procedure that defines the circumstances under which a recall of an active substance should be considered.

7.11   The recall procedure should designate who should be involved in evaluating the information, how a recall should be initiated, who should be informed about the recall and how the recalled material should be treated. The designated person (cf. Section 3.1) should be involved in recalls.

CHAPTER 8 SELF-INSPECTIONS

8.1   The distributor should conduct and record self-inspections in order to monitor the implementation of and compliance with these guidelines. Regular self-inspections should be performed in accordance with an approved schedule.

Annex

Glossary of terms applicable to these guidelines

Terms	Definition
Batch	A specific quantity of material produced in a process or series of processes so that it is expected to be homogeneous within specified limits. In the case of continuous production, a batch may correspond to a defined fraction of the production. The batch size can be defined either by a fixed quantity or by the amount produced in a fixed time interval.
Batch number	A unique combination of numbers, letters and/or symbols that identifies a batch (or lot) and from which the production and distribution history can be determined.
Brokering of active substances	All activities in relation to the sale or purchase of active substances that do not include physical handling and that consist of negotiating independently and on behalf of another legal or natural person.
Calibration	The demonstration that a particular instrument or device produces results within specified limits by comparison with those produced by a reference or traceable standard over an appropriate range of measurements.
Consignee	The person to whom the shipment is to be delivered whether by land, sea or air.
Contamination	The undesired introduction of impurities of a chemical or microbiological nature, or of foreign matter, into or onto a raw material, intermediate, or active substance during production, sampling, packaging or repackaging, storage or transport.
Distribution of active substances	All activities consisting of procuring, importing, holding, supplying or exporting of active substances, apart from brokering.
Deviation	Departure from an approved instruction or established standard.
Expiry date	The date placed on the container/labels of an active substance designating the time during which the active substance is expected to remain within established shelf life specifications if stored under defined conditions, and after which it should not be used.

Terms	Definition
Falsified active substance	Any active substance with a false representation of:
	(a) its identity, including its packaging and labelling, its name or its components as regards any of the ingredients and the strength of those ingredients;
	(b) its source, including its manufacturer, its country of manufacture, its country of origin; or
	(c) its history, including the records and documents relating to the distribution channels used.
Holding	Storing active substances.
Procedure	A documented description of the operations to be performed, the precautions to be taken and measures to be applied directly or indirectly related to the distribution of an active substance.
Procuring	Obtaining, acquiring, purchasing or buying active substances from manufacturers, importers or other distributors.
Quality risk management	A systematic process for the assessment, control, communication and review of risks to the quality of an active substance across the product lifecycle.
Quality system	The sum of all aspects of a system that implements quality policy and ensures that quality objectives are met (ICH Q9).
Quarantine	The status of materials isolated physically or by other effective means pending a decision on the subsequent approval or rejection.
Re-test date	The date when a material should be re-examined to ensure that it is still suitable for use.
Supplying	All activities of providing, selling, donating active substances to distributors, pharmacists or manufacturers of medicinal products.
Signed (signature)	The record of the individual who performed a particular action or review. This record can be initials, full handwritten signature, personal seal, or authenticated and secure electronic signature.
Transport (transportation)	Moving active substances between two locations without storing them for unjustified periods of time.
Validation	A documented programme that provides a high degree of assurance that a specific process, method or system will consistently produce a result meeting predetermined acceptance criteria.

8

UK Guidance on the Manufacture, Importation and Distribution of Active Substances

Contents

Introduction

The Human Medicines Regulations 2012 (SI 2012/1916) lay down the rules for the manufacture, import, marketing and supply of medicinal products, and ensure the functioning of the internal market for medicinal products while safeguarding a high level of protection of public health in the UK.

The falsification of medicinal products is a global problem, requiring effective and enhanced international coordination and cooperation in order to ensure that anti-falsification strategies are more effective, in particular as regards sale of such products via the Internet. To that end, the National Competent Authorities are cooperating closely and supporting ongoing work in international fora on this subject.

Active substances are those substances which give a medicinal product its therapeutic effect. They are the Active Pharmaceutical Ingredient (API).

Falsified active substances and active substances that do not comply with applicable requirements of UK national legislation pose serious risks to public health. As such, guidelines are in place for good manufacturing practice and good distribution practice for active substances to minimise the risk to public health associated with falsification.

Registration

To provide a greater level of control, and transparency of supply for active substances, manufacturers, importers and distributors of active substances have to notify the MHRA of their activities and provide certain details. The MHRA will enter these details into a National Database (MHRA-GMDP) following the determination of a successful application for registration. The MHRA may then conduct inspections against the requirements of the relevant good practices before permitting such businesses to start trading. Manufacturers, importers and distributors of active substances will not only be subject to inspection on the basis of suspicions of non-compliance, but also on the basis of risk analysis.

MHRA-GMDP database: https://cms.mhra.gov.uk/mhra

Authorised manufacturers of medicinal products who also manufacture and/or import active substances, either for use in their own products or products manufactured by other companies, are not exempt from the requirement to register.

Persons who are requested to import an active substance from a third country that provide facilities solely for transporting the active substance, or where they are acting as an import agent, imports the active substance solely to the order of another person who holds a certificate of good manufacturing practice issued by the licensing authority, are not required to register.

The registration regime for manufacturers, importers and distributors of active substances will be subject to an application procedure, followed by a determination procedure completed by the MHRA.

The person applying for registration must notify the MHRA immediately of any changes that have taken place as regards the information in the registration form, where such changes may have an impact on quality or safety of the active substances that are manufactured, imported or distributed. These changes shall be treated as incorporated in the application form.

The MHRA must grant or refuse an application for registration within 60 working days beginning immediately after the day on which a valid application is received.

The MHRA will notify the applicant within 60 days of receipt of a valid application for registration whether they intend to undertake an inspection.

The applicant may not undertake any activity before either:

- 60 days have elapsed and the applicant has not been notified of the Agency's intention to inspect, or
- following inspection the Agency has notified the applicant that they may commence their activities.

Registration requirements for NI companies involved in the sourcing and supply of an active substance (AS) to be used in the manufacture of human medicines.

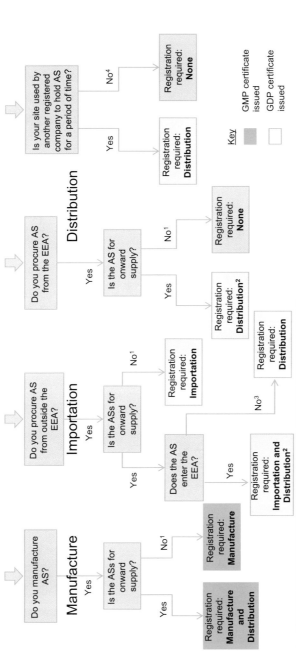

This flowchart may be used to determine the appropriate registration required for UK companies. Where more than one activity is carried out, the company should register for all activities that apply.

1. Site holds a Manufacturer's Licence and uses the AS in the manufacture of the finished dose form.
2. Where the registration holder contracts out the physical handling of the AS, the company that physically handles the product should be named as a 3rd party site on the registration if they hold the AS and this takes place in the UK.
   In addition, the company should hold its own registration. If the company are based in an approved country for import, they should be registered with the competent authority in that approved country.
3. AS is procured from a country other than an approved country for import and are supplied directly to customers based in a country other than an approved country for import.
4. AS is not held (stored) for any length of time and the company are simply contracted to transport the AS.

Figure 8.1 Registration requirements for UK companies involved in the sourcing and supply of active substances (ASs) to be used in the manufacture of human medicines.

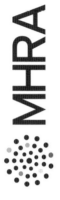

Registration requirements for GB companies involved in the sourcing and supply of active substance (AS) to be used in the manufacture of human medicines.

This flowchart may be used to determine the appropriate registration required for UK companies. Where more than one activity is carried out, the company should register for all activities that apply.

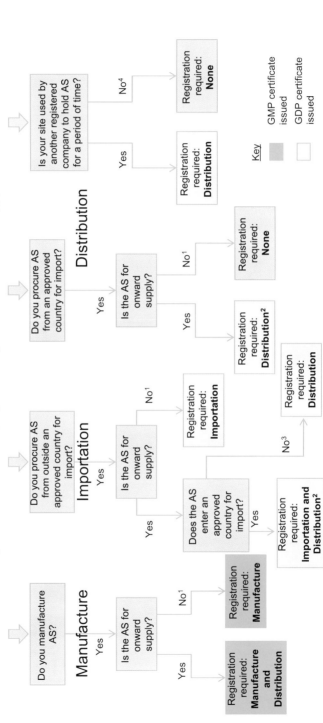

1. Site holds a Manufacturer's Licence and uses the AS in the manufacture of the finished dose form.
2. Where the registration holder contracts out the physical handling of the AS, the company that physically handles the product should be named as a 3rd party site on the registration if they hold the AS and this takes place in the UK.
   In addition, the company should hold its own registration. If the company are based in an approved country for import, they should be registered with the competent authority in that approved country.
3. AS is procured from a country other than an approved country for import are supplied directly to customers based in a country other than an approved country for import.
4. ASs is not held (stored) for any length of time and the company are simply contracted to transport the AS.

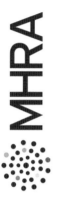

Registration requirements for companies involved in the sourcing and supply of active substance (AS) between GB and NI to be used in the manufacture of human medicines.

This flowchart may be used to determine the appropriate registration required for UK companies. Where more than one activity is carried out, the company should register for all activities that apply.

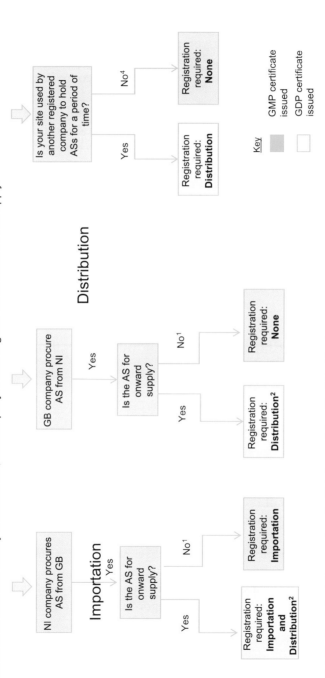

Importation

NI company procures AS from GB

Is the AS for onward supply?

Yes → Registration required: **Importation and Distribution²**

No¹ → Registration required: **Importation**

Distribution

GB company procure AS from NI

Is the AS for onward supply?

Yes → Registration required: **Distribution²**

No¹ → Registration required: **None**

Is your site used by another registered company to hold ASs for a period of time?

Yes → Registration required: **Distribution**

No⁴ → Registration required: **None**

Key

GMP certificate issued

GDP certificate issued

1. Site holds a Manufacturer's Licence and uses the ASs in the manufacture of the finished dose form.
2. Where the registration holder contracts out the physical handling of the AS, the company that physically handles the product should be named as a 3rd party site on the registration if they hold the ASs and this takes place in the UK.
   In addition, the company should hold its own registration. If the company are based in an approved country for import, they should be registered with the competent authority in that approved country.
3. ASs procured from a country other than an approved country for import are supplied directly to customers based in a country other than an approved country for import.
4. ASs are not held (stored) for any length of time and the company are simply contracted to transport the ASs.

UK GUIDANCE ON ACTIVE SUBSTANCES

After inspection, the MHRA will prepare a report and communicate that report to the applicant. The applicant will have the opportunity to respond to the report. Within 90 days of an inspection, the MHRA shall issue an appropriate good practice certificate to the applicant, indicating that the applicant complies with the requirements of the relevant good practices. Where an applicant is found to be non-compliant with the requisite standards, a statement of non-compliance will be issued by the MHRA.

If after 60 days of the receipt of the application form the MHRA has not notified the applicant of their intention to carry out an inspection, the applicant may commence their business activity and regard themselves as registered. The MHRA will issue a certificate to the applicant and enter the details into the national database, and for sites in Northern Ireland into the community database (EudraGMDP).

The database, which is publicly available, will enable competent authorities in other countries or other legal entities, to establish the bona fides and compliance of manufacturers, importers and distributors of active substances established in the UK. The MHRA will investigate concerns with regard to UK registrations of non-compliance.

Conditions of Registration as a Manufacturer, Importer or Distributor of an Active Substance

A person in the UK may not import, manufacture or distribute an active substance for use in a licensed human medicine unless they are registered with the MHRA in accordance with the Human Medicines Regulations 2012 and the respective conditions of those Regulations are met.

For registration the MHRA must have received a valid registration form from the applicant for import, manufacture or, as the case may be, distribution of the active substance.

Registration holders must submit to the MHRA an annual update of any changes to the information provided in the application or provide a statement there was no change. Any changes that may have an impact on the quality or safety of the active substance that the registrant is permitted to handle must be notified to the Agency immediately.

An annual compliance report will need to be submitted: by 30 April for the previous year.

For an active substance manufactured in the UK, the registered manufacturer must comply with good manufacturing practice in relation to that active substance.

Where principles and guidelines of good manufacturing practice have been published under, or apply by virtue of, regulation C17 of the Human

Medicines Regulations 2012 ("the Regulations"), which apply to an active substance manufactured in Great Britain, a manufacturer in Great Britain must comply with those principles and guidelines of good manufacturing practice in relation to that active substance.

Where the Commission has adopted principles and guidelines of good manufacturing practice under the third paragraph of Article 47 of the 2001 Directive which applies to an active substance manufactured in Northern Ireland, a manufacturer in Northern Ireland must comply with those principles and guidelines of good manufacturing practice in relation to that active substance.

Where principles and guidelines of good distribution practice have been published under, or apply by virtue of, regulation C17 of the Regulations, which apply to an active substance distributed in Great Britain, a distributor in Great Britain must comply with those principles and guidelines of good distribution practice in relation to that active substance.

Where the Commission has adopted principles and guidelines of good distribution practice under the fourth paragraph of Article 47 of the 2001 Directive, which applies to an active substance distributed in the Northern Ireland, a distributor in Northern Ireland must comply with those principles and guidelines of good distribution practice in relation to that active substance.

Where principles and guidelines of good manufacturing practice have been published under, or apply by virtue of, regulation C17, which apply to an active substance imported into the Northern Ireland and where an active substance is imported into Northern Ireland from a country other than an EEA State so imported:

- the importer must comply with good manufacturing practice and good distribution practice in relation to the active substance;
- the active substances must have been manufactured in accordance with standards that are at least equivalent to good manufacturing practice*; and
- the active substances must be accompanied by a written confirmation from the competent authority of the exporting country of the following:
  - the standards of manufacturing practice applicable to the plant manufacturing the exported active substance are at least equivalent to good manufacturing practice,
  - the manufacturing plant concerned is subject to regular, strict and transparent controls, and to the effective enforcement of standards of manufacturing practice at least equivalent to good manufacturing practice, including repeated and unannounced inspections, so as to ensure a protection of public health at least equivalent to that in Northern Ireland, and

– in the event of findings relating to non-compliance, information on such findings is supplied by the exporting country to the licensing authority without any delay.

Where principles and guidelines of good manufacturing practice have been published under, or apply by virtue of, regulation C17, which apply to an active substance imported into Great Britain other than from Northern Ireland and where an active substance is so imported:

- the importer must comply with good manufacturing practice and good distribution practice in relation to the active substance;
- the active substances must have been manufactured in accordance with standards that are at least equivalent to good manufacturing practice*; and
- the active substances must be accompanied by a written confirmation from the competent authority of the exporting country of the following:
  - the standards of manufacturing practice applicable to the plant manufacturing the exported active substance are at least equivalent to good manufacturing practice,
  - the manufacturing plant concerned is subject to regular, strict and transparent controls, and to the effective enforcement of standards of manufacturing practice at least equivalent to good manufacturing practice, including repeated and unannounced inspections, so as to ensure a protection of public health at least equivalent to that in Great Britain, and
  - in the event of findings relating to non-compliance, information on such findings is supplied by the exporting country to the licensing authority without any delay.

The criteria mentioned above marked with an "*" do not apply:

- where the country from where the active substance is exported is included in the list referred to in Article 111b of the 2001 Directive (in the case of an import into Northern Ireland) or paragraph (6) (in the case of an import into Great Britain); or
- for a period not exceeding the validity of the certificate of good manufacturing practice, where:
  - in relation to a plant where active substances are manufactured where the competent authority of a member State or licensing authority (in the case of an import into Northern Ireland) or licensing authority or an appropriate authority responsible for the licensing of medicinal products in a country included in a list under paragraph (6) (in the case of an import into Great Britain) has found, upon inspection, that a plant complies with the principles and guidelines of good manufacturing practice, and
  - the licensing authority is of the opinion that it is necessary to waive the requirement to ensure availability of the active substance.

All provisions apply regardless of whether an active substance is intended for export.

GMP for Active Substances

An "active substance" is defined as any substance or mixture of substances intended to be used in the manufacture of a medicinal product and that, when used in its production, becomes an active ingredient of that product intended to exert a pharmacological, immunological or metabolic action with a view to restoring, correcting or modifying physiological functions, or to make a medical diagnosis.

The manufacture of active substances should be subject to good manufacturing practice, regardless of whether those active substances are manufactured in the UK or imported. Where active substances are manufactured in third countries it should be ensured that such substances have been manufactured to the required standards of good manufacturing practice (GMP), so as to provide a level of protection of public health equivalent to that provided for by UK law.

A manufacturer or assembler of an active substance will have to comply with the principles and guidelines for GMP for active substances. Manufacture, in relation to an active substance, includes any process carried out in the course of making the substance and the various processes of dividing up, packaging and presentation of the active substance. Assemble, in relation to an active substance, includes the various processes of dividing up, packaging and presentation of the substance, and "assembly" has a corresponding meaning. These activities will be the subject of a GMP certificate.

Importers of an active substance from a third country have to comply with the guidelines for good distribution practice (GDP) in relation to the active substance. This activity will be the subject of a GDP certificate.

Distributors of an active substance within the UK that has been sourced from a manufacturer or an importer within the EU will have to comply with the guidelines for GDP for active substances. This activity will be the subject of a GDP certificate.

GDP for Active Substances

Since March 2015, guidelines on the principles of good distribution practices for active substances for medicinal products for human use have been published.

The guidelines set out the quality system elements for the procuring, importing, holding, supplying or exporting active substances. The scope of the guidelines exclude activities consisting of re-packaging, re-labelling or dividing up of active substances that are manufacturing activities and as such are subject to the guidelines on GMP of active substances. The guidelines, which can be found in Chapter 7 of this guide, cover:

- Quality system
- Personnel
- Documentation
- Orders
- Procedures
- Records
- Premises and equipment
- Receipt
- Storage
- Deliveries to customers
- Transfer of information
- Returns
- Complaints and recalls
- Self-inspections.

Written Confirmation

UK legislation requires importers of active substances for use in the manufacture of authorised medicinal products to obtain written confirmations from competent authorities in third countries that the standards of manufacture of active substances at manufacturing sites on their territory are equivalent to EU good manufacturing practice (EU GMP). These confirmations are required before importation of active substances into the UK.

Each shipment of active substance received should be accompanied by a written confirmation from the competent authority of the exporting third country, stating that the active substance has been:

- manufactured to GMP standards at least equivalent to those laid down in the Human Medicines Regulations;
- the third country manufacturing plant is subject to regular, strict and transparent inspections, and effective enforcement of GMP;
- in the event of non-conformance of the manufacturing site on inspection, such findings will be communicated to the UK without delay.

The European Commission's questions and answers document on this subject can be found on the Commission's website and has been reproduced in Appendix 5 of this guide.

The template for the written confirmation is reproduced here.

The MHRA will generate Written Confirmations for Active Substance manufacturers in Great Britain whether they intend to export Active Substances or not. For a distributor of Active Substances that the site/company did not manufacture, Written Confirmations will not be generated for these activities. If a Written Confirmation is required for a distributor for export activities of an Active Substance not manufactured by that distributor, it may be obtained from the appropriate issuing authority, or directly from the manufacturer.

Importation of Active Substances into Great Britain (England, Wales and Scotland) without a Written Confirmation is accepted from the following list of countries:

- European Economic Area (EEA) countries,
- USA,
- Japan,
- Republic of Korea,
- Brazil,
- Australia,
- Israel,
- Switzerland;

as well as from Northern Ireland.

Northern Ireland will also continue to align with all relevant EU rules relating to the placing on the market of manufactured goods.

Template for the "written confirmation" for active substances exported to the European Union for medicinal products for human use, in accordance with Article 46b(2)(b) of Directive 2001/83/EC

(1) Directive 2011/62/EU of the European Parliament and of the Council of 8 June 2011 amending Directive 2001/83/EC on the Community code relating to medicinal products for human use, as regards the prevention of the entry into the legal supply chain of falsified medicinal products (OJ L 174, 1.7.2011, p. 74) introduces EU-wide rules for the importation of active substances: According to Article 46b(2) of Directive 2001/83/EC, active substances shall only be imported if, inter alia, the active substances are accompanied by a written confirmation from the competent authority of the exporting third country which, as regards the plant manufacturing the exported active substance, confirms that the standards of good manufacturing practice and control of the plant are equivalent to those in the Union.

(2) The template for this written confirmation is set out in the annex.

ANNEX

Letterhead of the issuing regulatory authority

Written confirmation for active substances exported to the European Union (EU) for medicinal products for human use, in accordance with Article 46b(2)(b) of Directive 2001/83/EC

Confirmation no. (given by the issuing regulatory authority):

....

1. Name and address of site (including building number, where applicable):

....

2. Manufacturer's licence number(s):[3]

....

Regarding the Manufacturing Plant under (1) of the Following Active Substance(s) Exported to the EU for Medicinal Products for Human Use

Active substance(s):[4]	Activity(ies):[5]

The Issuing Regulatory Authority Hereby Confirms That:

The standards of good manufacturing practice (GMP) applicable to this manufacturing plant are at least equivalent to those laid down in the EU (= GMP of WHO/ICH Q7);

The manufacturing plant is subject to regular, strict and transparent controls and to the effective enforcement of good manufacturing practice, including repeated and unannounced inspections, so as to ensure a protection of public health at least equivalent to that in the EU; and

In the event of findings relating to non-compliance, information on such findings is supplied by the exporting third country without delay to the EU.[6]

---

[3] Where the regulatory authority issues a licence for the site. Record "not applicable" in the case where there is no legal framework for issuing of a licence.

[4] Identification of the specific active substances through an internationally agreed terminology (preferably international non-proprietary name).

[5] For example, "Chemical synthesis", "Extraction from natural sources", "Biological processes", "Finishing steps".

[6] qdefect@ema.europa.eu

Date of inspection of the plant under (1). Name of inspecting authority if different from the issuing regulatory authority:

....

This written confirmation remains valid until

....

   The authenticity of this written confirmation may be verified with the issuing regulatory authority.
   This written confirmation is without prejudice to the responsibilities of the manufacturer to ensure the quality of the medicinal product in accordance with Directive 2001/83/EC.

Address of the issuing regulatory authority:

....

Name and function of responsible person:

....

E-mail, Telephone no., and Fax no.:

....

Signature   Stamp of the authority and date

Written Confirmations for Export to EEA and Northern Ireland of Active Substances Manufactured in Great Britain

1.   Purpose of the Written Confirmation

A Written Confirmation confirms that, for a third country exporting Active Substances to the EEA:

- the standards of Good Manufacturing Practice (GMP) are equivalent to those in the EU/EEA;
- the manufacturing plant is subject to regular inspections (which may be both announced and unannounced);
- significant non-compliance events would be communicated to the EEA without delay.

   A template for the Written Confirmation can be found on the European Commission website.
   The requirement for the Written Confirmation is stated in Article 46b(2)(b) of Directive 2001/83/EC.

2. **"Third Country" status for Great Britain (England, Wales and Scotland) manufacturers of Active Substances**

Great Britain is recognised as a third country for the export of Active Substances for human use to the EEA. Active Substance manufacturers in Northern Ireland will continue to be recognised by the EEA.

A Written Confirmation will then be required for each shipment of Active Substance manufactured in Great Britain that is exported to the EEA and Northern Ireland.

3. **Generation of Written Confirmations for Active Substances manufactures in the UK**

You will not need to provide any information to the MHRA to allow the Written Confirmation to be generated. All the information required for the Written Confirmations is available within MHRA systems.

Written Confirmations will be generated for Active Substance manufacturers in Great Britain whether they intend to export Active Substances or not.

3.1   Biological products

Manufacture of biological active substance is considered to be partial manufacture of the biological medicinal product. These activities are recorded in section 1.3 of the UK Manufacturing Authorisation (MIA) and the associated GMP certificate issued following a satisfactory inspection "(EU Interpretation of the Union Format for Manufacturer/Importer Authorisation)".

If you hold an MIA that includes manufacture of biological active substance, separate registration as an Active Substance manufacturer is not required. No written confirmation will be issued, because this is already confirmed by the MHRA GMP certificate.

4. **Obtaining Written Confirmations for Active Substances manufactured in other third countries**

There will be no change to the requirements for obtaining Written Confirmations for importation of Active Substances from other "third countries". You will still need to obtain the Written Confirmations from the issuing authority in that country.

A Written Confirmation will not be required for the supply of Active Substance manufactured in Northern Ireland to Great Britain.

5. Requirements for distributors of Active Substances

If you are a Distributor of Active Substances that you did not manufacture, Written Confirmations will not be generated for your activities. If a Written Confirmation is required for export activities, it can be obtained from the appropriate issuing authority, or directly from the manufacturer.

6. Validity period of a Written Confirmation

A Written Confirmation is valid for the same period as the corresponding GMP certificate. Where required the MHRA will offer an assessment to reissue GMP certificates of Active Substance manufacturing sites in Great Britain, prior to 1 January 2021, to allow generation of Written Confirmations with an appropriate validity period.

Provision of Written Confirmations for Each Shipment of Active Substances Exported to the EEA and Northern Ireland

A "Questions and Answers" document on the EU expectations relating to Written Confirmations is available on the European Commission website. This document identifies how the Written Confirmation should be provided to the customer within the EEA.

8. Companies with confidential GMP certificates

If your company has a confidential GMP certificate due to the nature of the Active Substances manufactured, the Written Confirmation will not be published on the MHRA website. The Written Confirmation will be sent to the contact named on your Active Substance registration.

9. Requirement for both a GMP certificate and a Written Confirmation

Although similar information is contained in a GMP certificate and a Written Confirmation, both documents serve different purposes:

- UK law requires a GMP certificate to be issued after an inspection;
- EU regulations require a Written Confirmation for any import of Active Substances into the EEA by a third country.

If you export Active Substances made in Great Britain to the EEA or Northern Ireland, you are therefore required to have a valid GMP certificate and a valid Written Confirmation.

10.   Ongoing requirement for Written Confirmations

The need for Written Confirmations is expected to be an interim position. An application will be made to recognise Great Britain's GMP standards for the manufacture of Active Substances in Great Britain as equivalent to those in the EU.

Once a country has been accepted as having equivalent GMP standards, they are added to a "White List" and Written Confirmations are then no longer required.

Short-term Holding of Active Substances

The MHRA has a long-established policy in respect of the licensing of sites undertaking the short-term holding of medicinal products. As with medicinal products, Active Substances should be stored only on premises that are covered by an Active Substance Registration. However, there are certain cases where active substances are held for short periods of time during transportation and prior to onward shipment, e.g. in overnight freight depots. In such instances it has been determined that, as a matter of policy, a site is not required to be registered where:

- Active Substances subject to "ambient" storage temperature require-ments remain for less than 36 hours;
- "cold-chain" Active Substances are transported and stored overnight in continuously refrigerated vehicles or in qualified packaging; vehicles must be "in transit" and the active substance is not unloaded at the site (e.g. moved from the vehicle into a fridge or cold store).

As a matter of policy, a site must be registered where:

- ambient storage active substances are held in excess of 36 hours;
- Active Substances requiring refrigeration are placed in a cold store; even when this is for less than 36 hours;
- activities that can be registered, other than storage, are being carried out. This includes the handling of returned goods and where decisions are made regarding suitability for re-sale, as well as the usual activities of picking against orders;
- ownership has been transferred.

Where transportation is performed by a third party and they are hold-ing product, then they require an Active Substance Registration in their own right, naming the relevant sites. Whether the licensed sites require naming as third parties on the supplying registration holder will depend on the nature of the commercial and GDP contracts. In general, if the product is "in transit", the transport site is not required to be named as a third party on the supplier's registration.

Use of Third-party Storage and Distribution Sites

Where an Active Substance registration holder uses a third-party storage and/or distribution provider ("3PL"), the 3PL must have an Active Substance Registration in its own right if it is undertaking activities that can be registered, naming all the sites at which these activities (manufacture, importation or distribution) take place. Any 3PL site that carries out activities that can be registered should be named on the Active Substance Registration of the contract giver.

A Wholesale Dealer's Licence is not relevant to the manufacture, importation or distribution of Active Substances, as a Wholesale Dealer's Licence relates to the procurement, holding or supply of medicinal products (the finished dosage form in the packaging intended for placing on the market). Where a 3PL holds a Wholesale Dealer's Licence, it may give the contract giver some reassurance that the contract acceptor is familiar with the general principles of Good Distribution Practice, because there are a number of parallels between the minimum standards described in Good Distribution Practice for medicinal products and those described for Active Substances; however, this does not lift the requirements of Regulation 45M of the Human Medicines Regulations 2012, as amended, in that the contract giver and contract acceptor both require Active Substance Registrations in their own right.

As required by Section 6.2 of Good Distribution Practice for Active Substances, a contract should be in place between the parties clearly defining responsibilities and the transfer of relevant information. There should be a process of information transfer between the parties that ensures that relevant information is kept up to date across the Active Substance Registrations, such as the range of Active Substances stored/distributed on the contract giver's behalf and the naming of key personnel.

Historically it has been possible for the holder of an Active Substance Registration to use third-party storage and distribution sites located within the European Economic Area (EEA); these sites have never been named on the face of a UK Active Substance Registration, but will hold Active Substance Registrations in their own right in the relevant territory. This MHRA policy continues to be implemented following the UK's exit from the European Union. As with the use of a 3PL in the United Kingdom, there should be a contract in place clearly defining responsibilities and the transfer of information between the contract giver and the contract acceptor.

UK GUIDANCE ON
ACTIVESUBSTANCES

Segregation of Medicinal Products and Active Substances

Sub-sections 5.1 and 6.7 of Good Distribution Practice for Active Substances require that:

"Premises and equipment should be suitable and adequate to ensure proper storage, protection from contamination, e.g. narcotics, highly sensitising materials, materials of high pharmacological activity or toxicity, and distribution of active substances. They should be suitably secure to prevent unauthorised access ...

Active substances should be stored under the conditions specified by the manufacturer, e.g. controlled temperature and humidity when necessary, and in such a manner to prevent contamination and/or mix up ..."

Sub-section 5.5 of Good Distribution Practice for medicinal products requires that:

"Medicinal products and, if necessary, healthcare products should be stored separately from other products likely to alter them ...

Medicinal products should be handled and stored in such a manner as to prevent spillage, breakage, contamination and mix-ups ..."

Where a site holds or distributes both medicinal products and Active Substances, there should be adequate segregation of the relevant activities to prevent contamination of one type of product by the other. This is particularly relevant where either the medicinal products or active substances are radioactive materials and other hazardous products, as well as products presenting special safety risks of fire or explosion. Adequate and appropriate security measures should be in place, if necessary restricting personnel who have access to either medicinal product or active substance storage areas if all staff have not received relevant training relating to both product types.

Customer Qualification

Good Distribution Practice for Active Substances requires that supplies of active substances are only made to "... other distributors, manufacturers or to dispensing pharmacies". Key to the supply of an active substance is the definition of an active substance contained in Regulation 8 of the Human Medicines Regulations 2012, as amended:

"'active substance' means any substance or mixture of substances intended to be used in the manufacture of a medicinal product and that, when used in its production, becomes an active ingredient of that product intended to exert a pharmacological, immunological or metabolic action with a view to restoring, correcting or modifying physiological functions or to make a medical diagnosis;"

One important aspect of this definition is that the substance "...is intended to be used in the manufacture of a medicinal product ..."; in relation to the holding of an Active Substance Registration the medicinal product referred to in this definition is a medicinal product for human use. There is currently no comparable registration regime for active substances intended for the manufacture of veterinary medicinal products, and the controls on active substance manufacture and distribution for veterinary medicinal products are achieved by other means.

It is not uncommon for persons manufacturing and/or distributing active substances to be involved in the supply of substances for other purposes, e.g. foodstuffs, cosmetics or industrial chemicals. It is important for the distributor to establish which of the materials they distribute are subject to controls under UK medicines legislation and those that are subject to different controls, because those materials considered to be Active Substances, rather than falling into some other product type, are subject to particular requirements in legislation and Good Distribution Practice.

In qualifying a customer and their authority to receive a particular substance, the use of "end-user declarations" can be helpful in establishing the legal basis of supply, identifying to what use the customer will be putting the substance they intend procuring. This is particularly relevant to the arena of medicinal products for human use as different controls apply to active substances and excipients. This can help a registration holder focus their resources on the appropriate management of their product portfolio and supplements other customer bona fide checks, such as licence or registration verification against authoritative sources of information.

UK GUIDANCE ON
ACTIVESUBSTANCES

Annual Reports and Registration Variations

Regulation 45P of the Human Medicines Regulations 2012, as amended, requires that Active Substance Registration Holders must provide the Licensing Authority with an annual report on or before 30 April each year. This report must contain certain information:

- a declaration that the registration holder has an appropriate system in place to ensure compliance with the requirements of Regulations 45N (Registration in relation to Active Substances) and 45O (Requirements for registration as an importer, manufacturer or distributor of an active substance) of the same regulations.

• a description of the system that the registration holder has in place to manage compliance with the regulations.

Regulation 45P then goes on the require that the registration holder must without delay notify the licensing authority of any changes to that system that could affect compliance with the requirements relating to the holding of an Active Substance Registration.

Regulation 45T provides the process for applying for a variation to the scope of an Active Substance Registration. An application for a variation has the effect of changing the scope of the granted Active Substance Registration, e.g. a change in named personnel or the addition or removal of certain active substances manufactured, imported or distributed under the registration. Registration variations should be submitted to the Licensing Authority in a timely manner, and may trigger an inspection dependent on the nature of the change(s) applied for.

From this it can be seen that there is a difference between the scope of an annual report made under Regulation 45P and a registration variation made under Regulation 45T. A registration holder is required to submit an annual report every year, whether or not the scope of the registration changes over time. The processes for the submission of the annual report and submission of a registration variation should be captured in the registration holders quality system, and naturally link in with processes such as change control and deviation management.

There are fees applied to both the submission of an annual report and registration variation, these can be found on the MHRA website[4] (www.gov.uk/mhra). Both annual reports and registration variations are submitted electronically through the MHRA's Process Licensing Portal (https://pclportal.mhra.gov.uk).

The Role of the "Designated Person" for Active Substance Importers and Distributors

Sub-section 3.1 of Good Distribution Practice for Active Substances requires that:

"The distributor should designate a person at each location where distribution activities are performed who should have defined authority and responsibility for ensuring that a quality system is implemented and maintained. The designated person should fulfil his responsibilities personally. The designated person can delegate duties but not responsibilities."

---

[4] https://www.gov.uk/government/publications/mhra-fees/current-mhra-fees.

On the face of a UK Active Substance Registration, and within the MHRA Process Licensing Portal, this person is referred to as "Person responsible for Importation, Storage or Distribution Activities".

Within the scope of a Wholesale Dealer's Licence is the "Responsible Person". Sub-section 2.2 of Good Distribution Practice for medicinal products requires that:

"The wholesale distributor must designate a person as responsible person. ...

... The responsible person should fulfil their responsibilities personally and should be continuously contactable. The responsible person may delegate duties but not responsibilities. ...

... The written job description of the responsible person should define their authority to take decisions with regard to their responsibilities. The wholesale distributor should give the responsible person the defined authority, resources and responsibility needed to fulfil their duties. ...

The responsibilities of the responsible person include:

(i) ensuring that a quality management system is implemented and maintained; ..."

In this respect the Designated Person and Responsible Person can be seen to be comparable in their role of ensuring that the compliance of the registration or licence holder with the requirements of legislation and Good Distribution Practice is maintained at an appropriate standard that protects public health.

Although the responsibilities of the Designated Person are less clearly defined in Good Distribution Practice for active substances than those for the Responsible Person in Good Distribution Practice for medicinal products, there are some activities that the MHRA's Good Distribution Practice Inspectorate consider key to the implementation and maintenance of an effective quality system:

- ensuring that importation/distribution activities under the registration are in accordance with the scope of the registration, including the submission of annual reports and applications for registration variations;
- ensuring that roles and responsibilities are clearly defined and understood, and that personnel have received appropriate training and are demonstrably competent;
- ensuring that records are accurate, complete and being generated and maintained contemporaneously;
- ensuring that Active Substances are stored under appropriate conditions and evaluating the impact of departures from the required storage conditions, whether those relate to temperature, humidity, light or other aspects.

UK GUIDANCE ON ACTIVE SUBSTANCES

- having oversight of customer complaints, particularly those relating to product quality;
- ensuring that Active Substances that are subject to recall action have been withdrawn from the market when required and that relevant information relating to Active Substance quality has been provided to customers and the relevant Competent Authorities;
- ensuring that active substances are sourced only from and supplied to appropriately authorised persons;
- having oversight of activities contracted out to third parties, particularly where those activities can be registered;
- carrying out timely, objective and comprehensive self-inspection activities in assessing the compliance of the registration holder's activities;
- having oversight of changes to or deviations from the company's established operations, particularly where there is potential impact on the importation or distribution of Active Substances, including the application of quality risk management;
- ensuring that the quality system is sufficiently comprehensive in respect of the registration holder's activities and that any other relevant requirements in legislation (e.g. in relation to safety, radioactive substances or Controlled Drugs) have been incorporated into the quality system and are complied with.

As with the Responsible Person, the Designated Person should maintain their competence in and awareness of Good Distribution Practice for Active Substances and the relevant UK legislation by way of on-going training; such training should be documented and demonstrate how relevant learning has been applied to the registration holder's operations. An assessment of the knowledge, awareness and competence of the Designated Person forms part of every inspection of an Active Substance Registration holder; where a Designated Person is not considered to be fulfilling their responsibilities regulatory action may be taken against the registration holder.

For further information on the role and responsibilities of the Responsible Person, please refer to Chapter 3 of this publication.

Appendices

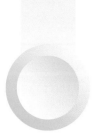

Appendix 1

HUMAN AND VETERINARY MEDICINES AUTHORITIES IN EUROPE

Austria

Austrian Medicines and Medical Devices
Agency – Austrian Federal Office for Safety in
Health Care
Traisengasse 5
A-1200 Vienna
Austria
Phone   +43 50 555 36111
E-mail BASG-AGESMedizinmarktaufsicht@
ages.at
Website(s) http://www.basg.gv.at

Belgium

DG Enterprise and Industry – F/2 BREY
10/073
Avenue d'Auderghem 45
B-1049 Brussels
Belgium

Federal Agency for Medicines and Health
Products
Avenue Galilée 5
031210 Brussels
Belgium
Phone   +32 2 528 40 00
Fax   +32 2 528 40 01
E-mail welcome@fagg-afmps.be
Website(s) http://www.fagg-afmps.be/en/

Bulgaria

Bulgarian Drug Agency
8, Damyan Gruev Str.
1303 Sofia
Bulgaria
Phone   +359 2 8903 555
Fax   +359 2 8903 434

E-mail bda@bda.bg
Website(s) http://www.bda.bg

Bulgarian Food Safety Agency
15A, Pencho Slaveiko Blvd
1606 Sofia
Bulgaria
Phone   +359 2 915 98 20
Fax   +359 2 954 95 93
E-mail cvo@bfsa.bg
Website(s) http://www.babh.government.bg

Croatia

Croatian Agency for Medicinal Products and
Medical Devices
Ksaverska c.4
10000 Zagreb
Croatia
Phone   +385 1 4884 100
Fax   +385 1 4884 110
E-mail halmed@halmed.hr
Website(s) http://www.halmed.hr

Ministry of Agriculture, Veterinary and Food
Safety Directorate
Planinska Street 2a
10000 Zagreb
Croatia
Phone   +385 6443 540
Fax   +385 6443 899
E-mail veterinarstvo@mps.hr
Website(s) http://www.veterinarstvo.hr

Cyprus

Pharmaceutical Services – Ministry of Health
7 Larnacos Ave
15 Polyphimou, Stravolos Industrial Area

2033 Nicosia
Cyprus
Phone   +357 22 608 607
Fax   +357 22 339 623
E-mail lpanagi@phs.moh.gov.cy
Website(s) http://www.moh.gov.cy

Czech Republic

State Institute for Drug Control
Srobárova 48
CZ-100 41 Praha 10
Czech Republic
Phone   +420 272 185 111
Fax   +420 271 732 377
E-mail posta@sukl.cz
Website(s) http://www.sukl.eu

Institute for State Control of Veterinary Biologicals and Medicaments
Hudcova Str. 56A
CZ-621 00 Brno-Medlánky
Czech Republic
Phone   +420 541 518 211
Fax   +420 541 210 026
E-mail uskvbl@uskvbl.cz
Website(s) http://www.uskvbl.cz/

Denmark

Danish Medicines Agency
Axel Heides Gade 1
2300 Copenhagen S
Denmark
Phone   +45 44 88 95 95
Fax   +45 44 88 95 99
E-mail dkma@dkma.dk
Website(s) http://www.Imst.dk

European Commission

DG Enterprise F2 Pharmaceuticals
Rue de la Loi 200
B-1049 Brussels
Belgium

DG Health and Consumers: Unit D6: Medicinal Products – Quality, Safety and Efficacy
Rue de la Loi 200
B-1049 Brussels
Belgium
Phone   +32 2 299 11 11

E-mail: sanco-pharmaceuticals-d6@ec.europa.eu
Website(s) http://ec.europa.eu/health/human-use/index_en.htm

European Medicines Agency (EMA)
Domenico Scarlattilaan 6
1083 HS Amsterdam
The Netherlands
Phone   +31 (0)88 781 6000
E-mail info@ema.europa.eu
Website(s) http://www.ema.europa.eu/

Estonia

State Agency of Medicines
1 Nooruse Street
EE-50411 Tartu
Estonia
Phone   +372 737 41 40
Fax   +372 737 41 42
E-mail info@ravimiamet.ee
Website(s) http://www. ravimiregister.ravimiamet.ee/en/default.aspx

Finland

Finnish Medicines Agency
PO Box 55
FI-00034 Fimea Helsinki
Finland
Phone   +358 29 522 3341
Fax   +358 29 522 3001
E-mail registry@fimea.fi
Website(s) http://www.fimea.fi/

France

French National Agency for Medicines and Health Products Safety (ANSM)
143-147 bd
Anatole France
FR-93285 Saint Denis Cedex
France
E-mail ANSM@ansm.sante.fr
Website(s) http://www.ansm.sante.fr

Agence Nationale du Médicament Vétérinaire (ANMV)/Agence nationale de sécurité sanitaire de l'alimentation, de l'environnement et du travail (Anses)
14 rue Claude Bourgelat, Parc d'Activités de la Grande Marche, Javené -CS

70611-35306 Fougères Cedex
France
Phone   +33 (0) 2 99 94 78 71
E-mail sylvie.goby@anses.fr
Website(s) http://www.anses.fr

Germany

Federal Institute for Drugs and Medical Devices
(BfArM)
Kurt-Georg-Kiesinger-Allee 3
53175 Bonn
Germany
Phone   +49 (0)228-207-30
Fax   +49 (0)228-207-5207
E-mail poststelle@bfarm.de
Website(s) http://www.bfarm.de

Federal Office of Consumer Protection and
Food Safety
Mauerstraße 39–42
D-10117 Berlin
Germany
Phone   +49 30 1 84 44-000
Fax   +49 30 1 84 44-89 999
E-mail poststelle@bvl.bund.de
Website(s) http://www.bvl.bund.de
(pharmaceuticals)

Paul-Ehrlich Institut (Federal Institute for
Vaccines and Biomedicines)
Paul-Ehrlich-Straße 51–59
63225 Langen
Germany
Phone   +49 6103 77 0
Fax   +49 6103 77 1234
E-mail pei@pei.de
Website(s) http://www.pei.de
(vaccines, blood products, sera)

Greece

National Organization for Medicines
Messogion Avenue 284, cholargos
GR-15562 Athens
Greece
Phone   +30 213 2040 384
Fax   +30 213 2040 569
E-mail inter.rel@eof.gr
Website(s) http://www.eof.gr/
(pharmaceuticals and immunologicals)

Hungary

National Institute of Pharmacy and Nutrition
Zrínyi U. 3
H-1051 Budapest
Hungary
Website(s) http://www.ogyei.hu/

National Food Chain Safety Office, Directorate
of Veterinary Medicinal Products
Szállás utca 8
H-1107 Budapest 10.Pf. 318
Hungary
Phone   +36 1 433 03 30
Fax   +36 1 262 28 39
E-mail ati@nebih.gov.hu
Website(s) http://www.nebih.gov.hu

Iceland

Icelandic Medicines Agency
Vinlandsleid 14
IS-113 Reykjavik
Iceland
Phone   +354 520 2100
Fax   +354 561 2170
E-mail ima@ima.is
Website(s) http://www.ima.is

Ireland

Health Products Regulatory Agency (HPRA)
Kevin O'Malley House
Earlsfort Centre
Earlsfort Terrace
Dublin 2
Ireland
Phone   +353 1 676 4971
Fax   +353 1 676 7836
E-mail info@hpra.ie
Website(s) http://www.hpra.ie

Department of Agriculture and Food
Kildare St
Dublin
Ireland
Phone   +353 1 607 20 00
Fax   +353 1 661 62 63
E-mail info@agriculture.gov.ie
Website(s) http://www.agriculture.gov.ie

HUMAN AND VETERINARY
MEDICINES AUTHORITIES
IN EUROPE

Italy

Italian Medicines Agency
Via del Tritone, 181
I-00187 Rome
Italy
Phone   +39 6 5978401
Fax   +39 6 59944142
E-mail forenamefirstletter.surename@aifa.gov.it
Website(s) http://www.agenziafarmaco.it/

Laboratorio di Medicina Veterinaria, Istituto Superiore di Sanità
Viale Regina Elena 299
I-00161 Rome
Italy
Phone   +39 6 49 38 70 76
Fax   +39 6 49 38 70 77

Ministero della Salute, Direzione Generale della Sanità Animale e dei Farmaci Veterinari, Uff. 4
Viale Giorgio Ribotta
5I-00144 Rome
Italy
Phone   +39 06 59 94 65 84
Fax   +39 06 59 94 69 49
Website(s) http://www.salute.it/

Latvia

State Agency of Medicines
15 Jersikas iela
LV-1003 Riga
Latvia
Phone   +371-7078424
Fax   +371-7078428
E-mail info@zva.gov.lv
Website(s) http://www.zva.gov.lv/

Food and Veterinary Service
Peldu St 30
LV-1050 Riga
Latvia
Phone   +371 67095271
Fax   +371 67095270
E-mail nrd@pvd.gov.lv
Website(s) http://www.pvd.gov.lv

Liechtenstein

Office of Health/Medicinal Products Control Agency
Äulestr 512
FL-9490 Vaduz
Liechtenstein
Fax   +423 236 73 50
E-mail pharminfo@llv.li
Website(s) www.llv.li/

Lithuania

State Medicines Control Agency
Žirmūnų str. 139A
LT-09120 Vilnius
Lithuania
Phone   +370 5 263 92 64
Fax   +370 5 263 92 65
E-mail vvkt@vvkt.lt
Website(s) http://www.vvkt.lt

National Food and Veterinary Risk Assessment Institute
J. Kairiukscio str. 10
LT-08409 Vilnius
Lithuania
Phone   +370 5 2780470
Fax   +370 5 2780471
E-mail nmvrvi@vet.lt
Website(s) http://www.nmvrvi.lt

State Food and Veterinary Service
Siesiku str. 19
LT-07170 Vilnius
Lithuania
E-mail info@vmvt.lt
Website(s) http://www.vmvt.lt

Luxembourg

Ministry of Health
Allée Marconi
L-2120 Luxembourg
Luxembourg
Phone   +352 24785593
Fax   +352 24795615
E-mail luxdpm@ms.etat.lu
E-mail vet marc.schmit@ms.etat.lu
Website(s) http://www.ms.etat.lu

Malta

Medicines Authority
Sir Temi Zammit Buildings, Malta Life Sciences Park
SGN 3000 San Gwann

Malta
Phone   +356 23439000
Fax   +356 23439161
E-mail info.medicinesauthority@gov.mt
Website(s) www.medicinesauthority.gov.mt

Veterinary Medicines Section within the National Veterinary Laboratory of the Veterinary and Phytosanitary Regulation Department
Abattoir Square
Albert Town
MRS 1123 Marsa
Malta
Phone   +356 22925375
E-mail veterinarymedicine@gov.mt
Website(s) http://agriculture.gov.mt/en/nvl/Pages/missionStatement.aspx

Netherlands

Medicines Evaluation Board
Graadt van Roggenweg 500
NL-3531 AH Utrecht
The Netherlands
Phone   +31 (0) 88 - 224 80 00
Fax   +31 (0) 88 - 224 80 01
Website(s) http://www.cbg-meb.nl/

Norway

Norwegian Medicines Agency (NOMA)
Postboks 240 Skøyen
0213 Oslo
Norway
Phone   +47 22 89 77 00
Fax   +47 22 89 77 99
E-mail post@noma.no
Website(s) http://www.legemiddelverket.no/

Poland

Chief Pharmaceutical Inspectorate
12 Senatorska str.
00-082 Warsaw
Poland
Phone   +48 (22) 831 21 31
Fax   +48 (22) 831 02 44
E-mail gif@gif.gov.pl
Website(s) http://www.gif.gov.pl

Office for Registration of Medicinal Products, Medical Devices and Biocidal Products
Al. Jerozolimskie 181C
02-222 Warsaw
Poland
Phone   +48 22 492 11 00
Fax   +48 22 492 11 09
Website (s) www.urpl.gov.pl

Portugal

INFARMED - National Authority of Medicines and Health Products, IP
Av. do Brasil 53
P-1749-004 Lisbon
Portugal
Phone   +351 217987100
Fax   +351 217987316
E-mail infarmed@infarmed.pt
Website(s) http://www.infarmed.pt/portal/page/portal/INFARMED

Food and Veterinary Directorate General
Campo Grande, n.º 50
1349-018 Lisboa
Portugal
Phone   +351 21 323 96 55
Fax   +351 21 346 35 18
E-mail dirgeral@dgav.pt
Website(s) http://www.dgv.pt

Romania

National Agency for Medicines and Medical Devices
48, Av. Sanatescu
011478 Bucharest
Romania
Phone   +4021 317 11 00
Fax   +4021 316 34 97
Website(s) http://www.anm.ro/en/

Institute for Control of Biological Products and Veterinary Medicines
Str. Dudului 37, sector 6
060603 Bucharest
Romania
Phone   +40 21 220 21 12
Fax   +40 21 221 31 71
E-mail icbmv@icbmv.ro
Website(s) http://www.icbmv.ro/

Slovakia

State Institute for Drug Control
Kvetná 11
SK-825 08 Bratislava 26
Slovakia
Phone   +421 2 5070 1111
Fax   +421 2 5556 4127
E-mail sukl@sukl.sk
Website(s) http://www.sukl.sk/

Institute for State Control of Veterinary
Biologicals and Medicaments
Biovetská 34
PO Box 52c
SK-949 01 Nitra
Slovakia
Phone   +421 37 6515506
Fax   +421 37 6517915
E-mail uskvbl@uskvbl.sk
Website(s) http://www.uskvbl.sk/

Slovenia

Javna agencija Republike Slovenije za zdravila
in medicinske pripomočke
Ptujska ulica 21
Slovenčeva ulica 22
Sl-1000 Ljubljana
Slovenia
Phone   +386 8 2000 500
Fax   +386 8 2000 557
E-mail info@jazmp.si
Website(s) http://www.jazmp.si

Spain

Spanish Agency of Medicines and Medical
Devices
Parque Empresarial Las
Mercedes Edificio 8C
Campezo, 1
E-28022 Madrid
Spain
Phone   +34 91 8225997
Fax   +34 91 8225128
E-mail internacional@aemps.es
Website(s) www.agemed.es

Sweden

Medical Products Agency
Dag Hammarskjölds väg 42 / Box 26
SE-751 03 Uppsala
Sweden
Phone   +46 (0) 18 17 46 00
Fax   +46 (0) 18 54 85 66
E-mail registrator@mpa.se
Website(s) www.lakemedelsverket.se

United Kingdom

Medicines and Healthcare products Regulatory
Agency
10 South Colonnade
Canary Wharf
London
E14 4PU
United Kingdom
Phone   +44 (0)20 3080 6000
Fax   +44 (0)203 118 9803
Website(s) www.mhra.gov.uk

National Institute for Biological Standards and
Control
Blanche Lane
South Mimms
Potters Bar
EN6 3QG
United Kingdom
Phone   +44(0) 1707 641000
Fax   +44 (0) 1707 641050
E-mail enquiries@nibsc.org
Website https://www.nibsc.org/

Veterinary Medicines Directorate (VMD)
Woodham Lane
New Haw
Addlestone
KT15 3LS
United Kingdom
Phone   +44 1932 33 69 11
Fax   +44 1932 33 66 18
E-mail postmaster@vmd.defra.gsi.gov.uk
Website(s) www.vmd.defra.gov.uk

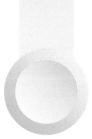

Appendix 2

LIST OF PERSONS WHO CAN BE SUPPLIED WITH MEDICINES BY WAY OF WHOLESALE DEALING (HUMAN MEDICINES REGULATIONS 2012)

Contents

All Medicines

- Doctors and dentists
- Persons lawfully conducting a retail pharmacy business within the meaning of section 69 of the Medicines Act 1968
- Holders of wholesale dealer's licences or persons to whom the restrictions imposed by regulation 18(1) of the Human Medicines Regulations do not apply because of an exemption in those Regulations
- Authorities or persons carrying on the business of:
  (a) An independent hospital, independent clinic or independent medical agency, or
  (b) A hospital or health centre which is not an independent hospital or independent clinic
  (c) A nursing home in Northern Ireland
- Ministers of the Crown and Government Departments
- Scottish Ministers
- Welsh Ministers
- Northern Ireland Ministers
- A person other than an excepted person (in this context a pharmacist) who carries on a business consisting (wholly or partly) of the supply

or administration of medicinal products for the purpose of assisting the provision of health care by or on behalf of, or under arrangements made by:

(a) A police force in England, Wales or Scotland,
(b) The Police Service of Northern Ireland,
(c) A prison service, or
(d) Her Majesty's Forces

- A person other than an excepted person (in this context a pharmacist) who carries on a business consisting (wholly or partly) of the supply or administration of medicinal products for the purpose of assisting the provision of health care by or on behalf of, or under arrangements made by:

(a) NHS trust or NHS foundation trust
(b) The Common Services Agency
(c) A local authority in the exercise of public health functions (within the meaning of the NHS Act 2006)
(d) A health authority or special health authority
(e) A clinical commissioning group
(f) NHS England
(g) A local authority

Health professionals may order medicines using a doctor or dentist's letter of authority. The letter should be clear that the health professional is authorised to order medicines on the doctor or dentist's behalf for delivery to that doctor or dentist.

Pharmacy Medicines

- Pharmacy medicines that are for the purpose of administration in the course of a business can be supplied to a person carrying on that business.

General Sale List Medicines

- Any person who requires GSL medicines for the purpose of selling, supplying or administering them to human beings in the course of a business carried on by that person.

Other Relevant Provisions

- Under medicines legislation, the general rule is that prescription-only medicines may only be sold or supplied on a retail basis against a prescription on registered pharmacy premises by or under the supervision of a pharmacist. There are exemptions from these restrictions for certain persons in respect of specific medicines that are contained in Schedule 17 to the Human Medicines Regulations 2012. The Regulations allow people who have exemptions to be sold the prescription only medicines relevant to their particular exemption on a wholesale basis. **See Schedule 17.**

- Similarly, the general rule for pharmacy medicines is that they may only be sold or supplied by or under the supervision of a pharmacist on registered pharmacy premises. Again, there are exemptions from these restrictions for certain persons in respect of specific medicines contained in Schedule 17 of the Human Medicines Regulations 2012 and the Regulations allow for the sale of the P medicines on the same basis as for POMs (above). **See Schedule 17.**

Additional Provisions for Optometrists and Dispensing Opticians not Included in Schedule 17

- The Human Medicines Regulations also contain other provisions that allow wholesale sales in certain circumstances:
  (a) Registered optometrists can obtain a range of medicines on a wholesale basis for sale or supply in the course of their professional practice. In addition to these arrangements, they may also obtain prescription only medicines containing the following substances for administration:
    – Amethocaine hydrochloride
    – Lidocaine hydrochloride
    – Oxybuprocaine hydrochloride
    – Proxymetacaine hydrochloride
  (b) Additional Supply Optometrists can be sold a product that is only classed as a POM because it contains thymoxamine hydrochloride
  (c) Dispensing opticians can obtain the following which are required for use by a registered optometrist or doctor attending their practice:
    – Amethocaine hydrochloride
    – Chloramphenicol
    – Cyclopentolate hydrochloride
    – Fusidic acid
    – Lidocaine hydrochloride
    – Oxybuprocaine hydrochloride
    – Proxymetacaine hydrochloride
    – Tropicamide
  (d) Dispensing opticians can also obtain medicines that are required in the course of their professional practice as a contact lens specialist that contain one or more of the following substances:
    – Lidocaine hydrochloride
    – Oxybuprocaine hydrochloride
    – Proxymetacaine hydrochloride

SCHEDULE 17 Exemption for Sale, Supply or Administration by Certain Persons

PART 1 Exemption from restrictions on sale or supply of prescription-only medicines

Persons exempted	Prescription-only medicines to which the exemption applies	Conditions
1 Persons selling or supplying prescription-only medicines to universities, other institutions concerned with higher education or institutions concerned with research.	1 All prescription-only medicines.	1 The sale or supply shall be: (a) subject to the presentation of an order signed by the principal of an institution concerned with educational research or the appropriate head of department in charge of a specified course of research stating: (i) the name of the institution for which the prescription only medicine is required, and (ii) the purpose for which the prescription only medicine is required, and (iii) the total quantity required; and (b) for the purpose of the education or research with which the institution is concerned.
2 Persons selling or supplying prescription-only medicines to any of the following: (a) a public analyst appointed under section 27 of the Food Safety Act 1990 or article 27 of the Food Safety (Northern Ireland) Order 1991; (b) an authorised officer within the meaning of section 5(6) of the Food Safety Act 1990; (c) a sampling officer within the meaning of article 38(1) of the Food (Northern Ireland) Order 1989; (d) an inspector acting under regulations 325 to 328; (e) a sampling officer within the meaning of Schedule 31.	2 All prescription-only medicines.	2 The sale or supply shall be subject to the presentation of an order signed by or on behalf of any person listed in column 1 stating the status of the person signing it and the amount of prescription-only medicine required, and shall be only in connection with the exercise by those persons of their statutory functions.
3 Persons selling or supplying prescription-only medicines to any person employed or engaged in connection with a scheme for testing the quality and checking the amount of the drugs and appliances supplied under the National Health Service Act 2006, the National Health Service (Scotland)	3 All prescription-only medicines.	3 The sale or supply shall be: (a) subject to the presentation of an order signed by or on behalf of the person so employed or engaged stating the status of the person signing it and the amount of the prescription-only medicine required; and

Persons exempted	Prescription-only medicines to which the exemption applies	Conditions
Act 1978, the National Health Service (Wales) Act 2006 and the Health and Personal Social Services (Northern Ireland) Order 1972, or under any subordinate legislation made under those Acts or that Order.		(b) for the purposes of a scheme referred to in column 1 in this paragraph.
4 Registered midwives.	4 Prescription-only medicines containing any of the following substances: (a) Diclofenac; (b) Hydrocortisone acetate; (c) Miconazole; (d) Nystatin; (e) Phytomenadione.	4 The sale or supply shall be only in the course of their professional practice.
5 Persons lawfully conducting a retail pharmacy business within the meaning of section 69 of the Medicines Act 1968.	5 Water for injection.	5 The sale or supply is to a person: (a) for a purpose other than parenteral administration; or (b) who has been prescribed dry powder for parenteral administration but has not been prescribed the water for injection that is needed as a diluent.
6 Persons lawfully conducting a retail pharmacy business within the meaning of section 69 of the Medicines Act 1968.	6 Items that are: (a) prescription-only medicines that are not for parenteral administration and that (i) are eye drops and are prescription-only medicines by reason only that they contain no more than 0.5 per cent of chloramphenicol, or (ii) are eye ointments and are prescription-only medicines by reason only that they contain no more than 1.0 per cent chloramphenicol, or (iii) are prescription-only medicines by reason only that they contain any of the following substances: (aa) cyclopentolate hydrochloride, (bb) fusidic acid, (cc) tropicamide; (b) the following prescription only medicines: (i) amorolfine hydrochloride cream where the maximum strength of the amorolfine in the cream does not exceed 0.25 per cent by weight in weight, (ii) amorolfine hydrochloride lacquer where the maximum strength of amorolfine in lacquer does not exceed 5 per cent by weight in volume,	6 The sale or supply shall be subject to the presentation of an order signed by: (a) a registered optometrist for a medicine listed under item (a) in column 2; (b) a registered chiropodist or podiatrist for a medicine listed under item (b) in column 2.

Persons exempted	Prescription-only medicines to which the exemption applies	Conditions
	(iii) amoxicillin,	
	(iv) co-codamol,	
	(v) co-dydramol 10/500 tablets,	
	(vi) codeine phosphate,	
	(vii) erythromycin,	
	(viii) flucloxacillin,	
	(ix) silver sulfadiazine,	
	(x) tioconazole 28%,	
	(xi) topical hydrocortisone where the maximum strength of hydrocortisone in the medicinal product does not exceed 1 per cent by weight in weight.	
7 Registered optometrists.	7 Prescription-only medicines listed in item (a) of paragraph 6 column 2.	7 The sale or supply shall be only: (a) in the course of their professional practice, and (b) in an emergency.
8 Persons lawfully conducting a retail pharmacy business within the meaning of section 69 of the Medicines Act 1968.	8 Medicinal products not for parenteral administration that are prescription-only medicines by reason only that they contain any of the following substances: (a) acetylcysteine, (b) atropine sulphate, (c) azelastine hydrochloride, (d) diclofenac sodium, (e) emedastine, (f) homotropine hydrobromide, (g) ketotifen, (h) levocabastine, (i) lodoxamide, (j) nedocromil sodium, (k) olopatadine, (l) pilocarpine hydrochloride, (m) pilocarpine nitrate, (n) polymyxin b/bacitracin, (o) polymyxin b/trimethoprim, (p) sodium cromoglycate.	8 The sale or supply shall be subject to the presentation of an order signed by an additional supply optometrist.
9 Additional supply optometrists.	9 Prescription-only medicines specified in paragraph 8 column 2.	9 The sale or supply shall be only: (a) in the course of their professional practice, and (b) in an emergency.
10 Holders of UK marketing authorisations, EU marketing authorisations, product licences or manufacturer's licences.	10 Prescription-only medicines referred to in those authorisations or licences.	10 The sale or supply shall be only: (a) to a pharmacist, (b) so as to enable that pharmacist to prepare an entry relating to the prescription-only medicine in question in a tablet or capsule identification guide or similar publication, and

Persons exempted	Prescription-only medicines to which the exemption applies	Conditions
		(c) of no greater quantity than is reasonably necessary for that purpose.
11 Registered chiropodists or podiatrists against whose names are recorded in the relevant register annotations signifying that they are qualified to use the medicine specified in column 2.	11 The following prescription-only medicines: (a) amorolfine hydrochloride cream where the maximum strength of the amorolfine in the cream does not exceed 0.25 per cent by weight in weight, (b) amorolfine hydrochloride lacquer where the maximum strength of amorolfine in lacquer does not exceed 5 per cent by weight in volume, (c) amoxicillin, (d) co-codamol, (e) co-dydramol 10/500 tablets, (f) codeine phosphate, (g) erythromycin, (h) flucloxacillin, (i) silver sulfadiazine, (j) tioconazole 28%, (k) topical hydrocortisone where the maximum strength of hydrocortisone in the medicinal product does not exceed 1 per cent by weight in weight.	11 The sale or supply shall be only in the course of their professional practice.
12 Persons selling or supplying prescription-only medicines to a school.	12 Prescription-only medicines comprising: (a) an inhaler containing salbutamol; or (b) an auto-injector containing adrenaline.	12 The sale or supply shall be: (a) subject to the presentation of an order signed by the principal or head teacher at the school concerned stating: (i) the name of the school for which the medicinal product is required, (ii) the purpose for which that product is required, and (iii) the total quantity required, and (b) for the purpose of supplying (or administering) the medicinal product to pupils at the school in an emergency.
13 Registered orthoptists (against whose names are recorded in the relevant register annotations signifying that they are qualified to sell or supply the medicine specified in column 2).	13 The following prescription-only medicines: (a) atropine, (b) cyclopentolate, (c) tropicamide, (d) lidocaine with fluorescein, (e) oxybuprocaine, (f) proxymetacaine, (g) tetracaine, (h) chloramphenicol, (i) fusidic acid.	13 The sale or supply shall be only in the course of their professional practice.

LIST OF PERSONS WHO CAN BE SUPPLIED WITH MEDICINES

PART 2 Exemption from the restriction on supply of prescription-only medicines

Persons exempted	Prescription-only medicines to which the exemption applies	Conditions
1 Royal National Lifeboat Institution and certified first aiders of the Institution.	1 All prescription-only medicines.	1 The supply shall be only so far as is necessary for the treatment of sick or injured persons in the exercise of the functions of the Institution.
2 The owner or master of a ship that does not carry a doctor on board as part of the ship's complement.	2 All prescription-only medicines.	2 The supply shall be only so far as is necessary for the treatment of persons on the ship.
3 Persons authorised by licences granted under regulation 5 of the Misuse of Drugs Regulations 2001 or regulation 5 of the Misuse of Drugs Regulations (Northern Ireland) 2002 to supply a controlled drug.	3 Such prescription-only medicines, being controlled drugs, as are specified in the licence.	3 The supply shall be subject to such conditions and in such circumstances and to such an extent as may be specified in the licence.
4 Persons employed or engaged in the provision of lawful drug treatment services.	4 Ampoules of sterile water for injection that contain no more than 2 ml of water each.	4 The supply shall be only in the course of provisions of lawful drug treatment services.
4a Persons employed or engaged in the provision of drug treatment services provided by, on behalf of or under arrangements made by one of the following bodies: (a) an NHS body; (b) a local authority; (c) Public Health England; or (d) Public Health Agency.	4a A prescription-only medicine ... containing naloxone hydrochloride but no other substance that is classified as a product available on prescription only.	4a The supply shall be only in the course of provisions of lawful drug treatment services and only where required for the purpose of saving life in an emergency.
5 Persons requiring prescription-only medicines for the purpose of enabling them, in the course of any business carried on by them, to comply with any requirements made by or in pursuance of any enactment with respect to the medical treatment of their employees.	5 Such prescription-only medicines as may be specified in the relevant enactment.	5 The supply shall be: (a) for the purpose of enabling them to comply with any requirements made by or in pursuance of any such enactment, and (b) subject to such conditions and such circumstances as may be specified in the relevant enactment.
6 Persons operating an occupational health scheme.	6 Prescription-only medicines sold or supplied to a person operating an occupational health scheme in response to an order in writing signed by a doctor or a registered nurse.	6 The supply of the prescription-only medicine shall be: (a) in the course of operating an occupational health scheme, and (b) made by: (i) a doctor, or (ii) a registered nurse acting in accordance with the written directions of a doctor as to the circumstance in which such medicines are to be used in the course of an occupational health scheme.

Persons exempted	Prescription-only medicines to which the exemption applies	Conditions
6a An NHS body or a local authority operating an occupational health scheme and occupational health vaccinators employed or engaged by them.	6b A prescription-only medicine used for vaccination or immunisation against coronavirus or influenza virus (of any type) sold or supplied to a person operating an occupational health scheme mentioned in entry 6a in response to an order in writing signed by a doctor or an occupational health vaccinator.	6c The supply of the medicine is in the course of an occupational health scheme mentioned in entry 6a and is made, if not by a doctor, by an occupational health vaccinator acting in accordance with the written directions of a doctor as to the circumstances in which such medicines are to be used.
7 The operator or commander of an aircraft.	7 Prescription-only medicines that are not for parenteral administration and that have been sold or supplied to an operator or commander of an aircraft in response to an order in writing signed by a doctor.	7 The supply shall be only so far as is necessary for the immediate treatment of sick or injured persons on the aircraft and shall be in accordance with the written instructions of a doctor as to the circumstances in which prescription-only medicines of the description in question are to be used on the aircraft.
8 Persons employed as qualified first-aid personnel on offshore installations.	8 All prescription-only medicines.	8 The supply shall be only so far as is necessary for the treatment of persons on the installation.
9 Persons who hold a certificate in first aid from the Mountain Rescue Council of England and Wales, or from the Northern Ireland Mountain Rescue Co-ordinating Committee.	9 Prescription-only medicines supplied to a person specified in column 1 in response to an order in writing signed by a doctor.	9 The supply shall be only so far as is necessary for the treatment of sick or injured persons in the course of providing mountain rescue services.
10 Persons ("P") who are members of Her Majesty's armed forces.	10 All prescription-only medicines.	10 The supply shall be: (a) in the course of P undertaking any function as a member of Her Majesty's armed forces; and (b) where P is satisfied that it is not practicable for another person who is legally entitled to supply a prescription-only medicine to do so; and (c) only in so far as is necessary: (i) for the treatment of a sick or injured person in a medical emergency, or (ii) to prevent ill-health where there is a risk that a person would suffer ill-health if the prescription-only medicine is not supplied.
11 A person ("P") carrying on the business of a school who is trained to administer the relevant medicine.	11 A prescription-only medicinal product comprising an inhaler containing salbutamol.	11 The supply shall be: (a) in the course of P carrying on the business of a school; (b) where supply is to a pupil at that school who is known to suffer from asthma; and (c) where the pupil requires the medicinal product in an emergency.
12 Registered midwives.	12 Prescription-only medicines for parenteral administration that contain: (a) diamorphine, (b) morphine, (c) pethidine hydrochloride.	12 The supply shall be only in the course of their professional practice.

PART 3 Exemptions from the restriction on administration of prescription-only medicines

Persons exempted	Prescription-only medicines to which the exemption applies	Conditions
1 Registered chiropodists or podiatrists against whose names are recorded in the relevant register annotations signifying that they are qualified to use the medicines specified in column 2.	1 Prescription-only medicines for parenteral administration that contain: (a) adrenaline, (b) bupivacaine hydrochloride, (c) bupivacaine hydrochloride with adrenaline where the maximum strength of adrenaline does not exceed 1 mg in 200 ml of bupivacaine hydrochloride, (d) levobupivacaine hydrochloride, (e) lidocaine hydrochloride, (f) lidocaine hydrochloride with adrenaline where the maximum strength of adrenaline does not exceed 1 mg in 200 ml of lignocaine hydrochloride, (g) mepivacaine hydrochloride, (h) methylprednisolone, (i) prilocaine hydrochloride, (j) ropivacaine hydrochloride.	1 The administration shall only be in the course of their professional practice and where the medicine includes a combination of substances in column 2, those substances shall not have been combined by the chiropodist or podiatrist.
2 Registered midwives and student midwives.	2 Prescription-only medicines for parenteral administration containing any of the following substances but no other substance that is classified as a product available on prescription only: (a) adrenaline, (b) anti-D immunoglobulin, (c) carboprost, (d) cyclizine lactate, (e) diamorphine, (f) ergometrine maleate, (g) gelofusine, (h) Hartmann's solution, (i) hepatitis B vaccine, (j) hepatitis immunoglobulin, (k) lidocaine hydrochloride, (l) morphine, (m) naloxone hydrochloride, (n) oxytocins, natural and synthetic, (o) pethidine hydrochloride, (p) phytomenadione, (q) prochloperazine, (r) sodium chloride 0.9%.	2 The medicine shall: (a) in the case of lidocaine and lidocaine hydrochloride, be administered only while attending on a woman in childbirth, and (b) where administration is: (i) by a registered midwife, be administered in the course of their professional practice; (ii) by a student midwife: (aa) be administered under the direct supervision of a registered midwife; and (bb) not include diamorphine, morphine or pethidine hydrochloride.

Persons exempted	Prescription-only medicines to which the exemption applies	Conditions
3 Persons who are authorised as members of a group by a group authority granted under regulations 8(3) or 9(3) of the Misuse of Drugs Regulations 2001 or, regulations 8(3) or 9(3) of the Misuse of Drugs Regulations (Northern Ireland) 2002, to supply a controlled drug by way of administration only.	3 Prescription-only medicines that are specified in the group authority.	3 The administration shall be subject to such conditions and in such circumstances and to such extent as may be specified in the group authority.
4 The owner or master of a ship that does not carry a doctor on board as part of the ship's complement.	4 All prescription-only medicines that are for parenteral administration.	4 The administration shall be only so far as is necessary for the treatment of persons on the ship.
5 Persons operating an occupational health scheme.	5 Prescription-only medicines that are for parenteral administration sold or supplied to the person operating an occupational health scheme in response to an order in writing signed by a doctor or a registered nurse.	5 The prescription only is administered in the course of an occupational health scheme, and the individual administering the medicine is: (a) a doctor, or (b) a registered nurse acting in accordance with the written instructions of a doctor as to the circumstances in which prescription-only medicines of the description in question are to be used.
5a An NHS body or a local authority operating an occupational health scheme and occupational health scheme vaccinators employed or engaged by them.	5b A prescription-only medicine used for vaccination or immunisation against coronavirus or influenza virus (of any type) sold or supplied to a person operating an occupational health scheme mentioned in entry 5a in response to an order in writing signed by a doctor or an occupational health vaccinator.	5c The administration of the medicine is in the course of an occupational health scheme mentioned in entry 5a, and the individual administering the medicine is, if not a doctor, an occupational health vaccinator acting in accordance with the written directions of a doctor as to the circumstances in which such medicines are to be used.
6 The operator or commander of an aircraft.	6 Prescription-only medicines for parenteral administration that have been sold or supplied to the operator or commander of the aircraft in response to an order in writing signed by a doctor.	6 The administration shall be only so far as is necessary for the immediate treatment of sick or injured persons on the aircraft and shall be in accordance with the written instructions of the doctor as to the circumstances in which prescription-only medicines of the description in question are to be used on the aircraft.
7 Persons employed as qualified first-aid personnel on offshore installations.	7 All prescription-only medicines that are for parenteral administration.	7 The administration shall be only so far as is necessary for the treatment of persons on the installation.
8 Persons who are registered paramedics.	8 The following prescription-only medicines for parenteral administration: (a) diazepam 5 mg per ml emulsion for injection, (b) succinylated modified fluid gelatin 4 per cent intravenous infusion,	8 The administration shall be only for the immediate, necessary treatment of sick or injured persons and in the case of prescription-only medicine containing heparin sodium shall be only for the purpose of cannula flushing.

Persons exempted	Prescription-only medicines to which the exemption applies	Conditions
	(c) medicines containing the substance ergometrine maleate 500 mcg per ml with oxytocin 5 iu per ml, but no other active ingredient,	
	(d) prescription-only medicines containing one or more of the following substances, but no other active ingredient:	
	(i) adrenaline acid tartrate,	
	(ii) adrenaline hydrochloride,	
	(iii) amiodarone,	
	(iv) anhydrous glucose,	
	(v) benzlypenicillin,	
	(vi) compound sodium lactate intravenous infusion (Hartmann's solution),	
	(vii) ergometrine maleate,	
	(viii) furosemide,	
	(ix) glucose,	
	(x) heparin sodium,	
	(xi) lidocaine hydrochloride,	
	(xii) metoclopramide,	
	(xiii) morphine sulphate,	
	(xiv) nalbuphine hydrochloride,	
	(xv) naloxone hydrochloride,	
	(xvi) ondansetron	
	(xvii) paracetamol,	
	(xviii) reteplase,	
	(xix) sodium chloride,	
	(xx) streptokinase,	
	(xxi) tenecteplase.	
9 Persons who hold the advanced life support provider certificate issued by the Resuscitation Council (UK).	9 The following prescription-only medicines for parenteral administration: (a) adrenaline 1:10,000 up to I mg; and (b) amiodarone.	9 The administration shall be only in an emergency involving cardiac arrest, and in the case of adrenaline the administration shall be intravenous only.
10 Persons ("P") who are members of Her Majesty's armed forces.	10 All prescription-only medicines.	10 The administration shall be: (a) in the course of P undertaking any function as a member of Her Majesty's armed forces; and (b) where P is satisfied that it is not practicable for another person who is legally entitled to administer a prescription only medicine to do so; and (c) only in so far as is necessary: (i) for the treatment of a sick or injured person in an emergency, or (ii) to prevent ill health where there is a risk that a person would suffer ill health if the prescription-only medicine is not administered.

Persons exempted	Prescription-only medicines to which the exemption applies	Conditions
11 A person ("P") carrying on the business of a school who is trained to administer the relevant medicine.	11 A prescription-only medicine comprising an auto-injector containing adrenaline.	11 The administration shall be: (a) in the course of P carrying on the business of a school; (b) where administration is to a pupil at that school who is known to be at risk of anaphylaxis; and (c) where the pupil requires the medicinal product in an emergency.

PART 4 Exemptions from the restrictions in regulations 220 and 221 for certain persons who sell, supply, or offer for sale or supply certain medicinal products

Persons exempted	Medicinal products to which exemption applies	Conditions
1 Registered chiropodists and podiatrists.	1 Medicinal products on a general sale list which are for external use and are not veterinary drugs and the following pharmacy medicines for external use: (a) potassium permanganate crystals or solution; (b) ointment of heparinoid and hyaluronidase; and (c) products containing, as their only active ingredients, any of the following substances, at a strength, in the case of each substance, not exceeding that specified in relation to that substance: (i) 9.0 per cent borotannic complex (ii) 10.0 per cent buclosamide (iii) 3.0 per cent chlorquinaldol (iv) 1.0 per cent clotrimazole (v) 10.0 per cent crotamiton (vi) 5.0 per cent diamthazole hydrochloride (vii) 1.0 per cent econazole nitrate (viii) 1.0 per cent fenticlor (ix) 10.0 per cent glutaraldehyde (x) 1.0 per cent griseofulvin (xi) 0.4 per cent hydrargaphen (xii) 2.0 per cent mepyramine maleate	

Persons exempted	Medicinal products to which exemption applies	Conditions
	(xiii) 2.0 per cent miconazole nitrate	
	(xiv) 2.0 per cent phenoxypropan-2-ol	
	(xv) 20.0 per cent podophyllum resin	
	(xvi) 10.0 per cent polynoxylin	
	(xvii) 70.0 per cent pyrogallol	
	(xviii) 70.0 per cent salicylic acid	
	(xix) 1.0 per cent terbinafine	
	(xx) 0.1 per cent thiomersal.	
2 Registered chiropodists and podiatrists against whose names are recorded in the relevant register annotations signifying that they are qualified to use the medicines in column 2.	2 (a) The following prescription-only medicines: (i) amorolfine hydrochloride cream where the maximum strength of the amorolfine in the cream does not exceed 0.25 per cent by weight in weight, (ii) amorolfine hydrochloride lacquer where the maximum strength of amorolfine in the lacquer does not exceed 5 per cent by weight in volume, (iii) amoxicillin, (iv) co-codamol, (v) co-dydramol 10/500 tablets, (vi) codeine phosphate, (vii) erythromycin, (viii) flucloxacillin, (ix) silver sulfadiazine, (x) tioconazole 28%, (xi) topical hydrocortisone where the maximum strength of the hydrocortisone in the medicinal product does not exceed 1 per cent by weight in weight; and (b) Ibuprofen, other than preparations of ibuprofen which are prescription-only medicines.	2 The sale or supply shall be only in the course of their professional practice, and the medicinal product must have been made up for sale or supply in a container elsewhere than at the place at which it is sold or supplied.
3 Registered optometrists.	3 All medical products on a general sale list, all pharmacy medicines and prescription-only medicines that are not for parenteral administration and that: (a) are eye drops and are prescription-only medicines by reason only that they contain no more than: (i) 30.0 per cent sulphacetamide sodium, or (ii) 0.5 per cent chloramphenicol, or (b) are eye ointments and are prescription-only medicines by reason only that they contain no more than:	3 The sale or supply shall be only: (a) in the case of medicinal products on a general sale list and pharmacy medicines, in the course of their professional practice; (b) in the case of prescription-only medicines, in the course of their professional practice and in an emergency.

Persons exempted	Medicinal products to which exemption applies	Conditions
	(i) 30.0 per cent sulphacetamide sodium, or	
	(ii) 1.0 per cent chloramphenicol, or	
	(c) are prescription-only medicines by reason only that they contain any of the following substances:	
	(i) cyclopentolate hydrochloride,	
	(ii) fusidic acid,	
	(iii) tropicamide.	
4 Additional supply optometrists.	4 Medicinal products that are prescription-only medicines by reason only that they contain any of the following substances: (a) acetylcysteine, (b) atropine sulphate, (c) azelastine hydrochloride, (d) diclofenac sodium, (e) emedastine, (f) homotropine hydrobromide, (g) ketotifen, (h) levocabastine, (i) lodoximide, (j) nedocromil sodium, (k) olopatadine, (l) pilocarpine hydrochloride, (m) pilocarpine nitrate, (n) polymyxin b/bacitracin, (o) polymyxin b/trimethoprim, (p) sodium cromoglycate.	4 The sale or supply shall be only in the course of their professional practice and only in an emergency.
5 Holders of manufacturer's licences where the licence in question contains a provision that the licence holder shall manufacture the medicinal product to which the licence relates only for a particular person after being requested by or on behalf of that person and in that person's presence to use their own judgement as to the treatment required.	5 Medicinal products on a general sale list that are for external use and are not veterinary drugs and pharmacy medicines that are for external use in the treatment of hair and scalp conditions and that contain any of the following: (a) not more than 5.0 per cent of boric acid, (b) isopropyl myristate or lauryl sulphate, (c) not more than 0.004 per cent oestrogens, (d) not more than 1.0 per cent of resorcinol, (e) not more than 3.0 per cent of salicylic acid, (f) not more than 0.2 per cent of sodium pyrithione.	5 The licence holder shall sell or supply the medicinal product in question only to a particular person after being requested by or on behalf of that person and in that person's presence to use their own judgement as to the treatment required.
6 Persons selling or supplying medicinal products to universities, other institutions concerned with	6 All medicinal products.	6 The sale or supply shall be: (a) Subject to the presentation of an order signed by the principal of

Persons exempted	Medicinal products to which exemption applies	Conditions
higher education or institutions concerned with research.		the institution concerned with education or research or the appropriate head of department in charge of the specified course of research stating: (i) the name of the institution for which the medicinal product is required, (ii) the purpose for which the medicinal product is required, and (iii) the total quantity required, and (b) for the purposes of the education or research with which the institution is concerned.
7 Persons selling or supplying medicinal products to organisations for research purposes.	7 All medicinal products.	7 The sale or supply is only for the purposes of research and shall be: (a) subject to the presentation of an order signed by the representative of the organisation concerned stating: (i) who requires the medicine, (ii) the purposes for which it is required, (iii) the quantity required, and (iv) the purposes of the research with which the organisation is concerned; and (b) not for administration to humans.
8 Persons selling or supplying medicinal products to any of the following: (a) a public analyst appointed under section 27 of the Food Safety Act 1990 or under article 27 of the Food Safety (Northern Ireland) Order 1991; (b) an agricultural analyst appointed under section 67 of the Agriculture Act 1970, (c) a person duly authorised by an enforcement authority under regulations 325 to 328, (d) a sampling officer within the meaning of Schedule 31.	8 All medicinal products.	8 The sale or supply is in connection with the exercise of any statutory function carried out by any person listed in sub-paragraphs (a) to (d) of column 1 provided that: (a) the medicinal products are requested on an order signed by or on behalf of a person listed in sub-paragraph (a) to (d) of column 1, and (b) the order gives: (i) the status of the person signing it, (ii) the amount of medicinal product required.
9 Holders of a UK marketing authorisation, EU marketing authorisation, a certificate of registration or a manufacturer's licence.	9 Medicinal product referred to in the UK marketing authorisations, EU marketing authorisation, certificate of registration or manufacturer's licence.	The sale or supply shall be only: (a) to a pharmacist, (b) so as to enable that pharmacist to prepare an entry relating to the medical product in question in a tablet or capsule identification guide or similar publication, and (c) of no greater quantity than is reasonably necessary for that purpose.

Persons exempted	Medicinal products to which exemption applies	Conditions
10 Registered dispensing opticians.	10 Pharmacy medicines for external use containing chloramphenicol at a strength not exceeding: (a) 0.5 per cent in eye drops; (b) 1 per cent in ointment.	10 The sale or supply shall only be in the course of their professional practice.
11 Operator or commander of an aircraft.	11 All medicinal products on a general sale list.	11 The medicinal product must: (a) have been made up for sale or supply in a container elsewhere than at the place at which it is sold or supplied; and (b) be stored in a part of the aircraft that the operator is able to close so as to exclude the public.
12 The operator of a train.	12 All medicinal products on a general sale list.	12 The medicinal product must: (a) have been made up for sale or supply in a container elsewhere than at the place at which it is sold or supplied; and (b) be stored in a part of the train which the operator is able to close so as to exclude the public.
13 Registered orthoptists (against whose names are recorded in the relevant register annotations signifying that they are qualified to sell or supply the medicine specified in column 2).	13 All medicinal products on a general sale list, all pharmacy medicines and the following prescription-only medicines: (a) atropine, (b) cyclopentolate, (c) tropicamide, (d) lidocaine with fluorescein, (e) oxybuprocaine, (f) proxymetacaine, (g) tetracaine, (h) chloramphenicol, (i) fusidic acid.	13 The sale or supply shall be only in the course of their professional practice.

PART 5 Exemptions from the restrictions in regulations 220 and 221 for certain persons who supply certain medicinal products

Persons exempted	Medicinal products to which exemption applies	Conditions
1 Royal National Lifeboat Institution and certificated first aiders of the Institution.	1 All medicinal products.	1 The supply shall be only so far as is necessary for the treatment of sick or injured persons.
2 British Red Cross Society and certificated first aid and certificated nursing members of the Society.	2 Pharmacy medicines and all medicinal products on a general sale list.	2 The supply shall be only so far as is necessary for the treatment of sick or injured persons.

LIST OF PERSONS WHO CAN BE SUPPLIED WITH MEDICINES

Persons exempted	Medicinal products to which exemption applies	Conditions
3 St John Ambulance Association and Brigade and certificated first aid and certificated nursing members of the Association and Brigade.	3 All pharmacy medicines and all medicinal products on a general sale list.	3 The supply shall be only so far as is necessary for the treatment of sick or injured persons.
4 St Andrew's Ambulance Association and certificated first aid and certificated nursing members of the Association.	4 All pharmacy medicines and all medicinal products on a general sale list.	4 The supply shall be only so far as is necessary for the treatment of sick and injured persons.
5 Order of Malta Ambulance Corps and certificated first aid and certificated nursing members of the Corps.	5 All pharmacy medicines and all medicinal products on a general sale list.	5 The supply shall be only so far as is necessary for the treatment of sick or injured persons.
6 Persons authorised by licences granted under regulation 5 of the Misuse of Drugs Regulations 2001 or regulation 5 of the Misuse of Drugs Regulations (Northern Ireland) 2002.	6 Such prescription-only medicines and such pharmacy medicines as are specified in the licence.	6 The supply shall be subject to such conditions and in such circumstances and to such an extent as may be specified in the licence.
7 Persons employed or engaged in the provision of lawful drug treatment services.	7 Ampoules of sterile water for injection that contain no more than 5 ml of water each.	7 The supply shall be only in the course of provision of lawful drug treatment services.
7a Persons employed or engaged in the provision of drug treatment services provided by, on behalf of or under arrangements made by one of the following bodies: (a) an NHS body; (d) a local authority; (c) Public Health England; or (d) Public Health Agency.	7a A medicinal product containing naloxone hydrochloride but no other substance that is classified as a product available only on prescription or as a product available only from a pharmacy.	7a The supply shall be only in the course of provisions of lawful drug treatment services and only where required for the purpose of saving life in an emergency.
8 Persons requiring medicinal products for the purpose of enabling them, in the course of any business carried on by them, to comply with any requirements made by or in pursuance of any enactment with respect to the medical treatment of their employees.	8 Such prescription-only medicines and such pharmacy medicines as may be specified in the relevant enactment and medicinal products on a general sale list.	8 The supply shall be: (a) for the purpose of enabling compliance with any requirement made by or in pursuance of any such enactment, and (b) subject to such conditions and in such circumstances as may be specified in the relevant enactment.
9 The owner or master of a ship that does not carry a doctor on board as part of the ship's complement.	9 All medicinal products.	9 The supply shall be only so far as is necessary for the treatment of persons on the ship.

Persons exempted	Medicinal products to which exemption applies	Conditions
10 Persons operating an occupational health scheme.	10 All pharmacy medicines, all medicinal products on a general sale list and such prescription-only medicines as are sold or supplied to a person operating an occupational health scheme in response to an order signed by a doctor or a registered nurse.	10 (a) The supply shall be in the course of an occupational health scheme. (b) The individual supplying the medicinal product, if not a doctor, shall be: (i) a registered nurse, and (ii) where the medicinal product in question is a prescription-only medicine, acting in accordance with the written instructions of a doctor as to the circumstances in which prescription-only medicines of the description in question are to be used in the course of an occupational health scheme.
10a An NHS body or a local authority operating an occupational health scheme and occupational health vaccinators employed or engaged by them.	10b A prescription-only medicine used for vaccination or immunisation against coronavirus or influenza virus (of any type) sold or supplied to a person operating an occupational health scheme mentioned in entry 10a in response to an order in writing signed by a doctor or an occupational health vaccinator.	10c The supply of the medicine is in the course of an occupational health scheme mentioned in entry 10a, and the individual supplying the medicine is, if not a doctor, an occupational health vaccinator acting in accordance with the written directions of a doctor as to the circumstances in which such medicines are to be used.
11 Persons carrying on the business of a school providing full-time education.	11 Pharmacy medicines that are for use in the prevention of dental caries and consist of or contain sodium fluoride.	11 The supply shall be: (a) in the course of a school dental scheme, and (b) if to a child under 16 only where the parent or guardian of that child has consented to such supply.
12 Health authorities or Primary Health Trusts.	12 Pharmacy medicines that are for use in the prevention of dental caries and consist of or contain sodium fluoride.	12 The supply shall be in the course of: (a) a pre-school dental scheme, and the individual supplying the medicinal product shall be a registered nurse, or (b) a school dental scheme, and if to a child under 16 only where the parent or guardian of that child has consented to such supply.
13 The operator or commander of an aircraft.	13 All pharmacy medicines, all medicinal products on a general sale list and such prescription-only medicines that are not for parenteral administration and that have been sold or supplied to the operator or commander of an aircraft in response to an order in writing signed by a doctor.	13 The supply shall be only so far as is necessary for the immediate treatment of sick or injured persons on the aircraft and, in the case of a prescription-only medicine, shall be in accordance with the written instructions of a doctor as to the circumstances in which the prescription-only medicines of the description in question are to be used on the aircraft.
14 Persons employed as qualified first-aid personnel on offshore installations.	14 All medicinal products.	14 The supply shall be only so far as is necessary for the treatment of persons on the installation.

Persons exempted	Medicinal products to which exemption applies	Conditions
15 A prison officer.	15 All medicinal products on the general sale list.	15 The supply shall only be so far as is necessary for the treatment of prisoners.
16 Persons who hold a certificate in first aid from the Mountain Rescue Council of England and Wales, or from the Northern Ireland Mountain Rescue Co-ordinating Committee.	16 All pharmacy medicines, all medicinal products on a general sale list and such prescription-only medicines which are sold or supplied to a person specified in column 1 of this paragraph in response to an order in writing signed by a doctor.	16 The supply shall be only so far as is necessary for the treatment of sick or injured persons in the course of providing mountain rescue services.
17 Her Majesty's armed forces.	17 All medicinal products.	17 The supply shall be only so far as is necessary for the treatment of a sick or injured person or the prevention of ill health.
18 A person ("P") carrying on the business of a school who is trained to administer the relevant medicine.	18 A prescription-only medicinal product comprising an inhaler containing salbutamol.	18 The supply shall be: (a) in the course of P carrying on the business of a school; (b) where supply is to a pupil at that school who is known to suffer from asthma; and (c) where the pupil requires the medicinal product in an emergency.
19 Persons supplying medicinal products under an off-site emergency plan prepared under the Radiation (Emergency Preparedness and Public Information) Regulations 2019.	19 Pharmacy medicines that contain any of the following substances but no other active ingredient: (a) potassium iodide; (b) potassium iodate.	19 The supply shall be: (a) in accordance with the off-site emergency plan; and (b) only in the event that a radiation emergency has occurred or an event has occurred which could reasonably be expected to lead to a radiation emergency.
20 A person or body listed in Part 1 or 2 of Schedule 1 to the Civil Contingencies Act 2004.	20 Pharmacy medicines that contain any of the following substances but no other active ingredient: (a) potassium iodide; (b) potassium iodate.	20 The supply shall only be in response to the occurrence, or likely occurrence, of one of the following events: (a) an emergency within the meaning of section 1 of the Civil Contingencies Act 2004; (b) a (radiation) emergency within the meaning of regulation 24 of the Carriage of Dangerous Goods and Use of Transportable Pressure Equipment Regulations 2009.

Appendix 3

SOURCES OF USEFUL INFORMATION

The Medicines and Healthcare products Regulatory Agency regulates medicines, medical devices and blood components for transfusion in the UK:
https://www.gov.uk/government/organisations/medicines-and-healthcare-products-regulatory-agency

Register of authorised online sellers of medicines:
http://medicine-seller-register.mhra.gov.uk/

The Home Office plays a fundamental role in the security and economic prosperity of the United Kingdom:
https://www.gov.uk/government/organisations/home-office

The UK Border Force is a law enforcement command within the Home Office. It secures the UK border by carrying out immigration and customs controls for people and goods entering the UK:
https://www.gov.uk/government/organisations/border-force

In England, the Care Quality Commission monitors, inspects and regulates health and social care services:
http://www.cqc.org.uk/

The Regulation and Quality Improvement Authority is responsible for registering and inspecting independent hospitals, clinics and other care services in Northern Ireland:
http://www.rqia.org.uk/

Healthcare Improvement Scotland regulates independent specialist clinics and healthcare services in Scotland:
http://www.healthcareimprovementscotland.org

Healthcare Inspectorate Wales is the regulator of independent healthcare in Wales:
http://www.hiw.org.uk

The General Medical Council's register of doctors, including "Licence to practise" information:
http://www.gmc-uk.org/doctors/register/LRMP.asp

The General Pharmaceutical Council's register of pharmacy premises, pharmacists and pharmacy technicians:
http://www.pharmacyregulation.org/registers

The Pharmaceutical Society of Northern Ireland's register of pharmacy premises, pharmacists and pharmacy technicians:
http://www.psni.org.uk/search-register/

The Health & Care Professions Council register:
https://www.hcpc-uk.org/check-the-register/

The Royal College of Veterinary Surgeons' register:
http://www.rcvs.org.uk/registration/check-the-register/

The General Dental Council's register:
https://olr.gdc-uk.org/SearchRegister

Public Health England's "Green Book" relating to vaccines:
https://www.gov.uk/government/collections/immunisation-against-infectious-disease-the-green-book

UK legislation:
http://www.legislation.gov.uk/

European medicines legislation and guidelines:
https://ec.europa.eu/health/documents/eudralex_en

European Medicines Agency:
http://www.ema.europa.eu/ema/

EudraGMDP database:
http://eudragmdp.ema.europa.eu/inspections/displayWelcome.do

World Health Organization guidelines – distribution:
http://www.who.int/medicines/areas/quality_safety/quality_assurance/distribution/en/

World Health Organization "List of globally identified websites of medicines regulatory authorities" (as of November 2012):
http://www.who.int/medicines/areas/quality_safety/regulation_legislation/list_mra_websites_nov2012.pdf?ua=1

Pharmaceutical Inspection Convention and Pharmaceutical Inspection Co-operation Scheme (PIC/S):
http://www.picscheme.org/

MHRA-GMDP database relating to manufacturing and wholesale authorisations and certificates:
https://cms.mhra.gov.uk/mhra

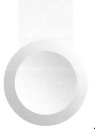

Appendix 4

IMPORTATION OF ACTIVE SUBSTANCES FOR MEDICINAL PRODUCTS FOR HUMAN USE – QUESTIONS AND ANSWERS

In June 2016 the Commission published a revised question and answer document responding to frequently asked questions in relation to the import of active substances. The revised document is produced here and includes the addition of Q&A 35 to clarify the requirements in case of importation of active substances released for sale before the expiration date of their written confirmation and minor editing of Q&A 10A and 29A and deletion of Q&A 29B.

The views expressed in this questions and answers document are not legally binding. Ultimately, only the European Court of Justice can give an authoritative interpretation of Union law.

This documents sets out frequently asked "questions and answers" regarding the new rules for the importation of active substances for medicinal products for human use.

These rules are contained in Articles 46b and 111b of Directive 2001/83/EC.

The "written confirmation" is addressed in Article 46b(2)(b) of Directive 2001/83/EC.

1. QUESTION: WHEN DO THE NEW RULES FOR THE WRITTEN CONFIRMATION APPLY?

Answer: They apply as of 2 July 2013. Any active substance imported into the EU from that date is subject to the rules on the written confirmation.

2. QUESTION: DO THE RULES ON THE WRITTEN CONFIRMATION ALSO APPLY TO ACTIVE SUBSTANCES FOR VETERINARY MEDICINAL PRODUCTS?

Answer: No. The rules apply only to active substances for medicinal products for human use.

2A. QUESTION: DO THE RULES ON THE WRITTEN CONFIRMATION ALSO APPLY TO BLOOD PLASMA?

Answer: No. However, processed derivatives of plasma having a pharmacological, immunological or metabolic action are considered as active substance and written confirmation is thus required.

3. QUESTION: DO THE RULES ON THE WRITTEN CONFIRMATION APPLY TO ACTIVE SUBSTANCES FOR MEDICINAL PRODUCTS INTENDED FOR RESEARCH AND DEVELOPMENT TRIALS?

Answer: Active substances imported to be used in the manufacture of non-authorised medicinal products intended for research and development trials are excluded from the rules.

Active substances imported to be used in the manufacture of authorised medicinal products intended for research and development trials are expected to fulfil the requirements of Directive 2001/83/EC and be accompanied by a written confirmation, unless there is proof that the full amount of the imported API will be used for the manufacture of batches/units of an authorised medicinal product exclusively intended for research and development trials. In the latter case, those batches/units of an authorised medicinal product fall outside the scope of Directive 2001/83/EC and the API used in their manufacture is exempted from the rules on the written confirmation.

4. QUESTION: DO THE RULES ON THE WRITTEN CONFIRMATION APPLY TO ACTIVE SUBSTANCES THAT ARE BROUGHT INTO THE EU WITHOUT BEING IMPORTED ("INTRODUCED" ACTIVE SUBSTANCES)? AN EXAMPLE IS THE INTRODUCTION OF AN ACTIVE SUBSTANCE WHICH IS SUBSEQUENTLY EXPORTED.

Answer: No. The rules on the written confirmation only apply to the import of active substances for medicinal products for human use.

5. QUESTION: WHAT IF, AT THE TIME OF EXPORT OF AN ACTIVE SUBSTANCE TO THE EU, IT IS NOT KNOWN WHETHER THE ACTIVE SUBSTANCE IS USED IN A MEDICINAL PRODUCT FOR HUMAN USE OR NOT?

Answer: If the consignment is not accompanied by a written confirmation, the active substance cannot be used in a medicinal product for human use.

6. QUESTION: IS THE WRITTEN CONFIRMATION EXPECTED TO CONFIRM COMPLIANCE WITH EU RULES?

Answer: No. The written confirmation has to confirm compliance with GMP rules "equivalent" to the rules applied in the EU.

7. QUESTION: IN MY NON-EU COUNTRY, THE APPLICABLE STANDARDS FOR MANUFACTURING OF ACTIVE SUBSTANCES ARE THE GOOD MANUFACTURING PRACTICES FOR ACTIVE SUBSTANCES OF THE WORLD HEALTH ORGANIZATION (WHO) – FORTY-FOURTH TECHNICAL REPORT, NO. 957, 2010, ANNEX 2. ARE THESE STANDARDS EQUIVALENT TO THOSE IN THE EU, AS REQUIRED ACCORDING TO EU LEGISLATION?

Answer: Yes.

8. QUESTION: IN MY NON-EU COUNTRY, THE APPLICABLE STANDARDS ARE ICH Q7. ARE THESE STANDARDS EQUIVALENT TO THOSE IN THE EU, AS REQUIRED ACCORDING TO EU LEGISLATION?

Answer: Yes.

9. QUESTION: DOES THE WRITTEN CONFIRMATION HAVE TO BE ISSUED BY A CENTRAL, REGIONAL OR LOCAL AUTHORITY?

Answer: Each non-EU country decides autonomously which body within that country issues the written confirmation. That non-EU country may decide to issue the written confirmation at central, regional or local level.

10. QUESTION: DO THE RULES APPLY ALSO TO ACTIVE SUBSTANCES CONTAINED IN AN IMPORTED FINISHED MEDICINAL PRODUCT?

Answer: No. Regarding finished medicinal products, the rules for importation of finished medicinal products (importation authorisation and batch release by a qualified person, see Articles 40(3) and 51 of Directive 2001/83/EC apply). These rules remain unchanged.

10A. QUESTION: IS WRITTEN CONFIRMATION ALSO REQUIRED FOR A STARTING MATERIAL OR AN INTERMEDIATE USED FOR THE PRODUCTION OF AN ACTIVE SUBSTANCE, FOR EXAMPLE BY WAY OF PURIFICATION OR FURTHER SYNTHESIS?

Answer: No. Such starting material or intermediate used for the production of an active substance does not fulfil the definition of Article 1(3a) of Directive 2001/83/EC.

11. QUESTION: IS THE WRITTEN CONFIRMATION ALSO REQUIRED FOR IMPORTED ACTIVE SUBSTANCES WHICH HAVE ALREADY BEEN MIXED WITH EXCIPIENTS, WITHOUT YET BEING THE FINISHED MEDICINAL PRODUCT?

Answer: No. Such partial manufacturing of the finished product is not included in the rules on the written confirmation.

IMPORTATION OF ACTIVE SUBSTANCES FOR MEDICINAL PRODUCTS

11A. QUESTION: IS THE WRITTEN CONFIRMATION ALSO REQUIRED WHERE THE FINISHED DOSAGE FORM MANUFACTURED IN THE EU IS DESTINED FOR EXPORTATION ONLY

Answer: Yes.

12. QUESTION: WHO CHECKS THAT THE IMPORTED ACTIVE SUBSTANCE IS ACCOMPANIED BY THE WRITTEN CONFIRMATION?

Answer: This should be checked by the receiving manufacturer of the finished medicinal product. It may also be checked by the importer of the active substance upon its importation.

The verification of whether such checks take place depends on the transposing law of the Member State where the active substance is imported. It may be verified:

- by the relevant authority upon importation; and/or
- in the context of an inspection of the importer of the active substance; and/or
- in the context of an inspection of the manufacturer of the medicinal product that uses the imported active substance.

13. QUESTION: HOW CAN I CHECK IF THE WRITTEN CONFIRMATION IS AUTHENTIC?

Answer: You should contact the manufacturer of the active substance or the issuing authority in the non-EU country.

14. QUESTION: IS THE WRITTEN CONFIRMATION SENT TO AN EU REGULATORY AGENCY?

Answer: No. The written confirmation accompanies the imported active substance.

15. QUESTION: DOES THE WRITTEN CONFIRMATION HAVE TO BE SUBMITTED WITH A REQUEST FOR AUTHORISATION OF A MARKETING AUTHORISATION OF A MEDICINAL PRODUCT?

Answer: No.

16. QUESTION: IS THE WRITTEN CONFIRMATION TO BE ISSUED FOR EACH BATCH/CONSIGNMENT?

Answer: No. The written confirmation is issued per manufacturing plant and the active substance(s) manufactured on this site.

17. QUESTION: DOES EACH IMPORTED CONSIGNMENT HAVE TO BE ACCOMPANIED BY THE WRITTEN CONFIRMATION?

Answer: Yes.

18. QUESTION: IS IT ACCEPTABLE THAT THE WRITTEN CONFIRMATION ACCOMPANYING THE IMPORTED CONSIGNMENT OF THE ACTIVE SUBSTANCE IS A COPY?

Answer: Yes, provided that the original written confirmation is still valid.

18A. QUESTION: REGARDING THE WRITTEN CONFIRMATION OF "EQUIVALENT" STANDARDS OF GOOD MANUFACTURING PRACTICE, CAN THE ISSUING AUTHORITY OF THE NON-EU COUNTRY BASE ITSELF ON INSPECTION RESULTS FROM EU AUTHORITIES OR OTHER AUTHORITIES APPLYING EQUIVALENT STANDARDS FOR GOOD MANUFACTURING PRACTICE, SUCH AS US FDA?

Answer: Yes. In this case, the written confirmation should indicate which authority has inspected the site.

18B. QUESTION: REGARDING THE WRITTEN CONFIRMATION OF "EQUIVALENT" STANDARDS OF GOOD MANUFACTURING PRACTICE, CAN THE ISSUING AUTHORITY OF THE NON-EU COUNTRY BASE ITSELF ON INSPECTIONS CONDUCTED IN THE PAST?

Answer: Yes. It is not necessary to conduct an inspection specifically for the purpose of issuing the "written confirmation".

19. QUESTION: WHAT IS THE VALIDITY PERIOD OF THE WRITTEN CONFIRMATION?

Answer: The validity of the written confirmation is established by the issuing authority of the non-EU country.

19A. THE WRITTEN CONFIRMATION REFERS TO "UNANNOUNCED INSPECTIONS". DOES THIS MEAN THAT AN UNANNOUNCED INSPECTION HAS TO HAVE BEEN CONDUCTED?

Answer: No. Rather, the system of supervision as a whole (including different types of inspections, such as unannounced inspections) has to ensure a protection of public health at least equivalent to that in the EU.

20. QUESTION: IF ACTIVE SUBSTANCES ARE MANUFACTURED IN A NON-EU COUNTRY "A", BUT IMPORTED IN THE EU VIA THE NON-EU COUNTRY "B", WHO HAS TO ISSUE THE WRITTEN CONFIRMATION?

Answer: The written confirmation accompanying the imported active substance has to be issued by the non-EU country where the active substance is manufactured (i.e. non-EU country "A").

IMPORTATION OF ACTIVE SUBSTANCES FOR MEDICINAL PRODUCTS

21. QUESTION: THE TEMPLATE FOR THE WRITTEN CONFIRMATION REFERS TO A "CONFIRMATION NUMBER". DOES THIS NUMBER HAVE TO BE A SEQUENTIAL NUMBER PER COUNTRY?

Answer: No. This number would be attributed by the issuing authority of the non-EU country.

22. QUESTION: THE TEMPLATE FOR THE WRITTEN CONFIRMATION REFERS TO A "RESPONSIBLE PERSON" IN THE ISSUING AUTHORITY. DOES THIS RESPONSIBLE PERSON HAVE TO HAVE A SPECIFIC QUALIFICATION?

Answer: No. The "responsible person" in this context is the person responsible within the administration for issuing the written confirmation.

23. QUESTION: ACCORDING TO THE TEMPLATE FOR THE WRITTEN CONFIRMATION, INFORMATION OF FINDINGS RELATING TO NON-COMPLIANCE ARE SUPPLIED TO THE EU. TO WHOM THIS INFORMATION SHOULD BE SENT TO?

Answer: The information should be sent to the European Medicines Agency (qdefect@ema.europa.eu).

24. QUESTION: IS THE WRITTEN CONFIRMATION ALSO REQUIRED WHERE THERE IS A "MUTUAL RECOGNITION AGREEMENT" BETWEEN A NON-EU COUNTRY AND THE EU?

Answer: Yes. The process of a written confirmation is independent of the existence of "mutual recognition agreements".

25. QUESTION: IF A MANUFACTURING PLANT IS LOCATED IN A NON-EU COUNTRY "A", CAN THE WRITTEN CONFIRMATION BE ISSUED BY AN AUTHORITY IN ANOTHER NON-EU COUNTRY (NON-EU COUNTRY "B")?

Answer: No.

26. QUESTION: ARE THERE EXCEPTIONS FROM THE REQUIREMENT OF A WRITTEN CONFIRMATION?

Answer: The Commission publishes a list of countries which, following their request, have been assessed and are considered as having equivalent rules for good manufacturing practices to those in the EU. Active substances manufactured in these countries do not require a written confirmation.

See also Questions 27 and 28.

27. QUESTION: WHERE CAN I FIND THE LIST OF NON-EU COUNTRIES TO WHICH THE REQUIREMENT OF A WRITTEN CONFIRMATION DOES NOT APPLY?

Answer: The list is published in the *Official Journal of the European Union* and also reproduced here: http://ec.europa.eu/health/human-use/quality/index_en.htm.

28. QUESTION: HOW MANY NON-EU COUNTRIES HAVE SO FAR REQUESTED TO BE LISTED?

Answer: A list of non-EU countries which have so far requested to be listed is available here: http://ec.europa.eu/health/human-use/quality/index_en.htm.

29. QUESTION: WHEN IS THE LIST GOING TO BE PUBLISHED BY THE COMMISSION?

Answer: The Commission is going to publish an additional non-EU country on the list once its equivalence assessment has been finalised. The equivalence assessment takes several months from the request from the non-EU country.

29A. QUESTION: HOW DOES A NON-EU COUNTRY REQUEST TO BE LISTED?

Answer: The request is made by way of a letter to the Director-General of DG SANTE. It should contain the relevant information for conducting the "equivalence assessment".

More information on the procedure and the documents to be submitted is available here: http://ec.europa.eu/health/human-use/quality/index_en.htm, under the section "Listing of third countries".

The relevant information can also be sent directly to the responsible service within the Commission (sante-pharmaceuticals-b4@ec.europa.eu).

30. QUESTION: DO I NEED A WRITTEN CONFIRMATION, EVEN THOUGH MY MANUFACTURING SITE HAS RECENTLY BEEN INSPECTED BY THE EUROPEAN DIRECTORATE FOR THE QUALITY OF MEDICINES (EDQM) OF THE COUNCIL OF EUROPE?

Answer: Yes. The process of a written confirmation is independent of such inspection activities. See also Question 31.

31. QUESTION: DO I NEED A WRITTEN CONFIRMATION, EVEN THOUGH MY MANUFACTURING SITE HAS RECENTLY BEEN INSPECTED BY AN EU MEMBER STATE?

Answer: Yes. The process of a written confirmation is independent of such inspection activities. However, exceptionally, and where necessary to ensure the availability of medicinal products, following inspections by an EU Member State, a Member State may decide to waive the need for a written confirmation for a period not exceeding the validity of the GMP certificate ("waiver").

32. QUESTION: I WOULD LIKE TO BE INSPECTED BY AN EU MEMBER STATE. WHERE DO I "APPLY" FOR SUCH AN INSPECTION?

Answer: You should address through:

IMPORTATION OF ACTIVE SUBSTANCES FOR MEDICINAL PRODUCTS

- any registered importer of the active substance;
- any holder of a manufacturing authorisation that uses the active substance;
- any holder of a marketing authorisation that lists the active substance manufacturer to the national competent authority of the EU Member State where they are established.

33. QUESTION: WHAT HAPPENS WHEN AN ACTIVE SUBSTANCE MANUFACTURING SITE COVERED BY A WRITTEN CONFIRMATION IS FOUND GMP NON-COMPLIANT FOLLOWING AN INSPECTION BY AN EU MEMBER STATE?

Answer: A statement of GMP non-compliance issued by a EU Member State for a specific site and API supersedes the corresponding written confirmation until the non-compliance is resolved.

34. QUESTION: WHERE CAN I FIND A LIST OF ACTIVE SUBSTANCE MANUFACTURING SITES THAT RECEIVED STATEMENTS OF GMP NON-COMPLIANCE?

Answer: Statements of GMP non-compliance are stored in the EudraGMDP database (http://eudragmdp.ema.europa.eu/inspections/logonGeneralPublic.do) and are publicly available.

35. QUESTION: CAN AN API BATCH MANUFACTURED DURING THE PERIOD OF VALIDITY OF A WRITTEN CONFIRMATION BE IMPORTED INTO THE EU ONCE THE WRITTEN CONFIRMATION IS EXPIRED?

Answer: Article 46(b)(2)(b) sets out that active substances can only be imported if manufactured in accordance with EU GMP or equivalent, and accompanied by a written confirmation from the competent authority of the exporting third country certifying, inter alia, that (1) the GMP standards applicable to the manufacturing plant are equivalent to those of the EU, and (2) the supervision of the plant compliance with GMP ensures a protection of public health equivalent to that of the EU.

It is legitimate to consider that the guarantees of equivalence provided by the written confirmation apply to any API batch in the scope of the written confirmation which was released for sale within the period of validity of the written confirmation, even if not exported in that time period.

Against this background, it can therefore be considered that the importation into the EU of an API accompanied by an expired WC is acceptable provided that the paperwork accompanying the consignment (1) unequivocally proves that the whole consignment has been manufactured and released for sale by the quality unit before the expiry date of the written confirmation; and (2) provides a solid justification of why a valid written confirmation is not available.

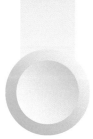

Appendix 5

SAFETY FEATURES FOR MEDICINAL PRODUCTS FOR HUMAN USE – QUESTIONS AND ANSWERS

Contents

In May 2021 the Commission published a revised question and answer document responding to frequently asked questions in relation to safety features for medicinal products. A revised Q&A 1.14 has been added.

The views expressed in this question and answer document are not a formal interpretation of Union law, nor are legally binding. Ultimately, only the European Court of Justice can give an authoritative interpretation of Union law.

This document aims at informing on the technical aspects of Commission Delegated Regulation (EU) 2016/161 with a view to facilitating its implementation. This document sets out frequently asked "questions and answers" regarding the implementation of the rules on the safety features for medicinal products for human use.

These rules are enshrined in Articles 47a, 54(o) and 54a of Directive 2001/83/EC, and in the Commission Delegated Regulation (EU) No 2016/161[1].

1. GENERAL

1.1. Question: What are the safety features?

Answer: The safety features consist of two elements placed on the packaging of a medicinal product:

(1) A unique identifier, a unique sequence carried by a two-dimensional barcode allowing the identification and authentication of the individual pack on which it is printed; and

(2) A device allowing the verification of whether the packaging of the medicinal product has been tampered with (anti-tampering device).

1.2. Question: When do the rules on the safety features apply?

Answer: They apply as of 9 February 2019. Belgium, Greece and Italy have the option of deferring the application of the rules by an additional period of up to 6 years.

Belgium has, however, formally renounced using this option and confirmed the application of the new rules as of 9 February 2019.

1.3. Question: Do the safety features need to be applied on all medicinal products for human use?

Answer: No. The safety features should only be applied on the packaging of the following medicinal products for human use:

(1) Medicinal products subject to prescription which are not included in the list set out in Annex I to of Commission Delegated Regulation (EU) 2016/161;

(2) Medicinal products not subject to prescription included in the list set out in Annex II of Commission Delegated Regulation (EU) 2016/161;

(3) Medicinal products to which Member States have extended the scope of the unique identifier or the anti-tampering device to in accordance with Article 54a(5) of Directive 2001/83/EC.

---

[1] Commission Delegated Regulation (EU) 2016/161 supplementing Directive 2001/83/EC of the European Parliament and of the Council by laying down detailed rules for the safety features appearing on the packaging of medicinal products for human use. OJ L 32, 9.2.2016, pp. 1–27.

1.4. Question: Are there exceptions from the requirements for certain medicinal products to bear or not the safety features?

Answer: Yes. The list of categories of medicinal products subject to prescription that shall not bear the safety features is set out in Annex I of Commission Delegated Regulation (EU) 2016/161, while the list of medicinal products not subject to prescription which shall bear the safety features is set out in Annex II of the same Regulation.

1.5. Question: Do the rules on the safety features also apply to veterinary medicinal products?

Answer: No. The rules apply only to medicinal products for human use.

1.6. Question: Do the rules on the safety features apply to medicinal products intended for research and development trials?

Answer: Medicinal products intended for research and development trials and not yet granted a marketing authorisation are excluded from the rules on the safety features.

Authorised medicinal products have to fulfil the requirements of Directive 2001/83/EC and Commission Delegated Regulation (EU) 2016/161 up to the moment it becomes known which batch/unit will be used for research and development trials. In practice, there are two possible situations:

1. The product is manufactured for known use in a clinical trial

An investigational medicinal product (IMP) that is manufactured in accordance with the marketing authorisation but is packaged for a clinical trial (not in the commercial presentation) is excluded from the rules on the safety features as it is solely manufactured and packed for the use in the clinical trial. The manufacturer would be required to hold a manufacturing and importation authorisation covering IMPs and the IMP certified under that authorisation in accordance with the clinical trial application noting that the clinical trial application must reflect these arrangements.

Authorised auxiliary medicinal products cannot be manufactured under a manufacturing and importation authorisation covering IMPs and must fulfil the requirements of a marketed pack bearing safety features and decommissioned appropriately (see below).

2. The product is authorised and sourced from the regulated supply chain

Medicines in their commercial presentations bearing safety features should be decommissioned in accordance with Articles 16 and 25(4)(c) of Commission Delegated Regulation (EU) 2016/161 before use as investigational medicinal products or authorised auxiliary medicinal products.

SAFETY FEATURES FOR MEDICINAL PRODUCTS

1.7. Question: Are the safety features required where the medicinal product manufactured in the EU is destined for exportation only?
Answer: No.

1.8. Question: In the case of a medicinal product bearing the safety features is brought into the territory of a Member State in accordance with Article 5(1) of Directive 2001/83/EC, do the rules on the safety features apply?
Answer: When a medicinal product is brought into the territory of a Member State in accordance with Article 5(1) of Directive 2001/83/EC, the rules on the safety features in principle do not apply, unless there is applicable national legislation requiring otherwise.

Member States can, however, use national legislation to regulate which provisions of Directive 2001/83/EC or of Commission Delegated Regulation (EU) 2016/16 apply to Article 5(1) products brought into their territory. Member States can, for example, require the mandatory verification/decommissioning of Article 5(1) products in accordance with Commission Delegated Regulation (EU) 2016/16.

In the absence of national legislation requiring otherwise, the rules on the safety features do not apply. The "importer" of a medicinal product brought into the territory of a Member State in accordance with Article 5(1) is not required, for example, to (re)place the safety features on its packaging (e.g. through labelling/re-labelling operations) or to upload the unique identifiers, if present, into the national repository of the new Member State of destination. The verification of the safety features and decommissioning of the unique identifiers of Article 5(1) products already bearing the safety features are also not mandatory.

Pharmacies, healthcare institutions and other relevant stakeholders in that Member State are nevertheless strongly encouraged to verify the authenticity of and decommission the medicinal product before supplying it to the public.

1.9. Question: Does an obligation to bear "the safety features" imply an obligation to bear both a unique identifier and an anti-tampering device?
Answer: Yes.

1.10. Question: Once Commission Delegated Regulation (EU) 2016/161 applies, can manufacturers place the safety features, on a voluntary basis, on medicinal products not required to bear the safety features?
Answer: No. Once Commission Delegated Regulation (EU) 2016/161 applies, manufacturers cannot place the safety features on medicinal products not required to bear the safety features, unless the Member States have extended the scope of application of the unique identifier or of the anti-tampering device to those medicinal products in accordance with Article 54a(5) of Directive 2001/83/EC.

1.11. Question: Certain medicinal products are currently bearing an anti-tampering device on a voluntary basis. Are those products allowed to maintain the anti-tampering device once Commission Delegated Regulation (EU) 2016/161 applies, if they are not required to bear the safety features?

Answer: Once Commission Delegated Regulation (EU) 2016/161 applies, medicinal products can only bear an anti-tampering device if they are in the scope of Article 54a(1) of Directive 2001/83/EC (i.e. if they are medicinal products subject to prescription or medicinal products listed in Annex II of Commission Delegated Regulation (EU) 2016/161) or if the Member State(s) where they are placed on the market extended the scope of the anti-tampering device to those medicinal products.

1.12. Question: Would it be possible to place a unique identifier on the packaging of a medicinal product during the 3-year period between the publication of Commission Delegated Regulation (EU) 2016/161 and its application?

Answer: Yes, on a voluntary basis. It is recommended that, whenever possible, unique identifiers are placed on the packaging only once a functional national/supranational repository allowing the storage, verification of the authenticity and decommissioning of those identifiers is in place. Unique identifiers which are placed on medicinal products before such repository is in place are expected to be uploaded in the repository as soon as it becomes operational.

1.13. Question: Will the mandatory changes to the packaging due to the placing of the unique identifier and of the anti-tampering device require the submission of variations to marketing authorisations?

Answer: The regulatory requirements to be followed to notify the EMA of the placing of the unique identifier and/or the anti-tampering device on centrally authorised products are detailed in an implementation plan developed by the EMA and the European Commission and published in the "product information templates" section of the EMA website: http://www.ema.europa.eu/docs/en_GB/document_library/Other/2016/02/WC500201413.pdf

The regulatory requirements for nationally authorised products are available on the HMA/CMDh website: http://www.hma.eu/fileadmin/dateien/Human_Medicines/CMD_h_/Falsified_Medicines/CMDh_345_2016_Rev00_02_2016_1.pdf

1.14. Question: Are there any mandatory specifications for the anti-tampering device?

Answer: In accordance with Article 54(o) of Directive 2001/83/EC and Article 3(2)(b) of Commission Delegated Regulation (EU) 2016/161, an anti-tampering device has to allow the verification of whether the packaging of the medicinal product has been tampered with.

There are no other mandatory specifications. The standard EN ISO 21976:2020 "Packaging – Tamper verification features for medicinal product packaging" is available for manufacturers to consider.

1.15. Question: Will the pharmaceutical companies receive any financial support (EU or national) for acquiring the instrumentation for applying the safety features on individual packages?

Answer: No, it is not currently foreseen that pharmaceutical companies will receive any financial support (EU or national) for acquiring the instrumentation for applying the safety features on individual packages.

1.16. Question: Who shall bear the financial responsibility for the covering the expenses of establishment and implementation of the repository system?

Answer: In accordance with Article 31(1) of Commission Delegated Regulation (EU) 2016/161, the repositories system shall be set up and managed by a non-profit legal entity or non-profit legal entities in the Union by manufacturer and marketing authorisation holders. The costs of the system shall be borne by the manufacturer of medicinal products bearing the safety features in accordance with Article 54a(2)(e) of Directive 2001/83/EC.

1.17. Question: Are radiopharmaceuticals required to bear the safety features?

Answer: No. All pharmaceutical forms and strengths of radiopharmaceuticals (as defined by Article 1(6) of Directive 2001/83/EC), radionuclide generators (as defined by Article 1(7) of Directive 2001/83/EC), radionuclide precursors (as defined by Article 1(9) of Directive 2001/83/EC) and kits (as defined by Article 1(8) of Directive 2001/83/EC) shall not bear safety features.

The wording of Article 54(o) of Directive 2001/83/EC ("medicinal products other than Radiopharmaceuticals") excludes radiopharmaceuticals, as defined by Article 1.6 of the said Directive, from the scope of the safety features. Consequently, any medicinal product fulfilling the definition of radiopharmaceutical shall not bear the safety feature. Since radiopharmaceuticals are outside of the scope of the safety features, their addition to Annex I of Commission Delegated Regulation (EU) 2016/161 is unnecessary.

1.18. Question: Concerning pandemic–influenza vaccines, the EMA mock-up procedure allows a vaccine to be developed and authorized in advance of a pandemic, containing a strain of flu virus that few people

have been exposed to but that could potentially cause a pandemic. These can be modified into pandemic–influenza vaccines in a future pandemic case. After a pandemic has been declared there is an emergency procedure for the final vaccine. Are there exceptions from the requirements for pandemic–influenza vaccines to bear or not the safety features?

Answer: No, as pandemic influenza vaccines are not included in Annex I of Commission Delegated Regulation (EU) 2016/161. Pandemic–influenza vaccines authorised via the mock-up procedure should bear the safety features in accordance with the said Regulation.

1.19. Question: In case of a bundle of several single packs sold as one unit, should the anti-tampering device and unique identifier be placed on the bundle packaging or on each single pack?

Answer: Whether a manufacturer needs to place the safety features on the bundle packaging or on each single pack within the bundle depends on how the medicinal product is described in its marketing authorisation dossier – regardless of what is the commercial sellable unit.

If, in the marketing authorisation dossier, the product presentation is described as a "multi-pack", the outer packaging as that of the bundle and the single packs as not for individual sale (the text "can't be sold separately" or equivalent is present on the packs), then both the UI and the ATD need to be placed on the bundle packaging. The outer packaging must include, in addition to the unique identifier and ATD, all applicable labelling requirements as laid down in Article 54 of Directive 2001/83/EC.

If, however, the marketing authorisation dossier of the medicinal product describes the product presentation as a single pack and the text "can't be sold separately" or equivalent is not present on the packs, then each pack within the bundle needs to be serialised and have an anti-tampering device. In this case, the bundle packaging should not bear a unique identifier, but it may bear an aggregated code containing the information on all unique identifiers within the bundle.

1.20. Question: If a pack bearing the safety features is lawfully opened (e.g. by parallel traders/manufacturers replacing the leaflet under the supervision of national competent authorities), can it be resealed (e.g. by applying a new ATD on top of the old, broken ATD)?

Answer: In certain circumstances, based on the assessment of the national competent authority in the destination Member State.

Parallel traders/manufacturers that wish to reseal packages must provide the competent authority in the destination Member State with sufficient information to allow an informed assessment of equivalence of the new anti-tampering device (description, explanation, mock-ups, pictures, etc., of both the original and replacement ATD). The newly placed ATD can only be considered equivalent if, inter alia, it is equally effective in

SAFETY FEATURES FOR MEDICINAL PRODUCTS

enabling the verification of authenticity of the medicinal product and in providing evidence of tampering.

An anti-tampering device (ATD) placed on top of an older, broken ATD can be considered as effective in providing evidence of tampering as an ATD placed on an intact outer packaging only if:

(a) The new ATD completely seals the pack and covers any visible sign of the original, broken ATD;

(b) The replacement of the ATD is conducted in accordance with applicable good manufacturing practice for medicinal products and is subject to supervision by the competent authority; and

(c) The manufacturer placing the equivalent ATD has verified the authenticity of the unique identifier and the integrity of the ATD on the original pack before breaking the ATD/opening the original pack, in accordance with Article 47a(1)(a) of Directive 2001/83/EC.

1.21. Question: Is it possible for manufacturers/wholesalers/parallel traders to market/supply medicinal products with a packaging showing visible signs of opening/intrusion, but where the ATD has been replaced by a new ATD in accordance with Article 47a of Directive 2001/83/EC?

Answer: No. If the pack has been opened lawfully (see Q&A 1.20), the manufacturer placing an equivalent ATD should ensure the pack is perfectly re-sealed and no signs of the original, broken ATD are visible.

It should be noted that Articles 24 and 30 of Commission Delegated Regulation (EU) 2016/161 prohibit wholesalers and persons authorised or entitled to supply who receive a medicinal products having a packaging showing signs of tampering from supplying that product.

1.22. Question: In case of parallel-traded packs, can parallel traders cover or remove the safety features of the original pack?

Answer: Parallel traders covering or removing the existing safety features are required to place equivalent safety features in accordance with Article 47a of Directive 2001/83/EC (see also Q&A 1.20).

The new unique identifier should comply with the requirements of the Member State where the medicine is intended to be placed on the market (Article 17 of Commission Delegated Regulation (EU) 2016/161).

Furthermore, if the product code and/or batch number of the parallel-traded product change compared to the original product, parallel traders must place a new unique identifier after first decommissioning the original one. Centrally authorised products that are subject to the covering or removing of existing safety features are expected to display the original manufacturer's batch number.

When placing an equivalent unique identifier, parallel traders are required to fulfil, inter alia, the obligations laid down in Articles 33, 40 and 42 of Commission Delegated Regulation (EU) 2016/161 concerning the uploading and keeping up to date of the information on the new unique identifier into the repositories system.

In all cases, traceability must be maintained in the repository system in accordance with Article 35(4).

1.23. Question: Is it possible to place a transparent sticker used as an ATD over the human readable codes or the 2D Data Matrix, even if opening the pack might lead to the human-readable data and/or the 2D barcode being damaged and unreadable?

Answer: It is acceptable to place a transparent sticker, used as an ATD, over the 2D Data Matrix, provided that it does not impact its readability (e.g. if the sticker is reflective), and the Data Matrix does not contain information intended for the patient or included in accordance with the recommendation in Q&A 2.12 (e.g. content previously included in a QR code).

Concerning the human-readable code, the human-readable batch number and expiry date are relevant information for the patient and should remain readable after the pack is opened. Hence, it is not acceptable to place a transparent sticker, used as an ATD, over the human-readable batch number and expiry date if it risks damaging this information when the pack is opened.

1.24. Question: In some cases a medicinal product may carry more than one batch number, typically when the product consists of an active component and a solvent. Which batch number(s) should be encoded in the medicines verification system in that case?

Answer: Only the batch number of the active substance needs to be encoded in the medicines verification system.

1.25. Question: When re-packaging or re-labelling a pack for the purpose of using it as authorised investigational medicinal product or authorised auxiliary medicinal product according to Article 16(2) of Commission Delegated Regulation (EU) 2016/161, the unique identifier should be decommissioned. What status of decommissioning should the pack have?

Answer: Until there is a specific status for these medicines in the EMVS system, the pack should be decommissioned as "SUPPLIED" when re-packaging or re-labelling for use as an authorised investigational medicinal product or authorised auxiliary medicinal product.

1.26. Question: During the transitional period, do manufacturers located in the EU/EEA need to place safety features on medicines intended for the Greek or Italian market?

Answer: No. Greece and Italy have decided to defer the entry into application of the safety features in line with Article 2(2)(b) of Directive

2011/62/EU. Medicines produced exclusively for the Greek or Italian market, regardless of their place of manufacture, are therefore not required to bear safety features before the entry into application of the new rules in Greece or Italy.

1.27. Question: During the transitional period, can manufacturers located in Greece or Italy place unique identifiers on medicines intended for the rest of the EU/EEA? What about uploading data to the EU hub?

Answer: Yes. There are no geographic restrictions on the placing of safety features by manufacturers. Please see Q&A 7.19 regarding data upload.

1.28. Question: Is there an obligation for direct suppliers to healthcare institutions to offer aggregation services?

Answer: No. The Delegated Regulation does not require hospital suppliers to provide aggregation services. Direct suppliers may, however, offer the service on a voluntary basis, providing the safeguards outlined in the *Expert Group paper on implementation of the Falsified Medicines Directive in the hospital settings are met*[2].

2. TECHNICAL SPECIFICATIONS OF THE UNIQUE IDENTIFIER

2.1. Question: Does Commission Delegated Regulation (EU) 2016/161 limit the length of the unique identifier to 50 characters?

Answer: No. Only the length of the product code, one of the data elements of the unique identifier, is limited to 50 characters.

2.2. Question: Would it be possible to include, on a voluntary basis, a two-dimensional barcode on the packaging of medicinal products for human use not having to bear the safety features if the information carried by the barcode does not serve the purposes of identification and authentication of the medicinal product and does not include a unique identifier?

Answer: Yes, provided that the relevant labelling provisions of Title V of Directive 2001/83/EC are complied with. Examples may include two-dimensional barcodes encoding price indications, reimbursement conditions, etc.

2.3. Is it possible to keep one-dimensional barcodes on the packaging of medicinal products for human use having to bear the safety features, when adding the two-dimensional barcode carrying the unique identifier?

Answer: Yes, provided that the presence of both barcodes does not negatively impact the legibility of the outer packaging. In order to avoid

---

[2] https://ec.europa.eu/health/sites/health/files/files/falsified_medicines/2018_hospitalsetting_en.pdf

incorrect scanning by end-users, if possible, the barcodes should not be placed in proximity to each other.

2.4. Question: Is a printing quality of 1.5 according to ISO/IEC 15415 mandatory?

Answer: No. Manufacturers are required to use a printing quality that ensures the accurate readability of the Data Matrix throughout the supply chain until at least 1 year after the expiry date of the pack or 5 years after the pack has been released for sale or distribution in accordance with Article 51(3) of Directive 2001/83/EC, whichever is the longer period. The use of a printing quality of 1.5 or higher gives a presumption of conformity, i.e. manufactures using a printing quality of 1.5 or higher will be presumed to have fulfilled the requirement mentioned in the first paragraph without need to prove that it is actually the case. If a printing quality lower than 1.5 is used, manufacturers may be asked to prove that requirements mentioned in the first paragraph are met.

2.5. Can manufacturers, on a voluntary basis, place the human readable code on medicinal products with packaging having the sum of the two longest dimensions equal or less than 10 centimetres?

Answer: Yes.

2.6. Are medicinal products with packaging having the sum of the two longest dimensions equal or less than 10 centimetres exempted from bearing the two-dimensional barcode carrying the unique identifier?

Answer: No, Article 7(2) only provides for an exemption from bearing the unique identifier in human readable format. The unique identifier in machine-readable format – the 2D barcode – is still required.

2.7. Question: Is it compulsory to print the national reimbursement number in human-readable format?

Answer: The national reimbursement number or other national number should be printed in human readable format only if required by the national competent authorities of the relevant Member State and not printed elsewhere on the packaging. It should be printed adjacent to the 2D barcode if the dimensions of the packaging allow it.

2.8. Question: Is it compulsory for the human-readable data elements of the unique identifier to be placed adjacent to the two-dimensional barcode?

Answer: Yes, whenever the dimensions of the packaging allow it.

SAFETY FEATURES FOR
MEDICINAL PRODUCTS

2.9. Question: What is the smallest font size that can be used to print the unique identifier in human-readable format?

Answer: The font size of the unique identifier should be in accordance with the "Guideline on the readability of the labelling and package leaflet of medicinal products for human use" published in EudraLex – Notice to Applicants – Volume 2C (http://ec.europa.eu/health/files/eudralex/vol2/c/2009_01_12_readability_guideline_final_en.pdf).

2.10. Question: When encoded in the 2D Data Matrix or printed on the packaging in human-readable format, should the data elements of the unique identifier follow the order laid down in Articles 4(b) or 7(1), respectively, of Commission Delegated Regulation (EU) 2016/161?

Answer: No. Manufacturers can choose the order of the data elements provided that all data elements required by national legislation and Article 4(b) (for the 2D Data Matrix) or Article 7 (for the human-readable format) are present.

2.11. Question: Commission Delegated Regulation (EU) 2016/161 does not mention batch number and expiry date as mandatory components of the human readable code. Is it mandatory to print the batch number and the expiry date in a human-readable format and adjacent to the two dimensional barcode?

Answer: Batch number and expiry date are mandatory components of the labelling of all medicinal products – regardless of whether they bear the safety features – and should be printed on the packaging in accordance with Article 54(h) and (m) of Directive 2001/83/EC. There is no obligation to place batch number and expiry date adjacent to the 2D barcode.

2.12. Question: Is it allowed to place a QR code on the packaging of a medicinal product bearing the safety features?

Answer: Commission Delegated Regulation (EU) 2016/161 does not prohibit the placing of a QR code as far as it is not used for the purposes of identification and authentication of medicinal products. Marketing authorisation holders are, however, encouraged, wherever technically feasible, to exploit the residual storage capacity of the Data Matrix to include the information they would otherwise include in the QR code (see also Q&A 2.16). This would minimise the number of visible barcodes on the packaging and reduce the risk of confusion as regard the barcode to be scanned for verifying the authenticity of the medicinal product. Furthermore, in order to avoid incorrect scanning by end users, if possible, the QR code should not be placed in proximity of the Data Matrix.

2.13. Question: Where on the packaging should the unique identifier be placed?

Answer: The Delegated Regulation does not specify where on the outer packaging the safety features should be placed. The placement of the safety features is therefore to be supervised by competent authorities in accordance with current practice for labelling requirements.

2.14. Question: Can the graphics on the containers of the medicinal products be printed separately and the Data Matrix added at the final packaging stage – or are there digital printing technologies where all packaging graphics and the UI can be printed in one step?

Answer: The Delegated Regulation does not specify how the safety features should be applied to the outer packaging. The placement of the safety features is therefore to be supervised by competent authorities in accordance with current practice for labelling requirements. The specifics of the technologies used to apply the UI will be for the individual manufacturer to decide and for them to select the most appropriate model suitable for their needs. According to Annex 16 of the EU GMP Guidelines paragraph 1.7.21, affixing the UI to the packaging of a medicinal product is the responsibility of the Qualified Person. Any outsourcing of this activity to a third party by the manufacturer of the finished medicinal product must be in accordance with the principles described in Chapter 7 of Part I of the EU GMP Guidelines.

2.15. Question: Upon the medicinal product being supplied to the public, the UI is decommissioned and the package is no longer active in the repository. However, the 2D Data Matrix can still be read out, e.g. by a consumer using a smartphone application. Will the possibility to verify the authenticity of the product via the Data Matrix be extended to the end user (patient)?

Answer: The Delegated Regulation does not provide for verification of the authenticity of the product by the end user. Nevertheless, the verification conducted by the person authorised to supply to the public guarantees that the product is not falsified.

2.16. Question: After the UI data has been encoded, can any residual storage capacity in the Data Matrix be used to store other information?

Answer: The Delegated Regulation states in Article 8 that manufacturers may include information additional to the information contained within the unique identifier in the 2D barcode, where permitted by the competent authority in accordance with article 62 of Title V of the Directive 2001/83/EC. That information should be consistent with the summary of product characteristics, useful for the patient and may not contain promotional elements. The amount of residual storage capacity of the Data

Matrix after the UI data has been encoded will depend upon the size of the Data Matrix as selected by the individual manufacturers responsible for the placing of the UI on the packaging.

2.17. Question: Do human-readable headers (PC, SN, Lot, EXP, NN) have to be placed adjacent to the respective data elements, on the same line, or is some flexibility possible?

Answer: Human-readable headers are not required to be placed adjacent/on the same line as the respective data element. Headers can be placed in any position that allows the unequivocal identification of the human-readable data element.

2.18. Question: For products bearing the human-readable code, is it acceptable to place data elements in multiple locations across the packaging?

Answer: It depends on the data elements and dimensions of the packaging. The product code and serial number should be placed on the same surface, where space allows, so to facilitate manual decommissioning of the unique identifier. Concerning the other data elements, an effort should be made to place them on the same surface as the product code and serial number. Should the packaging dimensions not allow it, however, it is acceptable to place the other data elements as close to the product code and serial number as possible (e.g. adjacent sides).

2.19. Question: Is it acceptable to use a 2D Data Matrix that is rectangular (rather than square) or printed white on black (rather than black on white)?

Answer: Yes. Manufactures can choose to encode the unique identifier in a 2D Data Matrix that is rectangular and/or printed white on black, provided that it fulfils the technical requirement laid down in Article 5 of Commission Delegated Regulation (EU) 2016/161.

2.20. Question: Is it mandatory to include Application/Data Identifiers as part of the human-readable headers or data elements?

Answer: No. Manufacturers can choose whether to include the Application/Data Identifiers as part of the human-readable headers/data elements.

2.21. Question: Is it acceptable to use stickers to place the unique identifier on the outer/immediate packaging?

Answer: The unique identifier should be printed on the packaging along with all other information required under article 54 of Directive 2001/83/EC, in accordance with Article 5(3) of Commission Delegated Regulation (EU) 2016/161.

Placing the unique identifier by means of stickers can be accepted in the following circumstances:

- no legal and/or technically feasible alternative exists (e.g. safeguard of trademark rights; glass/plastic immediate packaging without outer packaging; etc.); or
- national competent authorities authorise it due to the marketing authorisation, including for parallel import, or to safeguard public health and ensure continued supply.

In cases where placing the unique identifier by means of stickers is authorised by national competent authorities under the circumstances mentioned above, the following conditions should be met:

- the sticker on which the unique identifier is printed should become one with the outer packaging/immediate packaging, i.e. the sticker should be tamper-evident and it should not be possible to remove it without damaging the packaging or the sticker itself or leaving visible signs;
- the sticker on which the unique identifier is printed should be placed by a manufacturer under GMP conditions; and
- the outer/immediate packaging on which the sticker is placed includes, in addition to the unique identifier, all applicable labelling requirements as laid down in Article 54 of Directive 2001/83/EC.

Notwithstanding the above, placing the unique identifier by means of stickers should never be allowed when:

- It impairs readability. Article 56 of Directive 2001/83/EC requires that "the particulars referred to in article 54, 55 and 62 shall be easily legible, clearly comprehensible and indelible"; or
- The sticker on which the unique identifier is printed can be detached from the packaging without damaging the packaging or the sticker itself or leaving visible signs; or
- The sticker on which the unique identifier is printed is intended to be placed on top of an existing sticker, as this could engender confusion and suspicions of tampering.

2.22. Question: Do human-readable headers (PC, SN, Lot, EXP, NN) have to comply with the provisions of the QRD template?

Answer: Yes, preferably. According to version 10 of the QRD-template[3], the product code, serial number and national reimbursement number in the human readable code should be preceded by the letters "PC", "SN" and "NN". Batch number and expiry date should follow the abbreviations laid out in Appendix IV of the QRD-template[4].

---

[3] https://www.ema.europa.eu/documents/template-form/qrd-product-information-annotated-templateenglish-version-10_en.pdf

[4] https://www.ema.euopa.eu/documents/regulatory-procedural-guideline/appendix-iv-terms-abbreviationsbatch-number-expiry-date-be-used-labelling-human-medicinal-products_en.pdf

2.23. Question: Are there specific requirements for the characters used in batch and serial numbers?

Answer: No. However, in order to reduce the risk of false alerts due to end-user scanner misconfigurations, manufacturers are strongly encouraged to follow the recommendations below. Serial and batch numbers should preferably:

- contain only uppercase letters;
- not include special characters (e.g. hyphens, question marks, etc.); and
- avoid the use of the letters "I", "O", "Y" and "Z".

3. GENERAL PROVISION ON THE VERIFICATION AND DECOMMISSIONING OF THE SAFETY FEATURES

3.1. Question: How should the unique identifier be decommissioned if the two-dimensional barcode is unreadable or deteriorated?

Answer: The unique identifier in human readable format should be recorded by any suitable method allowing the subsequent manual querying of the repository system in order to verify and decommission the unique identifier.

3.2. Question: Where the barcode carrying the unique identifier cannot be read, or in case the verification of the unique identifier is temporarily impeded, is it possible to supply the medicinal product to the public?

Answer: Article 30 of Commission Delegated Regulation (EU) 2016/161 prohibits supply to the public if there is reason to believe that the packaging of the medicinal product has been tampered with, or the verification of the safety features of the medicinal product indicates that the product may not be authentic. In all other cases, the supply of medicinal products to the public is regulated by national legislation. Without prejudice to national legislation, in the case where it is permanently impossible to read the unique identifier and verify the authenticity of the medicinal product, for example because both the Data Matrix and the human readable code are damaged, it is recommended that the medicinal product is not supplied to the public.

3.3. Question: Can a medicinal product that cannot be authenticated be returned, and to whom? Who should pay for the return?

Answer: Commission Delegated Regulation (EU) 2016/161 does not change the national provisions in place regulating returns of medicines from persons authorised or entitled to supply medicinal products to the public (e.g. pharmacies and hospitals). The regulation of returns of medicinal products, including their financial aspects, remains a national competence.

3.4. Question: Is the use of aggregated codes to simultaneously verify the authenticity of or decommission multiple unique identifiers permitted?

Answer: Recital 20 of the Delegated Regulation gives the possibility of giving aggregated codes allowing the simultaneous verification of multiple Unique Identifiers, provided that the requirements of Commission Delegated Regulation (EU) 2016/161 are complied with. However, since aggregation is not regulated in the Delegated Regulation any action in that sense from manufacturers/wholesalers/parallel traders (or any actor in the supply chain, for the matter) is only voluntary and needs to be agreed upon by the stakeholders.

3.5. Question: Is it possible to reverse the decommissioned status of a medicinal product that has been physically exported to third countries, when such a product is brought back into the EU?

Answer: No. When a medicinal product is physically exported outside of the EU, its unique identifier must be decommissioned in accordance with Article 22(a) of Commission Delegated Regulation (EU) 2016/161. If the exported product is subsequently re-imported onto the EU territory (e.g. because it is returned), it is considered an "import" and must be imported by a manufacturing import authorisation (MIA) holder (not a wholesaler) and is subject to the import requirements laid down in Article 51 of Directive 2001/83/EC (batch testing, batch release, etc.). The imported medicinal product should also be given a new unique identifier containing a new batch number and expiry date, if applicable, before it is released for sale and distribution in the EU.

3.6. Question: Can a medicine with only one of the safety features (either the UI or ATD) that has been released for sale before 9 February 2019 remain on the market?

Answer: Yes, a medicine with either a UI or ATD that has been released for sale before 9 February 2019 and has not been re-packaged or re-labelled may remain on the market until its expiry date.

3.7. Question: Who should verify and decommission medicines with safety features that are to be used in clinical trials as investigational medicinal products or authorised auxiliary medicinal products?

Answer: According to Articles 16, 23 and 25(4)(c) of Commission Delegated Regulation (EU) 2016/161, the unique identifier on medicines in their commercial presentations bearing safety features should be verified and decommissioned either by manufacturers, wholesalers or persons entitled or authorised to supply to the public before use as authorised investigational medicinal products (IMPs) or authorised auxiliary medicinal products. For medicines re-packaged or re-labelled for use in clinical trials, the manufacturer holding the manufacturing and importation authorisation covering IMPs should verify and decommission the unique identifier before they re-package or re-label the medicine. For medicines that are not re-packaged or re-labelled, the person entitled or authorised to supply to the public who supplies the medicinal product for subsequent use in a clinical trial should verify and decommission the unique identifier. In some cases, Member States may require wholesalers to verify and decommission unique identifiers on medicines supplied for clinical trials on behalf of certain entities under Article 23.

4. VERIFICATION OF THE SAFETY FEATURES AND DECOMMISSIONING OF THE UNIQUE IDENTIFIER BY MANUFACTURERS

4.1. Question: Do the records referred to in Article 15 of Commission Delegated Regulation (EU) 2016/161 have to be stored in the repositories system?

Answer: No. The manufacturers can decide how and where to keep the records of every operation they perform with or on the unique identifier.

4.2. Question: Article 18 requires that, in case of suspected falsification or tampering, the manufacturer should inform the competent authorities. Should he also inform the holder of the marketing authorisation for the medicinal product?

Answer: Yes, Article 46 of Directive 2001/83/EC requires manufacturers to inform the competent authority and the marketing authorisation holder immediately if they obtain information that medicinal products that come under the scope of their manufacturing authorisation are, or are suspected of being, falsified.

4.3. Question: Articles 18, 24 and 30 of Commission Delegated Regulation (EU) 2016/161 require that manufacturers, wholesalers and persons authorised or entitled to supply medicinal products to the public immediately inform national competent authorities in case of suspected falsification of medicinal products. How should this information be notified by manufacturers?

Answer: It is recommended that manufacturers contact national competent authorities, since the procedure to follow for such notification is a national competence. If they exist, national guidelines should be followed.

4.4. Question: Can a manufacturer use outer packaging carrying a unique identifier that has been placed by a packaging materials provider?

Answer: Yes. Art. 14 of Commission Delegated Regulation (EU) 2016/161 requires that the manufacturer responsible for placing the safety features on the medicinal product verifies that the 2D barcode carrying the unique identifier complies with Articles 5 and 6 of the said Regulation, is readable and contains the correct information before releasing the medicinal product for sale and distribution.

Where pre-printed cartons are used, the outsourcing of the pre-printing of the UI to a packaging material provider should be done in accordance with Chapter 7 of Part I of the EU GMP Guidelines, including the signature of a written agreement among the parties establishing the corresponding responsibilities. The packaging materials provider should be audited and qualified. The manufacturer releasing the product for sale and distribution (see Q&A 7.13) should verify the capacity of the contracted packaging materials provider to perform the task in accordance with the requirements of the Regulation and in compliance with applicable GMP. Upon receipt of the pre-printed packaging materials, the manufacturer of the finished medicinal product is expected to perform appropriate checks on the quantity and quality of the UIs in line with EU-GMP principles.

4.5. Question: Are manufacturers responsible for ensuring unique identifiers are readable and complete?

Answer: Yes. Manufacturers must check that the 2D barcode is readable and contains the correct information (Article 14 of Commission Delegated Regulation (EU) 2016/161). Furthermore, manufacturers must work closely with marketing authorisation holders to ensure that all relevant information on unique identifiers has been uploaded correctly to the repository system and corresponds to the information encoded in the unique identifier before they release medicines for sale or distribution (Article 33(2) of Commission Delegated Regulation (EU) 2016/161).

4.6. Question: Can a manufacturer outsource the placing of the safety features on a packaged medicinal product to another manufacturer?

Answer: Yes. The outsourcing of the placing of the safety features on a packaged medicinal product can be contracted to another manufacturer in line with Chapter 7 of Part I of the EU GMP Guidelines, as long as they have a manufacturing authorisation (MIA). The contracting manufacturer must also make a statement confirming compliance with Annex 16 Appendix 1 of the EU GMP Guidelines available to the Qualified Person certifying the final product. The contracted manufacturer must be included in the marketing authorisation.

SAFETY FEATURES FOR
MEDICINAL PRODUCTS

5. VERIFICATION OF THE SAFETY FEATURES AND DECOMMISSIONING OF THE UNIQUE IDENTIFIER BY WHOLESALERS

5.1. Question: How should the expression "the same legal entity" referred to in Articles 21(b) and 26(3) of Commission Delegated Regulation (EU) 2016/161 be interpreted?

Answer: This expression should be interpreted in accordance with national legislation. As general guidance, and without prejudice to national legislation, a legal entity may be considered the same when, e.g., it has the same registration number in the national company registry or, if no national registration is required, the same number for tax purposes (i.e. VAT number).

5.2. Question: Member States may hold stocks of certain medicinal products for the purpose of public health protection. How should the unique identifiers on those products be verified and decommissioned?

Answer: In accordance with Article 23(f) of the Delegated Regulation, Member States may request wholesalers to verify the safety features of and decommission the unique identifier of medicinal products which are supplied to governmental institutions maintaining stocks of medicinal products for the purposes of civil protection and disaster control.

5.3. Question: Articles 18, 24 and 30 of Commission Delegated Regulation (EU) 2016/161 require that manufacturers, wholesalers and persons authorised or entitled to supply medicinal products to the public immediately inform national competent authorities in case of suspected falsification of medicinal products. How should this information be notified by wholesalers?

Answer: It is recommended that wholesalers contact national competent authorities, since the procedure to follow for such notification is a national competence. If they exist, national guidelines should be followed.

5.4. Question: Articles 20, 21 and 22 require wholesalers to verify the authenticity and/or decommission the unique identifier only. Do wholesalers need to verify the integrity of the anti-tampering device when complying with those Articles?

Answer: No, wholesalers do not need to (but can) verify the integrity of the anti-tampering device when complying with Articles 20, 21 and 22.

5.5. Question: Article 22(a) requires a wholesaler to verify the authenticity of and decommission the unique identifier of all medicinal products they intend to distribute outside of the Union. Is it necessary to decommission the unique identifier if the medicinal product is sold to a party established

outside the EU but that product does not physically leave the wholesaler's premises in the EU?

Answer: No. The purpose of Article 22(a) is to ensure the decommissioning of unique identifiers on packs which leave the EU territory, in order to avoid that those active codes may be harvested by traffickers. In case the medicinal product is sold to a party established outside the EU but physically remains in the wholesaler's premises in the EU, the unique identifier on the product should not be decommissioned. If that medicinal product is subsequently imported (while physically remaining in the EU) by a holder of a manufacturing and import authorisation (a wholesaler cannot import medicinal products), no action from the wholesaler physically holding the product is required with regard to the safety features.

5.6. Question: Do wholesalers have the obligation to decommission the unique identifier of a medicinal product when they sell the product "business-to-business" to a company that buys it for the purpose of research?

Answer: Article 23(g) allows the decommissioning by wholesalers of medicinal products supplied for the purpose of research, except when supplied to healthcare institutions. Although the Article does not explicitly mention that it applies to the supply of products for the purpose of research to companies that are not universities or other higher-education establishments, it is desirable to include such a case in the scope of this Article (provided that those companies are not healthcare institutions) in order to guarantee the decommissioning of the unique identifiers on those products.

5.7. Question: Is wholesale distribution of medicinal products with a damaged/unreadable 2D Data Matrix code allowed, if there is no suspicion of falsification?

Answer: It depends on the human readable code. If the verification of the authenticity of the unique identifier (UI) can be performed using the human readable code, the product can be further distributed. If the verification of the authenticity of the UI cannot be performed (because the human readable code is damaged or absent), then the wholesaler should not further distribute the product with unreadable codes (Article 24 of Regulation No 2016/161). This requirement is independent of whether the verification was mandatory under Article 20 of Commission Delegated Regulation (EU) 2016/161 or voluntarily performed by wholesalers.

5.8. Question: Can a wholesaler request another wholesaler to verify the authenticity and decommission the unique identifiers for medicinal products they intend to distribute outside the EU on their behalf?

Answer: No. According to Article 22(a), the wholesaler who intends to distribute medicinal products outside the EU must verify their authenticity and decommission the unique identifiers. This obligation cannot be delegated to another wholesaler.

5.9. Question: During the transition period, can medicinal products destined for the rest of the EU (where safety features are mandatory) be distributed through the territory of Italy or Greece?

Answer: Yes. Directive 2001/83/EC and Commission Delegated Regulation (EU) 2016/161 do not prevent the distribution of medicines with safety features to Italy or Greece during the transition period.

5.10. Question: How can a wholesaler be sure that medicines they receive without safety features have been batch released prior to the entry into application of the safety features (9 February 2019)?

Answer: According to Commission Delegated Regulation (EU) 2016/161, marketing authorisation holders and manufacturers may only place medicines released before 9 February 2019 on the EU market without safety features. In principle, this means that products on the EU market without safety features must have been released before the entry into application of the safety features. Wholesalers may request that manufacturers include the batch release date in the delivery note of non-serialised medicines in order to confirm that the medicines were released before the safety features became mandatory.

5.11. Question: Should wholesalers be connected to the national repositories or can they be connected to the European hub?

Answer: A wholesaler physically holding products and performing activities related to wholesale outlined in Articles 20-23 Commission Delegated Regulation (EU) 2016/161 (such as the verification of returns or decommissioning for export) should be connected to and perform operations in the national repository where the activities take place. A connection to the national system is necessary to ensure that the audit trail is accurate and complete.

5.12. Question: Is it possible for a wholesaler with multiple locations to use a single NMVO connection and account to verify and decommission medicines?

Answer: No. In order to ensure compliance with Articles 13 and 35(1) (g) of Commission Delegated Regulation (EU) 2016/161, each physical location of the wholesaler must be uniquely identifiable when connecting to the NMVS and performing operations in the system.

5.13. Question: According to Article 20(b) Commission Delegated Regulation (EU) 2016/161, wholesalers must verify medicinal products they do not receive from the manufacturer, marketing authorisation holder or

wholesalers designated by the marketing authorisation holder. Is it necessary to verify the unique identifier of medicinal products sent directly from the manufacturer but purchased from a wholesaler who is neither the manufacturer, marketing authorisation holder or designated by the marketing authorisation holder?

Answer: No. The exemption in Article 20(b) refers to the physical transfer of medicines. Even if they have been purchased from a third party, medicines that have been shipped directly from the manufacturer, marketing authorisation holder or a designated wholesaler do not need to be verified in accordance with Article 20(b).

6. VERIFICATION OF THE SAFETY FEATURES AND DECOMMISSIONING OF THE UNIQUE IDENTIFIER BY PERSONS AUTHORISED OR ENTITLED TO SUPPLY MEDICINAL PRODUCTS TO THE PUBLIC

6.1. Question: In-patients in a hospital may be administered medicinal products during their stay, the costs of which may be charged to their insurer, which constitutes a sale. In this case, would the hospital (or any other healthcare institution) be allowed to verify the safety features and decommission the unique identifier of those products earlier than the time of supply to the public, in accordance with Article 25(2)?

Answer: Yes. In the case described, the charging of the medicinal products costs to the patient's insurer happens as a consequence of the administration of that product to the patient (regardless of whether the sale takes place before or after the actual administration). Consequently, it is considered that the charging of the cost of the medicinal product to the patient's insurer (or to the patient himself, for the matter) does not preclude hospitals from applying the derogation provided for in Article 25(2).

6.2. Question: How should the expression "the same legal entity" referred to in Articles 21(b) and 26(3) of Commission Delegated Regulation (EU) 2016/161 be interpreted?

Answer: See Q&A 5.1.

6.3. Question: Many hospitals and other healthcare institutions supply the contents of packages of a medicinal product to more than one patient. Where only part of a pack of a medicinal product is supplied, when should the decommissioning of the unique identifier be performed?

Answer: The unique identifier should be decommissioned when the packaging is opened for the first time, as required by Article 28 of Commission Delegated Regulation (EU) 2016/161.

6.4. Question: Does automated dose dispensing require the placing of new safety features on the individual patient doses/packs?

Answer: No. Automated dose dispensing falls in the scope of Article 28 of Commission Delegated Regulation (EU) 2016/161. Consequently, it is not necessary to place new safety features on the individual patient's dose/ pack.

6.5. Question: Is it possible for the wholesaler to scan the unique identifiers (UI) in a consignment before shipping the consignment to a hospital, store the UI information and then, once the hospital received the consignment, decommission the UIs using the stored information following an explicit request by the hospital?

Answer: No, the above process is not in line with the provisions of Commission Delegated Regulation (EU) 2016/161:

- Since the decommissioning would happen through the wholesaler's computer using the wholesaler's log-in ID, the decommissioning operation would be recorded in the system and in the audit trail as an operation performed by the wholesaler, and not by the hospital. This is not acceptable as the audit trail would not reflect the reality of the supply chain, as required by Article 35(1)(g) of the Regulation.
- Articles 23 and 26 of Commission Delegated Regulation (EU) 2016/161 are explicit about those cases where wholesalers are entitled to decommission the safety features on behalf of hospitals. Decommissioning on behalf of hospitals under other circumstances is therefore not allowed.

6.6. Question: Is it acceptable for hospitals/hospital pharmacies to subcontract their decommissioning obligations to wholesalers?

Answer: No. However, there are possible scenarios, compatible with Commission Delegated Regulation (EU) 2016/161, where wholesalers (including manufactures supplying their own products by wholesale) could facilitate the decommissioning operation of hospitals (illustrative examples only, list not exhaustive):

- Wholesalers could scan the packs in the hospital consignment to acquire the information on the UIs and encode such information into an aggregated code. Decommissioning would then be performed by the hospital by scanning the aggregated code. The only equipment needed for this operation would be a hand-held scanner and a computer (connected to the national repository).
- Wholesalers could acquire the information on the UIs in the hospital consignment and make this information available to the hospital, by secure means. The hospital would then use such information to perform the decommissioning (without having to physically scan the packs).

6.7. **Question: Articles 18, 24 and 30 of Commission Delegated Regulation (EU) 2016/161 require that manufacturers, wholesalers and persons authorised or entitled to supply medicinal products to the public immediately inform national competent authorities in case of suspected falsification of medicinal products. How should this information be notified by persons authorised or entitled to supply medicinal products to the public?**

Answer: It is recommended that persons authorised or entitled to supply medicinal products to the public contact national competent authorities, since the procedure to follow for such notification is a national competence. If they exist, national guidelines should be followed.

6.8. **Question: For persons authorised or entitled to supply medicinal products to the public operating within a healthcare institution, must the verification of the integrity of the anti-tampering device be done at the same time as the verification and decommissioning of the unique identifier?**

Answer: No. Article 25(2) of Commission Delegated Regulation (EU) 2016/161 outlines that verification of the safety features can be done at any time a medicine is in the physical possession of a healthcare institution as long as no sale takes place between delivery to the healthcare institution and supply to the public. Therefore, decommissioning of the UI and verification of the ATD can be done separately before supply to the public.

6.9. **Question: Is it possible for a pharmacy chain with multiple locations to use a single NMVO connection and account to verify and decommission medicines in different branches before dispense?**

Answer: No. In order to ensure compliance with Articles 13 and 35(1) (g) of Commission Delegated Regulation (EU) 2016/161, each physical location of a pharmacy chain must be uniquely identifiable when connecting to the NMVS and performing operations in the system.

7. ESTABLISHMENT, MANAGEMENT AND ACCESSIBILITY OF THE REPOSITORIES SYSTEM

7.1. **Question: How should the expression "manufacturers of medicinal products bearing the safety features", as used in Commission Delegated Regulation (EU) 2016/161, be interpreted?**

Answer: For the purposes of Commission Delegated Regulation (EU) 2016/161, "manufacturer" means the holder of a manufacturing authorisation in accordance with Article 40 of Directive 2001/83/EC. The expression "manufacturers of medicinal products bearing the safety features" encompasses any holder of the said authorisation performing partial or total manufacture of a medicinal product bearing the safety features.

7.2. Question: Article 31 of Commission Delegated Regulation (EU) 2016/161 allows wholesalers and persons authorised or entitled to supply medicinal products to the public to participate in the legal entity/ies setting up and managing the repositories system, at no costs. Can the terms of such participation be regulated by stakeholders, e.g. through the statutes of establishment or incorporation of the legal entity/ies?

Answer: Yes, it is possible, provided that the terms do not contradict what is enshrined in legislation. In case of discrepancy, the provisions of Commission Delegated Regulation (EU) 2016/161 and Directive 2001/83/EC prevail.

7.3. Question: What is a supranational repository?

Answer: In practice, a repository serving as "national" repository for more than one Member State.

7.4. Question: How should the expressions "application programming interface" or "graphical user interface" referred to in Articles 32(4) and 35(1) of Commission Delegated Regulation (EU) 2016/161 be interpreted?

Answer: The expression "application programming interface" refers to a software/software interface consisting of a set of programming instructions and standards used by a piece of software to ask another piece of software to perform a task. The 26 programming instructions and standards are set by the software being called upon. In the context of Commission Delegated Regulation (EU) 2016/161, the expression refers to the programming instructions and standards allowing the software of persons authorised or entitled to supply medicines to the public, wholesalers and national competent authorities to query the repository system. The expression "graphical user interface" (GUI) refers to a human/computer interface that allows users to interact with software or a database through graphical icons and visual indicators without the need of using complex programming language. The purpose of Article 35(1)(i) is to ensure that, in case of software failure, wholesalers and persons authorised/entitled to supply medicines to the public have an alternative way to connect to the national medicine verification system to verify the authenticity of/decommission the unique identifier. However, to avoid that wholesalers and persons authorised/entitled to supply medicines to the public rely routinely on the GUI to verify the authenticity of/decommission the unique identifiers on their products, Article 35(1)(i) limits the circumstances in which they are entitled (i.e. have the legal right) to use the GUI to the case of failure of their own software. The use of the GUI in any other circumstance is not prohibited but is subject to the agreement of the national medicine verification organisation owning the GUI. See also Q&A 7.18.

7.5. Question: Article 33(1), second subparagraph, requires that information referred to in paragraphs 2(a) to 2(d) of that article, with the exception of the serial number, is stored in the hub. Does this mean that the serial number cannot be uploaded to the hub?

Answer: No, the provision only regulates which information is to be stored in the hub.

7.6. Question: Articles 34(4), 35(4) and 36(n) refer to the linking of the information on unique identifiers removed or covered to the information on the equivalent unique identifiers placed for the purposes of complying with Article 47a of Directive 2001/83/EC. Is the linking required to be at the level of individual unique identifiers? How does the linking work in practice?

Answer: No, it is not necessary to link individual unique identifiers. The link can be made at batch level by linking the list of decommissioned unique identifiers in the "old" batch (the batch to be re-packed/re-labelled) and the list of new unique identifiers placed on packs in the "new" batch (the re-packed batch). The provision does not require the linking to be done at the level of individual unique identifiers, since the number of packs in the batch to be re-packed/re-labelled (and consequently the number of unique identifiers in that batch) may not correspond to the number of packs (and of unique identifiers) in the new batch – making a one-to-one link between unique identifiers impossible.

7.7. Question: In Article 35(1)(f), does the upper limit of 300 ms for a repository to respond to queries also apply when multiple repositories are implicated in the query, e.g. in case of cross-border verification?

Answer: 300 ms is the maximum response time of an individual repository. When the verification/decommissioning operation requires the querying of multiple repositories in 27 the repositories system, e.g. in case of cross-border verification, the maximum response time is obtained by multiplying the maximum response time of an individual repository (300 ms) by the number of repositories involved in the query – e.g. the maximum response time for a query involving national repository A, the hub and national repository B would be 900 ms. It should be noted that the system response time does not include the time needed by the query data to move from one repository to the other (which depends from the speed of the internet connection).

7.8. Question: How will the identity, role and legitimacy of the users of the repository system be verified?

Answer: It is the responsibility of the legal entity establishing and managing a repository to put in place appropriate security procedures ensuring that only verified users, i.e. users whose identity, role and legitimacy has been verified, are granted access to that repository.

7.9. Question: In Article 38(1), does the sentence "with the exception of the information referred to in Article 33(2)" refer to data access only, or also to data ownership?

Answer: It refers to data access only.

7.10. Question: In Article 38(1), what is the meaning of "information on the status of the unique identifier"?

Answer: The information on the status of the unique identifier includes whether the unique identifier is active or decommissioned, and in the latter case, the reasons for the decommissioning.

7.11. Question: What is the purpose of the exceptions laid out to in the second sentence of Article 38(1) concerning access to the information referred to in Article 33(2) and the information on the status of a unique identifier?

Answer: Article 38 of Commission Delegated Regulation (EU) 2016/161 regulates the ownership and the access of the data stored in the repositories system. It lays down the general rule and an exception to that rule. Since the purpose of Article 38 is, inter alia, to protect the confidentiality of data in the repositories system, including commercially confidential data, as required by Article 54a(3)(b) and (c) of Directive 2001/83/EC, the exception should be interpreted narrowly. In particular, the use of the exception should be limited to those cases where access to the data is necessary to perform the verification/decommissioning operations required by Commission Delegated Regulation (EU) 2016/161, as explained in recital 38.

7.12. Question: Is it possible to have multiple national repositories, multiple supranational repositories or a combination of national and supranational repositories serving the territory of a given Member State?

Answer: No. In accordance with Article 32, paragraphs 1 and 2, the territory of a given Member State should be served by the hub and either a national or a supranational repository connected to the hub.

7.13. Question: For the purposes of the application of Articles 33 and 48 of Commission Delegated Regulation (EU) 2016/161, what is understood for "medicinal products that have been released for sale or distribution"?

Answer: The text "medicinal products that have been released for sale or distribution" refer to products that have been batch released in accordance with Article 51 of Directive 2001/83/EC. According to Annex 16 of the EU Guidelines for Good Manufacturing Practice for Medicinal Products for

Human and Veterinary Use "Certification by a Qualified Person (QP) and Batch Release", the process of batch release comprises of:

(i)   The checking of the manufacture and testing of the batch in accordance with defined release procedures.
(ii) The certification of the finished product batch performed by a QP signifying that the batch is compliant with GMP and the requirements of its MA. This represents the quality release of the batch.
(iii) The transfer to saleable stock, and/or export of the finished batch of product which should account for the certification performed by the QP. If this transfer is performed at a site other than that where certification takes place, then the arrangement should be documented in a written agreement between the sites. Therefore, medicinal products that have been certified for release by a QP without including the safety features in their packaging before 9 February 2019, may be placed on the market, distributed and supplied to the public until their expiry date.

7.14. Question: How should the expression "marketing authorisation holder", as used in Commission Delegated Regulation (EU) 2016/161, be interpreted?

Answer: The term "marketing authorisation holder" is used in Commission Delegated Regulation (EU) 2016/161 to indicate holders of marketing authorisations in the sense of Article 6 of Directive 2001/83/EC.

7.15. Question: Are parallel importers/distributors required to comply with Article 33(1) and upload the information in Article 33(2) into the repository system? Should they also upload a list of designated wholesalers?

Answer: Parallel traders are obliged to comply with Article 33 and upload in the repositories system in the following two cases:

- If they hold a marketing authorisation in the sense of Article 6 of Directive 2001/83/EC, in which case they may also upload the list of wholesalers they have designated in accordance with Article 20(b) of Commission Delegated Regulation (EU) 2016/161; or
- If they re-pack/re-label and place new safety features or replace safety features in accordance with Article 47a of Directive 2001/83/EC on the medicinal products they supply. In this case, parallel traders who do not hold a marketing authorisation in the sense of Article 6 of Directive 2001/83/EC may not designate their own wholesalers and should not upload a list of wholesalers into the repository system. Parallel traders who re-pack/re-label their products and place new safety features or replace safety features in accordance with Article 47a of Directive 2001/83/EC on the medicinal products they supply have to comply with Articles 33, 40 and 42 of Commission Delegated Regulation (EU)

2016/161 as they are considered the "persons responsible for placing those medicinal products on the market" in that Member State.

7.16. Question: In accordance with Article 33(1), the information laid down in Article 33(2) must be uploaded in the repositories system before the product is released for sale and distribution. Does this mean that the upload needs to take place before the Qualified Person (QP) performs the batch certification and thus the safety feature information relative to any manufacturing waste should also be uploaded in the system?

Answer: No. The information laid down in Article 33(2) of Commission Delegated Regulation (EU) 2016/161 needs to be present in the system at the time the batch is released for sale and distribution (see Q&A 7.13 for what is understood for released for sale or distribution). It is acceptable to upload that information at such a time that the system is not burdened with information relative to manufacturing waste, i.e. (parts of) manufactured batches that have not been certified, provided that the upload takes place before the medicinal product is transferred to saleable stock.

7.17. Question: Does Article 37(d) require that a national medicine verification organisation (NMVO) directly alerts the relevant national competent authorities, the EMA and the Commission about a falsification? Is there is a time limit for such alerting?

Answer: The use of the term "provide for" in Article 37(d) of Commission Delegated Regulation (EU) 2016/161 means that an NMVO has to ensure that the national competent authorities, the EMA[5] and the Commission[6] are informed. The NMVO can fulfil this obligation either directly or by ensuring this task is performed by someone else. The NMVO should ensure authorities are informed as soon as it is clear that the alert triggered in accordance with Article 36(b) cannot be explained by technical issues with the repositories system, the data upload, the person performing the verification or similar technical issues.

7.18. Question: Does Article 35(1)(i) of Commission Delegated Regulation (EU) 2016/161 prohibit wholesalers and persons authorised or entitled to supply medicinal products to the public from using the national medicine verification system's graphical use interface (GUI) to verify/decommission the unique identifiers on their products when their own software is not broken?

Answer: No. The use of the GUI by wholesalers and persons authorised/entitled to supply medicines to the public in circumstances other than the failure of their own software is not prohibited but is subject to the

---

[5] By email to QDEFECT@ema.europa.eu
[6] By email to SANTE-PHARMACEUTICALS-B4@ec.europa.eu

agreement of the national medicine verification organisation owning the GUI (in the absence of entitlement, the agreement of the system owner is necessary). See also Q&A 7.4.

7.19. Question: Can a marketing authorisation holder delegate the uploading of the information laid down in Article 33(2) of Commission Delegated Regulation (EU) 2016/161?

Answer: Yes. Marketing authorisation holders (MAHs) may delegate the uploading of the information laid down in Article 33(2) to third parties by means of a written agreement between both parties. Please note that the MAHs can subcontract or delegate data uploading only to parties which perform the data upload by means of infrastructures, hardware and software that are physically located in the EEA. The MAH remains legally responsible for these tasks.

7.20. Question: What is meant by investigation of all potential incidents of falsification flagged in the system in Article 37(d) of Commission Delegated Regulation (EU) 2016/161?

Answer: The purpose of the investigation in Article 37(d) is to rule out that alerts triggered in the system have been caused for technical reasons, such as issues with the repository system, data upload, data quality, incorrect end-user scanning or other similar technical issues. As outlined in Q&A 7.17, national competent authorities, EMA and the European Commission should be informed as soon as it is clear that alert cannot be explained by technical reasons. On the basis of the information received, an investigation into the falsification incident will be launched by the authorities in line with European and national procedures.

8. OBLIGATIONS OF MARKETING AUTHORISATION HOLDERS, PARALLEL IMPORTERS AND PARALLEL DISTRIBUTORS

8.1. Question: Can marketing authorisation holders delegate the performing of their obligations under Articles 40 and 41 to a third party?

Answer: Marketing authorisation holders can (but are not obliged to) delegate part of their obligations under Articles 40 and 41 to a third party by means of a written agreement between both parties. However, marketing authorisation holders remain legally responsible for those tasks.

In particular, marketing authorisation holders can delegate the performing of their legal obligation under Article 40(a) and 40(b), as well as the decommissioning task in referred to in Article 41.

8.2. Question: Situations arise where, for the same batch of product, competent authorities from different Member States issue different levels of

recall, e.g. patient level vs wholesaler level, or no recall at all. How will Article 40 of Commission Delegated Regulation (EU) 2016/161 work in this type of scenario?

Answer: Article 40 of Commission Delegated Regulation (EU) 2016/161 would not apply to recalls at patient level as the scope of the Delegated Regulation does not extend beyond the supply of the medicinal product to the end consumer. Where a medicinal product is recalled at pharmacy level in a Member State and at wholesale level in another, the marketing authorisation holder should customise the information they need to provide in the relevant national/supranational repositories in accordance with Article 40(c).

8.3. Question: Certain Member States have national systems managing recalls and withdrawals of medicinal products in place. Would it be possible to interface those national systems with the repositories system for the verification of the safety features?

Answer: Commission Delegated Regulation (EU) 2016/161 does not provide for the connection between the national systems for recalls/withdrawal of medicinal product and the repositories system. Such connections may be considered by the legal entities managing the relevant repositories in the repositories system, on a voluntary basis.

8.4. Question: Are parallel importers/distributors required to comply with Articles 40 and 42 of Commission Delegated Regulation (EU) 2016/161?

Answer: Parallel traders are obliged to comply with Articles 40 and 42 of Commission Delegated Regulation (EU) 2016/161 in the following two cases:

- If they hold a marketing authorisation in the sense of Article 6 of Directive 2001/83/EC.
- If they re-pack/re-label and place new safety features or replace safety features in accordance with Article 47a of Directive 2001/83/EC on the medicinal products they supply.

Parallel traders who re-pack/re-label their products and place new safety features or replace safety features in accordance with Article 47a of Directive 2001/83/EC on the medicinal products they supply have to comply with Articles 33, 40 and 42 of Commission Delegated Regulation (EU) 2016/161 as they are considered the "persons responsible for placing those medicinal products on the market" in that Member State.

8.5. Question: In the case of free samples which are obliged by national law to include in their labelling the sentence "Free sample. Not to be sold", can the obligation to bear the safety features be waived?

Answer: No. Article 41 of Commission Delegated Regulation (EU) 2016/161 requires that marketing authorisation holder intending to supply any of his medicinal products as a free sample shall, where that product bears the safety features, indicate it as a free sample in the repositories system and ensure the decommissioning of its unique identifier before providing it to the persons qualified to prescribe it. Consequently, free samples are in the scope of the Regulation and have to bear the safety features.

8.6. Question: Can marketing authorisation holders upload in the repositories system serial numbers that are never actually used as data elements of unique identifiers?

Answer: No. The purpose of the repository system is so the information on the safety features is contained. Serial numbers that are not actually used as data elements in unique identifiers should not be uploaded and stored in the repositories system as they represent a security risk for the system.

8.7. Question: What are the obligations of operators who supply medicinal products on the ground of Article 126a (Cyprus clause) with regard to the safety features?

Answer: The term "marketing authorisation holder" is used in Commission Delegated Regulation (EU) 2016/161 and in Directive 2001/83/EC to indicate holders of marketing authorisations in the sense of Article 6 of the said Directive. Hence, the term does not apply to operators who distribute medicinal products on the ground of Article 126a. However, in order to handle medicinal products, those legal entities have to have a manufacturing authorisation and/or a wholesale distribution authorisation and/or a parallel import licence. They are therefore subject to the obligations laid down in Commission Delegated Regulation (EU) 2016/161 for manufacturers and/or wholesale distributors and/or parallel importers/distributors. In addition, should those operators place or replace the safety features in accordance with Article 47a of Directive 2001/83/EC on the medicinal products they supply, they need to comply with Articles 33, 40 and 42 of Commission Delegated Regulation (EU) 2016/161 as they are the "person responsible for placing those medicinal products on the market" in the Member State for which an authorisations in the sense of Article 126a was granted.

8.8. Question: In the case of replacement of the safety features by parallel traders, can the decommissioning of the original unique identifier be carried out by the wholesaler from whom they receive the product?

Answer: No. The decommissioning of the original unique identifier must be performed by the parallel trader holding the manufacturing authorisation and replacing the safety features (Article 16 of Commission Delegated Regulation (EU) 2016/161).

8.9. Question: Should marketing authorisation holders upload the unique identifiers for products with 2D barcodes released for sale or distribution before 9 February 2019?

Answer: Yes. According to Article 48 of Commission Delegated Regulation (EU) 2016/161, medicines released for sale or distribution before 9 February 2019 without a unique identifier may remain on the EU market until their expiry date, as long as they are not re-packaged or re-labelled after that date. If they are re-packaged or re-labelled after 9 February 2019, the manufacturer must place safety features in accordance with Directive 2001/83/EC and Commission Delegated Regulation (EU) 2016/161. This transitional measure does not apply for products that were released before 9 February 2019 with a unique identifier. The unique identifiers for such products should be uploaded to the system before the entry into application of the new rules (9 February 2019). This should help to avoid alerts for genuine products released before 9 February due to lack of data in the repository.

9. LISTS OF DEROGATIONS AND NOTIFICATIONS TO THE COMMISSION

9.1. Question: Can marketing authorisation holders submit their proposals for amendments to Annex I of Regulation (EU) No 2016/161 to the Commission?

Answer: Only Member States notifications are taken into account for the purpose of establishing Annex I and II of the delegated Regulation, in accordance with Article 54a(2)(c) of Directive 2001/83/EC. Concerning Annex I, Member States may inform the Commission of medicinal products that they consider not to be at risk of falsification (Article 54a(4) of Directive 2001/83/EC).

10. TRANSITIONAL MEASURES AND ENTRY INTO FORCE.

10.1. Question: For the purposes of the application of Article 48 of Commission Delegated Regulation (EU) 2016/161, what is understood for "medicinal products that have been released for sale or distribution"?

Answer: see Q&A 7.13.

11. ANNEX I

11.1. Question: How should the term "Kits" referred to in Annex I to Commission Delegated Regulation (EU) 2016/161 be interpreted?

Answer: The term "kit" is defined in Article 1(8) of Directive 2001/83/EC. It refers to "any preparation to be reconstituted or combined with radionuclides in the final radiopharmaceutical, usually prior to its administration".

11.2. Question: Are fat emulsions used for parenteral nutrition and having an ATC code beginning with B05BA exempted from bearing the safety features?

Answer: Yes. Fat emulsions having an ATC code beginning with B05BA are included in the category "solutions for parenteral nutrition" listed in Annex I to Commission Delegated Regulation (EU) 2016/161. Such emulsions are therefore exempted from the obligation to bear the safety features.

12. ANNEX II

12.1. Question: Are over-the-counter omeprazole products formulated as gastro-resistant tablets in the scope of Annex II and therefore required to bear the safety features?

Answer: No. Only over-the-counter medicinal products containing omeprazole 20 or 40 mg formulated as hard gastro-resistant capsules have to bear the safety features, as the two reported incidents of falsification that led to certain omeprazole products being added to Annex II concerned that specific pharmaceutical form of omeprazole.

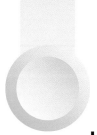

Index

B

Y

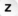

Z